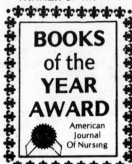
C0-ASC-201

# HOSPICALIZACION
## or
# *FREEDOM OF CHOICE IN CHILDBIRTH ?*

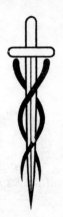

## VOL
## ONE

GOVERNMENT REGULATION
PERINATAL REGIONALIZATION
OBSTETRIC INTERVENTION
HOSPITAL PRACTICE

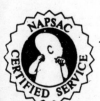

What is a NAPSAC Certified Maternity Service?
How Can Yours Qualify?
See Ch. 26, p. 269

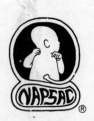

National
Association of
Parents & Professionals for
Safe
Alternatives in
Childbirth

STEWART &
STEWART
editors

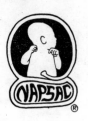

# COMPULSORY HOSPITALIZATION

# FREEDOM OF CHOICE IN CHILDBIRTH?

## VOL ONE

GOVERNMENT REGULATION
PERINATAL REGIONALIZATION
OBSTETRIC INTERVENTION
HOSPITAL PRACTICE

A
NAPSAC
PUBLICATION

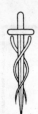First Printing, March 1979
Second Printing, January 1980

Library of Congress Catalogue Number: 77-92613
International Standard Book Numbers:
  Complete Set:  ISBN 0-917314-12-3
  Volume One:  ISBN 0-917314-13-1
  Volume Two:  ISBN 0-917314-14-X
  Volume Three: ISBN 0-917314-15-8

---

• Typeset by Thelma Pomeroy, Vicki Rotvic & Jeaneal
  Vandeven with the Generous Cooperation & Facilities of
  the Banner Press Newspaper, Lee & Joan Flor, Editors
  & Publishers, Marble Hill, Missouri, USA.

• Cover Printed by Missourian Litho & Printing Company,
  Cape Girardeau, Missouri, USA.

• Chief Printers/Bookmakers: Jonathan Stewart & Father.
• Chief Assistant Printer/Bookbinder:  Keith Irvin
• Chief Collator/Supervisor:  Lee Stewart
• Other Assistants:  Jamy Braun, Lora Lee Stewart,
                Keith Stewart, Ben Stewart, Anthony Stewart

• Produced, Printed, Designed & Bound by
  Napsac Reproductions, Marble Hill, Missouri, USA.

• Price:  $18/3 vol set plus $1.25 shipping or
          $7/individual vol plus 75¢ shipping
        Available from: NAPSAC, P.O. Box 267
                        Marble Hill, MO 63764

# PROCEEDS FROM NAPSAC BOOKS

Proceeds from the sale of this book go towards
accomplishing the goals of NAPSAC, the National
Association of Parents & Professionals for Safe
Alternatives in Childbirth--a non-profit, tax exempt
educational service organization. None of the authors
receive royalties. All have generously contributed
their time, insight, expertise, and work to produce
this anthology.

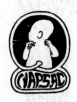

## ACKNOWLEDGEMENT

NAPSAC wishes to express its appreciation to
ANN GRAY
who carefully proofed the first printing of this volume and offered valuable suggestions. Ms. Gray
is the Editor/Publisher of an excellent periodical
called THE FEDERAL MONITOR which keeps its
subscribers posted of current legislative and legal
activities nationally, statewise, and locally in the
area of health care for women & children. Rates
are $8/year. Write to:  **THE FEDERAL MONITOR**
Drawer Q, McLean, VA 22101

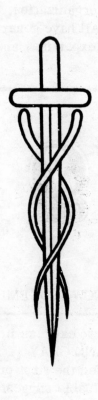

# About Volume One

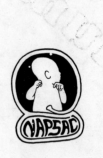

# SYNOPSIS OF VOLUME ONE

These volumes are intended to provide scientific, factual, inspirational, useful, and practical information for both parents and professionals seeking improvements in the delivery of maternity care -- either for themselves, for others, or both. They are an anthology of differing opinions, some even contradictory. There are those who favor 100 percent hospitalization (see Chapter 5 by Ryan in this volume, or The Great Debate or the Chapters by Sharp and Long, in Volume Two). There are those who favor fetal monitors, albeit with reservations (see Chapter 13 by Jarzembski). For the most part, the authors favor freedom of choice, including choices outside of the hospital with alternatives to doctors.

In addition to the 27 chapters of this particular volume, summarized in the following pages, there are some items at the end that will be helpful in reading this book. One is a list of selected abbreviations of organizations, agencies and degrees. For example, you probably know the meaning of "HEW" or "FDA." Right. Those would be the U.S. Department of Health, Education and Welfare and the U.S. Food and Drug Administration. But do you know the meaning of "SAC", "HSA", or "SHPDA"? If you want to have a say in the health programs of your area, programs that will be spending your tax dollars, you'd better find out. See the listing at the end of the book for the meanings, but also read Chapter Three by Diony Young to find out how you can do something.

Also at the end of the book is a listing of the addresses of all of the authors. You may have further questions or desire to write them for other reasons.

Reading these volumes will place you far ahead of most persons in the field in understanding current trends and how to become a more effective participant. NAPSAC also has some other books that compliment these volumes. They are described, along with where they can be obtained, at the end of the volume. You may wish to obtain a complete NAPSAC Library.

The NAPSAC publications strive to be on the frontier of thinking in research and trends in maternity care and serve the leadership in the childbirth reform movement--both professionals who provide and parents who participate by intelligently choosing the best alternatives for their own families.

The following is a brief description of each chapter intended to assist you in focusing on the aspects of this volume that can help you the most. For page numbers, see table of contents.

**Chapter One. Compulsory Hospitalization: How It Threatens You by David Stewart, PhD, & Lee Stewart.** Is the title of these volumes, "Compulsory Hospitalization...", accurate and justified? This chapter explains why it is and places content of volume one and the other two volumes into perspective. Warns both concerned consumers and caring providers about the conspiracies of organized medicine against all who disagree with them or who would stand in the way of their self-serving plans. Relates the volumes to their origin -- the 3rd NAPSAC Conference, May 19-21, 1978, in Atlanta, Georgia, which was attended by 1300 delegates from 45 states, 6 Canadian provinces, Mexico, England, and the Virgin Islands. Includes a reproduction of the proclamation by the Mayor of Atlanta declaring "Safe Alternatives in Childbirth" Day. Also contains reproduction, words and music, composed for and sung at the conference by Victor Berman, MD.

**Chapter Two. How Doctors Use Government to Maintain a Monopoly by Ann Gray.** Documents the historical origins of how our society's health care came within the grips of a single type of professional -- the physician -- to the virtual exclusion of all others. Gives specific and practical suggestions to those who wish to lessen the power of this monopoly, offer a greater spectrum of alternatives, and allow individuals greater freedom to assume more responsibility for themselves.

**Chapter Three. How Government Guidelines Originate by Robbi Pfeufer.** In October of 1977 an edict came down from the U.S. Department of HEW tantamount to a dictum that would close down all small Hospital Ob Departments (those with less than 2000 births a year). The edict was opposed by both consumers and professionals nationwide and was finally changed due to the outcry. This chapter investigates how such an arbitrary regulation came to be and finds that the process is not based upon valid consideration of science and is open to corruption by powers with vested interests.

**Chapter Four. Health Care Planning: Who is in Control? by Diony Young.** This excellent chapter summarizes the complex new set of laws and regulations that now determine the means by which health care planning is accomplished in the U.S. It offers many valuable suggestions on how consumers can become directly involved in such decision making--both on the local and regional levels of government. The laws are designed such that consumers can be in control if they would only learn what to do, and then become involved. This chapter is a must for consumers who desire to have a say in the way tax dollars are to be spent on area health programs.

**Chapter Five. Perinatal Regional Planning: What It Is & Why Doctors Recommend It by George Ryan, MD, MPH.** George Ryan is the Secretary of the Am. College of Obstetricians & Gynecologists (ACOG). The ACOG is the principle organization that opposes alternatives in childbirth outside of hospitals. This article expresses the official ACOG view and that of the majority of the nation's board certified obstetricians. This chapter favors compulsory hospitalization. 11 cited references.

**Chapter Six. Regionalization: A Model of Planned Neglect for Primary Care by Judy Norsigian.** This brief chapter points out one of the major flaws in most of the perinatal regionalization programs being initiated around the country -- namely, that all the money and all the concentration is on high risk care -- care that can only benefit less than 10 percent of mothers. The fallacy of this approach is that by ignoring primary care, care of the healthy and the low risk, a greater incidence of high risk is created.

**Chapter Seven. The Politics of Regionalization by Norma Swenson, MPH.** This chapter points out the fact that the users of maternity care are transients who pass through the system briefly and then leave. By contrast, the providers of maternity care are permanent figures who remain and who develop vested interests often contrary to the needs and interests of the users of their services. She points out how physicians, and particularly the ACOG, has learned how to exploit the current health planning regulations to their own financial and power ends. The regionalization model was conceived entirely by a committee of white, male physicians representing the

AMA, the AAP, the AAFP, and the ACOG. The Committee was funded by the March of Dimes. No nurses or midwives were invited to participate. There was no consumer input.

**Chapter Eight. A Mother's Response to Regionalization by Judith Dickson Luce.** Ms. Luce is a mother, but is also an educated and astute observer of current trends and regulations concerning maternity care. Her presentation includes a beautiful narrative of the birth of her own last child -- Damara -- born at home. In her words, "birth is one of the moments we are given to live by -- and it shouldn't be taken from anyone." In her view, regionalization enforces separations of the family and, thereby, robs families of the experience of birth.

**Chapter Nine. Regionalization of Maternity & Newborn Care: Facts, Fantasies, Flaws & Fallacies by Muriel Sugarman, MD.** A thorough, well-documented analysis of regionalization, point by point, with concrete suggestions for alternatives that would obtain better outcomes at less cost. Should be read and studied by everyone engaged in health planning as a member of an HSA or SAC. 47 cited references.

**Chapter Ten. Analysis & Critique of a Regionalization Proposal with Recommendations for Alternatives by Susan M. Basham, MA, Judith Dickson Luce, Judy Norsigian, Robbi Pfeufer, Muriel Sugarman, MD, and Norma Swenson, MPH.** Another excellent analysis of the problems of regionalization with constructive criticism and suggestions. This particular chapter focuses upon one particular regionalization proposal for the State of Massachusetts. This analysis and critique was submitted to the appropriate Health Systems Agencies of Massachusetts and due to the efforts of this group of concerned parents and professionals, Massachusetts has been spared the full assault of the negative aspects of regionalization. 76 cited references.

**Chapter Eleven. Fetal Monitoring: For Better or For Worse? by Madeleine H. Shearer, RPT.** Points out known dangers of monitoring -- infections, injuries, higher rates of cesarean, etc., as well as potential, but as yet unknown, dangers of ultrasound -- genetic alterations, damage to internal organs, etc. Points out the needlessness of monitoring in the presence of competent caring health professionals who simply stand by and give support while listening for fetal heart tones with a stethoscope. Points out flaws of current research that seems to support use of monitoring and identifies conflicts of interest for researchers finding in favor of the monitor (eg. some own stock in monitor companies, etc.). Also mentions monetary motives of proponents of monitors. 37 cited references.

**Chapter Twelve. Does Anyone Need Fetal Monitors? by Albert D. Haverkamp, MD.** This is a report on the classic and thoroughly rigorous scientific work of Haverkamp and associates who have shown that nurses with a stethoscope do as well or better, even with high risk mothers, than electronic monitors. While monitors showed no improvement in outcome, they showed a definite correlation with increased cesarean surgery and its attendant higher morbidities and mortalities. This chapter is a transcript of U.S. Senate Testimony by Dr. Haverkamp, April 17, 1978.

**Chapter Thirteen. Benefits, Limitations, Fallacies & Hazards of Electronic Monitoring of the Human Body by W.B. Jarzembski, PE, PhD.** Dr. Jarzembski is a professional engineer and designer of biomedical devices. Discusses the technical limitations of biomedical devices in general, with commentary about electronic fetal monitors. The greatest risk and limitation of electronic fetal monitors, in his view, is the ignorance of the physicians who think they know how to use them when, in fact, they have only the most elementary comprehension of the engineering capabilities of the device. Jarzembski does not feel that physicians, in general, are qualified to even choose between different brands of monitors, much less use them reliably. Even so, Jarzembski believes monitors have a place if properly used.

**Chapter Fourteen. Lasting Behavioral Effects of Obstetric Medications by Yvonne Brackbill, PhD.** The newborn human is poorly positioned for dealing with drugs. They cross the placenta rapidly. They lodge in developing brain structures. They are not readily transformed into nontoxic substances since the liver is immature and they are not easily excreted since the kidney does not function fully. From all these considerations, it would be small wonder if Ob medications did not inflict damage. As a behavioral psychologist, she discusses the long term effects on children -- including developmental disabilities and loss of I.Q. from commonly used Ob drugs. Points out that use of drugs in childbirth is on the increase in the U.S. and should be considered "at the head of the class in national health priorities." Documentation available: 168 references.

**Chapter Fifteen. Episiotomy: Facts, Fictions, Figures & Alternatives by Carol Brendsel, RN, Gail Peterson, MSSW, and Lewis Mehl, MD.** Destroys the old doctor's tales about how not doing episiotomies will lead to later weakening of pelvic muscles, frigidity, undue tearing, etc. Presents original data from a year's research. Finds that worse tearing occurs with episiotomy than without. Presents alternatives in the management of birth, such as a perineal massage, perineal support, maternal participation, etc., that reduces the incidence of tearing and the need for cutting

**Chapter Sixteen. Unnecessary Cesareans: Doctor's Choice, Parent's Dilemma by Susan G. Doering, PhD.** Presents analysis of current published works and original research. Explores causes of alarming increase in cesarean surgery over past few years – fetal monitors, fear of malpractice, chemical stimulants to labor, greater intervention, etc. Also mentions a curious diurnal variation in the rates of cesareans -- it seems that in some hospitals, they occur during the most convenient daylight hours, not randomly around the clock as births occur. Discusses hazards and complications of cesarean sections for both mother and baby. Dr. Doering has experienced a cesarean birth followed by a vaginal one. 61 cited references.

**Chapter Seventeen. What Every Pregnant Woman Should Know About Cesareans by Lynn R. Browne.** Ms. Browne was the victim of an unnecessary cesarean and has subsequently had vaginal births. Anywhere from 50 percent to 75 percent of all of today's cesareans are unnecessary (i.e. there was no real medical problem or the problem could have been prevented or corrected by alternative means). She lists the excuses doctors give to mothers for doing cesareans -- breech, CPD, no progress in labor, etc., and gives valuable information to assist parents in combatting the doctor's misinformation and misjudgment. Also lists practices that lead to higher incidences of cesarean – induction of labor, fetal monitors, etc. -- and how to avoid them. Above all--doubt your doctor. They may be well meaning, and may not, but all have received erroneous training and education in these matters.

Chapter Eighteen. Vaginal Birth After Previous Cesarean by J.R. Mc-Tammany, MD. Refutes the old doctor's dictum, "once a section, always a section." Dr. McTammany is Chief of Obstetrics & Gynecology in a community hospital and has successfully attended many vaginal births after previous cesareans. An excellent chapter for parents of previous sections desiring a vaginal birth as well as for physicians interested in learning how to safely carry out such a practice.

Chapter Nineteen. How Hospitals Disrupt the Process of Family Bonding by Sheila Kitzinger. Discusses the myriad disruptive routines of hospitals -- IV's, oxytocin, lithotomy position, fetal monitors, forceps, condescending attitudes of hospital personnel, rupturing membranes, face masks, immobility in labor, etc. -- that interfere with the normal bonding processes between baby, mother, father, and family. Points out that many hospitals claim to "understand bonding," and yet do not. They somehow mistakenly think it to be some sort of "magic glue" that affixes itself in the first hour after birth, not realizing that all of the events leading up to and following that hour are also relevant. Hospitals have succeeded in routinizing another spontaneous process--bonding.

Chapter Twenty. An In-Hospital Birthing Room: One Year's Experience by Richard B. Stewart, MD, Asher Galloway, MD, and Linda Goodman, CNM. Give philosophy and statistics on a successful birthing room in Douglasville, Georgia Hospital. Discusses interfacing with occasional need for high risk care measures – cesareans, etc. Financially successful, the birthing room is also a form of Ob practice that offers a great deal of personal gratification to the providers of the service – as well as to those who use it. While Stewart, Galloway & Goodman are not directly engaged in home birth practice, they do offer backup and prenatal care for home birth couples. This, too, is discussed. An excellent chapter for physicians and nurse midwives desiring to set up such a service.

Chapter Twenty One. Making Hospitals More Like Home: Opportunities for Innovative Research by James R. Allen, MD. A scholarly work that documents the medical safety and desirability of family-centered hospital care. Dr. Allen is with the U.S. Center for Disease Control, Hospital Infections Branch, and refutes the arguments that family-centered programs would increase infections or cause other such problems. 37 cited references.

Chapter Twenty Two. Family Centered Care for the High Risk by Murray Enkin, MD. If healthy mothers and babies need family-centered maternity care, then sick mothers and babies need it even more. That is the thesis of Dr. Enkin who not only discusses it in detail, but practices it with his colleagues, at McMaster University Medical Center. An excellent chapter for hospital practitioners who wish to offer kind, humane care to everyone -- including the high risk.

**Chapter Twenty Three. Blueprint for the Rehumanization of American Obstetrics: Costs, Personnel & Floor Plans by Loel Fenwick, MD.** Discusses how American obstetrics became dehumanized and how it can become more humane and family-centered. Presents arguments in favor of short stay, single room services--how it would save money, reduce the need for personnel, and, of course, be more acceptable to the public. Includes comparative floor plans between conventional service and childbearing center. Exactly the sort of thing a hospital needs to read if contemplating the adopting of such a service.

**Chapter Twenty Four. A Sociologic View of Birth; Physiologic Reality vs. People's Interpretations of that Reality by Barbara Katz Rothman.** A penetrating analysis of the cultural phenomena of birth and how different parties view it--parent, doctor, etc. Points out that even seemingly objective concepts--such as length of labor--are really subjective and arbitrary depending on one's sociologic position. A very helpful article to all who wish to obtain a better understanding of birth as it is and as it has come to be in modern culture. This chapter is in a class of its own and offers unique insight.

**Chapter Twenty Five. Synopsis of an Optimal Maternity Plan by David Stewart, PhD.** Takes the broad view of birth as part of life, and how education about birth and breastfeeding should begin, not with childbirth classes when one is pregnant, but in high school and earlier. Points out the failure of 100 percent hospitalization in reducing mortalities and morbidities and outlines an alternative plan that includes education, good nutrition, nonuse of drugs, tobacco and alcohol, training for expectant couples, family-centered maternity care for all, well-coordinated home birth programs with birth centers working with hospitals, availability of midwives for most, natural childbirth, no separation of family, universal breastfeeding, and postpartum follow-up at home. Points out that risk is something that cannot be eliminated regardless of where birth takes place or by whom attended.

**Chapter Twenty Six. What is a NAPSAC Certified Maternity Service & How Can Yours Qualify? by Penny Simkin, RPT.** Defines "NAPSAC Certification." Explains how a maternity service can qualify and how to apply for such certification. Lists the seven NAPSAC Principles of Maternity Care: Childbearing as a normal process, parent responsibility, cooperation between parents and birth attendants, informed consent, maintaining the family unit, limits of care and back-up, and the essential features of the maternity service itself.

**Chapter Twenty Seven. Forced Labor or Free Choice: Which Will It Be? by Robert S. Mendelsohn, MD.** This is a transcript of the closing address at the 1978 NAPSAC Conference. Begins with reference to the Old Testament account of the midwives who disobeyed the Egyptian pharaoh which ultimately led to the survival of Moses and the liberation of the Hebrews from bondage. Mentions Semmelweiss who stood against the doctors of his time and ultimately led to the lowering of the death rate of laboring mothers. Mentions the founding of La Leche League which has replaced "the stupidity of modern doctors with the sage advice of experienced mothers." Ends with mention of Martin Luther King, who preached in Atlanta, another leader who lead thousands to freedom and the message of NAPSAC that is leading "men and women from decades of bondage under forced labor and the tyranny of modern medicine." "As important as it is to be reborn," says Dr. Mendelsohn, "it is even more important to be born right the first time."

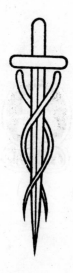

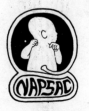

## AUTHORS OF
## VOLUME ONE

**COMPULSORY HOSPITALIZATION or**
**FREEDOM OF CHOICE IN CHILDBIRTH ?**

The following 32 authorities generously contributed their thoughts, research, and time to make this volume possible. If you would like to write to any of them individually, their addresses are given on p. 281 of this volume.

James R. Allen, MD, MPH
Susan M. Basham, MA
Victor Berman, MD
Yvonne Brackbill, PhD
Carol Brendsel, RN
Lynn R. Browne
Susan G. Doering, PhD
Murray Enkin, MD
Loel Fenwick, MD
Asher Galloway, MD
Linda Goodman, CNM
Ann Gray
Albert Haverkamp, MD
W.B. Jarzembski, PE, PhD
Sheila Kitzinger
Judith Dickson Luce

J.R. McTammany, MD
Lewis E. Mehl, MD
Robert Mendelsohn, MD
Judy Norsigian
Gail Peterson, MSSW
Robbie Pfuefer
Barbara Katz Rothman
George Ryan, MD, MPH
Madeleine Shearer, RPT
Penny Simkin, RPT
David Stewart, PhD
Lee Stewart
Richard Stewart, MD
Muriel Sugarman, MD
Norma Swenson, MPH
Diony Young

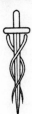

# COMPULSORY HOSPITALIZATION or
## CONTENTS
### VOLUME ONE

## ABOUT VOLUME ONE

## INTRODUCTION

## GOVERNMENT REGULATION

## PERINATAL REGIONALIZATION

continued on next page...

## OBSTETRIC INTERVENTION

## HOSPITAL PRACTICE

## MODEL MATERNITY PROGRAMS & OTHER TOPICS

## APPENDICES

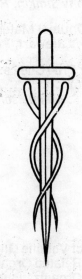

# Introduction

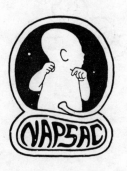

# CHAPTER ONE

## COMPULSORY HOSPITALIZATION: HOW IT THREATENS YOU

### by David and Lee Stewart

There is a movement among many medical professionals to force all births into hospitals. The movement is not new. It began, perhaps, nearly a hundred years ago — about the same time as the move among physicians to do away with midwives. Most professionals caught up in the movement have been well-meaning. They have sincerely believed that hospitals are the safest place for everyone to give birth. They have been led to believe by their educational institutions that the more technically trained the accoucheur the better.

However well intended, such belief is not supported by fact. There is no scientific basis — not now nor at any time in history — to support the belief that hospitals are best for everyone or that surgically skilled obstetricians are the safest attendants for most birthing mothers. All available valid scientific data, current and historic, in the United States and other industrialized countries indicates the opposite: i.e. the lowest mortality and morbidity rates for both mothers and newborns are in maternity care systems that emphasize nutrition, employ a high proportion of nurses or midwives, encourage universal breastfeeding, practice effective methods of prenatal screening, promote natural childbirth, and offer systems of good home birth programs working with hospitals and birth centers. None of the items in this list are typical of American maternity care and, predictably, the United States ranks very poorly in outcomes among industrialized countries.

While it is true that the American perinatal mortality rates have fallen during the past century while rates of hospitalization and specialization of obstetricians have increased, these are apparently coincidences. One can just as easily correlate the growth in automobile sales or the consumption of hamburgers. No valid statistical study has demonstrated a good correlation between improving outcomes of pregnancy and proliferation of hospitals and-or specialists. Such improvements have, it seems, occurred in spite of these developments, not because of them

While the movement to take over birth by doctors and hospitals is not new, it has recently taken a new twist: Perinatal Regionalization. Now, not only do they want to force mothers and babies into hospitals under doctor treatment, but they want to tell you which hospital and what kind of doctor. The enormous cost of such hospitals, along with the high fees of the average hospital obstetrician, are yet another compulsory component of this movement.

At the same time as one segment of the population drives toward technology and institutionalized birth, the home birth movement and the trend toward out-of-hospital birth centers is accelerating like never before. While the over-all incidence of home births is low in the United States (probably less than 2 percent nationwide), the rate has doubled in many states every year for the past 4 - 5 years. At the same time, the interest in out-of-hospital birth centers grows exponentially. In 1972 there was only one such center — Su Clinica in Raymondville, Texas. In 1975 three more started — Nachis in Culver City, California, the Southwest Maternity Center in Albuquerque, New Mexico, and the Maternity Center Association in New York City. In 1978, three years later, there were over 50 such centers and countless others in the process of organizing. In spite of increasing numbers of doctors who refuse prenatal care and hospital back-up to couples desiring home birth and who fight the practice of midwifery and the formation of free-standing birth centers, the movement grows. Out-of-hospital birth is here to stay. It will continue with or without the approval of the medical community. Medical societies can pass resolutions to make it less safe, they can lobby for legislation to outlaw midwifery and home birth. They can make it illegal, but they cannot stop it. There is no indication that anything will reverse the trend.

And why should it reverse? Many enlightened parents and professionals are awakening to the fact that ultra-technology and ultra-specialization are not the answer to optimal maternity care. They have become, in fact, a major obstacle to optimal maternity care. Most mothers could have healthy home births if they were given the correct prenatal advice on nutrition, had natural childbirth, breastfed their babies, and if their care was by experts in health and normality. Hospitals and obstetricians, in general, are not experts in health and normality. Most know little about health and normality. Their special expertise is in sickness and abnormality.

Most of the apparent need for hospitalization in birth is created by the hospital itself and the greatest cause for needing obstetrical intervention is obstetricians. By use of IV's and oxytocin they create fetal distress; they then intervene. By use of fetal monitors and lack of skill in handling breech presentations, they set up a crisis calling for cesarean surgery; they then do the surgery. By polluting the maternal blood stream with analgesic and anesthetic drugs and by impatience in third stage, they cause hemorrhages; they have a ready blood bank to take care of it. By inducing labors by chemicals or breaking the bag of waters, they increase the incidence of prematurity and respiratory distress syndrome in newborns; they have a neonatologist and an intensive care unit to handle it. By frequent, unnecessary internal exams in labor, by use of internal fetal monitors, and because hospitals house concentrations of harmful germs not found anywhere except in hospitals, they cause infections in both mother and baby; they have the antibiotics to attack it. And so on. Doctors and hospitals place mothers and babies at risk routinely under the misconception that they have the means to mend the damages without permanent effect. And sadly, families subjected to this sort of risk are grateful afterwards to those who rescued them from such complications, not realizing that it was their "rescuers" who were the cause of the complications in the first place.

The point of this set of volumes is to help both parents and professionals to realize the truth about current medical practices and that the political activities of such organizations as the AMA, ACOG, AAP, NAACOG and others to limit the choices of parents to hospitals only is not in the best interest of the parents, their babies, or their families — medically, emotionally, or economically. It does serve the best interests of these organizations — in terms of money and power. We are not saying that the motives of these organizations are "money and power." We are merely pointing out the simple fact, observable to all, that the efforts of these organizations to universalize hospital birth would, regardless of their motives, serve to enhance their financial status and power position.

Is it fair to label this movement "compulsory hospitalization?" Yes, it is both fair and accurate. When doctors and hospitals make it difficult or impossible for midwives, home birth programs or free standing birth centers to function — the choices of parents are reduced to a doctor-dominated hospital or a medically unattended home birth. What kind of a choice is this? For most couples, it is tantamount to "compulsory hospitalization." Although out-of-hospital birth is still legal in all of the United States, medical organizations in several states are attempting to bring about legislation to make hospitalization compulsory in legal fact by outright outlawing home birth and making it impossible for professionals to practice outside of hospitals.

We are not suggesting that hospitals have no place in birth nor that the surgical specialty of obstetrics be discarded. 5 - 10 percent of mothers truly need such care. Another 10 - 20 percent may need such care on stand-by basis. But the majority do not. Hospitals and obstetrical specialists have their place, but in the interest of safety and optimal care, it must be a minor place — not the dominant one. If left obstetrically unhampered normality dominates the birth experience. Therefore, the dominant specialists of birth must be midwives and physicians skilled in healthful practices, and the dominant site of birth must be the most healthful and normal — the home.

Actions by organized medicine to keep themselves and their institutions in power via perinatal regionalization must be considered a major threat to the health and welfare of the nation's families. The conspiracy must be broken by educated parents and enlightened professionals. Perinatal regionalization may have some good points in theory, but it cannot be accepted as it is currently being promoted. In the interest of mothers and babies the world over the movement toward compulsory hospitalization in all forms must be stopped. We must come to understand that compulsory hospitalization implies much more than the simple site of birth. Compulsory hospitalization also commonly means compulsory IV's, compulsory electronic fetal monitoring, compulsory oxytocin, compulsory analgesia, compulsory surgery (episiotomy or cesarean), together with compulsory compliance to hospital authority including compulsory payment of all charges for services rendered whether desired, necessary or not. Compulsory hospitalization takes birth away from those to whom it rightfully belongs — families.

We are not saying that IV's, electronic fetal monitoring, oxytocin, analgesia, episiotomy, cesareans, etc., are intrinsically bad. They all have their place in a small percent of cases and are sometimes beneficial. But analgesia and oxytocin are not substitutes for human support and freedom of mobility in labor. Cesarean sections are no substitute for skill in handling breech or other problems of labor. Episiotomy is no substitute for patient, gentle assistance in second stage. And electronic fetal monitoring is no substitute for good midwifery or adequate nursing. In short, when scientific studies have shown that existing hospital obstetrical services fare better with IV's, drugs and surgery, these studies have not proven the necessity of such procedures but have only demonstrated how bad existing hospital obstetrical services really are. When medical staff have to rely upon drugs to stimulate labor or to support a mother under stress, this merely proves their misunderstanding of the situation. When medical doctors have to rely upon episiotomy to prevent tearing most of the time, it only demonstrates the errors of their manner of delivery. When doctors resort to cesareans for 10 percent, 15 percent, even 25 - 30 percent of mothers, they have only proven their training and experience deficient to handle such situations in an alternative and better way. When fetal monitors prove better than doctors or nurses at determining fetal conditions and improving outcomes, it has only proven the lack of proper attention by those particular doctors or nurses because with good nursing and attentive doctors fetal monitors do not improve outcomes. With proper prenatal care (in which most physicians today are not trained), and with kind, continuous human attentiveness at birth, all of these procedures prove unnecessary most of the time. Technology, which has come to disrupt and destroy the meaningfulness of the birth for the family, has also crippled the professional such that they can no longer function without it. Doctors no longer believe themselves — they believe the machines, the computers, the laboratory tests. Both parents and professionals have become the victims of technology. Compulsory hospitalization would only make the victimization worse.

Can normal birth occur in a hospital? The simple entry of a laboring couple into the hospital environment can warp the process and change the course of labor from what it would have been in more familiar surroundings. It is a clinical fact that when people enter strange settings such as hospitals, blood pressures are altered and bodily hormones and blood chemistry are changed. Hospital nurses can tell of many incidences of mothers, having begun labor at home, come into the hospital only to have it stop. Sometimes they are advised to return home, at which time labor begins again. Sometimes obstetrical intervention is required to force the body to do in a hospital what it would have been able to do easily and without complication at home. Therefore hospitals, per se, can be a risk in childbirth. And while family-centered programs in hospitals can help reduce this risk, no amount of family-centeredness can completely eliminate it. Unless it is clearly evident that a particular pregnant couple is at greater risk by not going to a hospital, they should not be compelled to go there. They may choose to go there even without definite indications, but it should be their choice, not something forced upon them by others.

Believers in total hospitalization point out the lack of immediately available technology as a disadvantage in out-of-hospital birth. A fact not yet generally recognized is the intrinsic disadvantage of having immediately available technology. We are not referring to the unnecessary over-use of technology, rampant in today's hospitals, which is another type of risk associated with technology, but a theoretically correctable one. We are referring to a much more subtle form of risk that has to do with the presence of technology rather than its use. Such presence can have a powerful paralyzing effect upon a laboring mother's mind and body.

Childbirth educators are all too familiar with the situation where a laboring mother is actually doing quite well, despite stress and pain. Then a well-intentioned nurse or doctor enters and offers medication for immediate relief and makes comments like, "You don't have to be a martyr," or "How about some Demerol to take the edge off." The effect is to demoralize the mother. She thought she was coping, but now she is not sure. After all, there is ready help available, so why not take it. Finding no human support to continue to endure her efforts, and now feeling no longer able to cope, she accepts the medication. Since no such medications are safe for babies, they should never be used unless absolutely necessary. If, in the same situation, the mother were given sympathetic, understanding support or, as in the case of a home birth, she knew that no such relief were readily available, she would muster up the will and have her baby naturally and safely.

This example is fairly obvious in how the presence of technology can reduce a mother's will to work with her labor. Even more subtle, yet of more profound consequence, is the fact that if a laboring mother knows that all manner of technologic support is at hand, her mind and body may cease to function as effectively as they would under "do it or else" circumstances without technology. The presence of too much technology weakens the will and the resolve of the mother. Her body, no longer given a mental mandate to carry out its necessary functions, lets up in its exertion, labor does not progress as it would have and technology, the silent culprit in the first place, rushes in for the rescue. The aftermath is usually a set of grateful parents and pleased professionals, neither realizing the true cause of the crisis.

This is an extremely important point. Those bent upon compulsory hospitalization do not realize it, and even those who have sensed the intrinsic dangers of hospital technology and opted for a birth elsewhere may not have been able to verbalize what they have sensed. Professionals who realize this fundamental truth often support out-of-hospital birth and try to practice in as unobtrusive a manner as possible. They do not flaunt their professionalism, which, like technology, can paralyze a mother's ability to give birth. While they keep their technology nearby, it is hidden away and not allowed to contaminate the scene and warp the progress of normal labor.

No one is proposing 100 percent out-of-hospital birth, but 100 percent hospital birth is equally illogical and unfounded. Freedom of choice in childbirth is essential to any optimal maternity system. Lately freedom of choice has been so narrowly restricted that today's hospitals are not usually safe places to be born. It is clear that one needs good hospitals working in close cooperation to provide back-up and to handle those few who are justifiably screened out of a home birth option. Equally true, but not so clear, is the fact that to insure safe hospitals, it is essential to have good home birth programs. Without home births, hospitals have no standard of normality by which to measure and model their practice. For lack of good home birth programs, our hospitals have become unsafe. The failure of perinatal regionalization programs to recognize the necessary inclusion of home birth is a major fundamental flaw to the whole idea — a flaw that must, for the welfare of babies and families, be corrected.

This set of three volumes is the result of a major conference held in Atlanta, Georgia, U.S.A., May 19 - 21, 1978, at the Marriott Hotel. Over 1300 persons attended from 45 states, 6 provinces of Canada, England, Mexico, and the Virgin Islands. About half were health care providers — midwives, doctors, nurses — while the rest were parents, childbirth educators, lawyers, journalists, La Leche League Leaders, sociologists, government officials and others.

It was a grand event. Members of President Jimmy Carter's family spoke there — Miss Lillian, his mother, Sybil, his sister-in-law, and Billy, his brother. Their comments are published in Volume 2 of this set. Shiela Kitzinger, from England spoke along with the over 90 other speakers, which included George Annas, Tom and Gail Brewer, Tonya Brooks, Mayer Eisenstein, Murray Enkin, Ina May and Stephen, Doris Haire, Rhondda Hartman, Marjie and Jay Hathaway, Esther Herman, Lewis Mehl, Robert Mendelsohn, Judy Norsigian, Gail Peterson, George Ryan, Madeleine Shearer, Penny Simkin, Norma Swenson, Marian Tompson, Fran Ventre, Gregory White and many others pioneering in the field. The leadership of the childbirth reform movement was there — both on the podium and in the audience.

Those who were fortunate enough to be there also felt the genuine warmth of the real southern hospitality that is Atlanta. The Mayor of Atlanta declared it "Safe Alternatives in Childbirth Day" and signed a proclamation reproduced here. NAPSAC shall always be grateful to Atlanta APSAC, who hosted the conference, as well as H.O.M.E. of Atlanta and CEA of Atlanta without whose assistance the conference would never have been.

It was the largest NAPSAC conference to that date and one of the two or three

# FREEDOM OF CHOICE

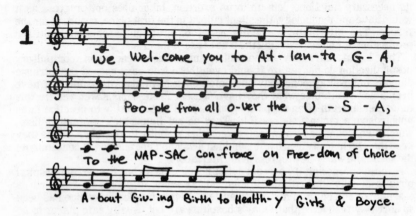

**1**

We wel-come you to At-lan-ta, G-A,

Peo-ple from all o-ver the U-S-A,

To the NAP-SAC con-f'rence on Free-dom of Choice

A-bout Giv-ing Birth to Health-y Girls & Boyce.

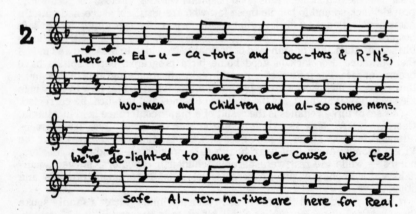

**2**

There are Ed-u-ca-tors and Doc-tors & R-N's,

Wo-men and Child-ren and al-so some mens.

We're de-light-ed to have you be-cause we feel

safe Al-ter-na-tives are here for Real.

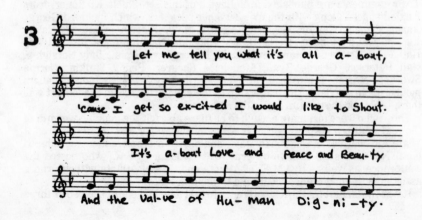

**3**

Let me tell you what it's all a-bout,

'cause I get so ex-cit-ed I would like to Shout.

It's a-bout Love and Peace and Beau-ty

And the Val-ue of Hu-man Dig-ni-ty.

words & music written & performed
## by Vic Berman, MD
on the Occassion of the 3rd NAPSAC Conference, May 19-21, 1978, Atlanta

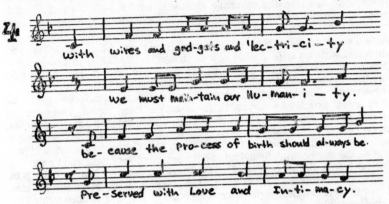

with wires and grd-gets and 'lec-tri-ci-ty

we must main-tain our Hu-man-i-ty.

be-cause the Pro-cess of birth should al-ways be.

Pre-served with Love and In-ti-ma-cy.

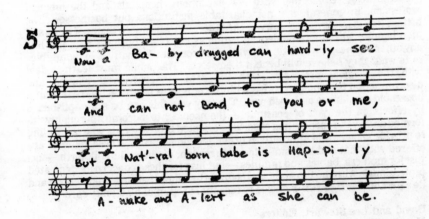

Now a Ba-by drugged can hard-ly see

And can not Bond to you or me,

But a Nat'-ral born babe is Hap-pi-ly

A-wake and A-lert as she can be.

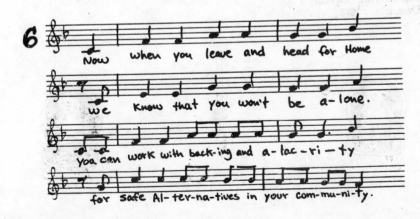

Now when you leave and head for Home

we know that you won't be a-lone.

you can work with back-ing and a-lac-ri-ty

for safe Al-ter-na-tives in your com-mu-ni-ty.

largest conventions of the childbirth reform movement in history. The gamut of topics and emotions was there. It was more than a meeting — it was an experience. And to make the coverage complete, on the last morning, Victor Berman appeared on stage before the whole assembly and sang the song reproduced here which he had just written for the occasion.

Vic is a member of NAPSAC's Consultant Board, an M.D., A.C.O.G., and co-director, with his wife, Sallee, of a birth center (NACHIS) in Culver City, California. It was one of the first birth centers in the nation. We are told that before his days as a physician, Vic was an entertainer and musician.

These volumes contain articles by various participants at that conference, as well as a few articles by non-participants on pertinent topics. The over 100 contributors to these volumes have shared a wealth of expertise and experience from every aspect of childbirth. This anthology, along with NAPSAC's previous volumes (Safe Alternatives in Childbirth and 21st Century Obstetrics Now!) comprise the most complete and up-to-date compilation of data and thought on childbirth trends available in print today. There are original data, new slants on old data, and new ideas. There are philosophical articles, scientific articles, and how-to-do-it articles. Written for the public at large, it is documented for the professional.

People must realize that with few exceptions, hospitals and the medical profession, in general, are not charitable institutions but businesses. The bottom line is money — one way or the other. They promote their services and merchandise with the same determination as any other business and, just like any other business, have little motivation to promote alternatives to themselves or to what they believe will benefit themselves. The public must learn to deal with the medical profession with the same independence, caution and discrimination they now exercise with the purchase of groceries, real estate, household appliances and used cars. The only way this can be accomplished is by efforts on the part of consumers, themselves, to become thoroughly informed and by the cooperation of service-oriented professionals who are willing to provide choices and alternatives to suit individual needs. These volumes are offered with that end in mind — toward freedom of choice in childbirth — not just for mothers, babies and families — but also for those concerned, dedicated professionals with the foresight and courage to follow their own convictions and be a part of that freedom of choice so essential to optimal maternity care.

David and Lee Stewart, Editors
Marble Hill, Missouri
December, 1978

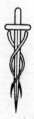

## Proclamation

# CITY OF ATLANTA
## Office of the Mayor

WHEREAS THE NATIONAL ASSOCIATION OF PARENTS AND PROFESSIONALS FOR SAFE ALTERNATIVES IN CHILDBIRTH (NAPSAC) IS A NATIONAL, NON-PROFIT GROUP DEDICATED TO FINDING SAFE, CONSUMER-ORIENTED METHODS FOR CHILDBIRTH; AND

WHEREAS TODAY'S PARENTS ARE TAKING ON A NEW AWARENESS AND CONCEPT ABOUT THE AWESOME, INDESCRIBABLE OCCASION OF GIVING BIRTH TO A CHILD AND ARE MAKING EFFORTS TO MAKE THIS SPECIAL TIME EVEN MORE MEANINGFUL; AND

WHEREAS NAPSAC CONDUCTS MEDICAL RESEARCH IN THE AREAS OF OBSTET-RICS AND PEDIATRICS WITH SPECIAL CONCERN FOR THE HEALTH AND SAFETY OF MOTHER AND CHILD; AND

WHEREAS OUR CITY IS IN THE FOREFRONT OF THIS CONSUMER-ORIENTED CHILDBIRTH MOVEMENT, WITH PARENTS AND PROFESSIONALS WORKING TOGETHER TO CREATE A MORE COMPASSIONATE, HUMANE, FAMILY-CENTERED METHOD OF MATERNITY CARE:

NOW, THEREFORE, I, MAYNARD JACKSON, MAYOR OF THE CITY OF ATLANTA, HEREBY DO PROCLAIM FRIDAY, MAY 19, 1978, AS

### SAFE ALTERNATIVES IN CHILDBIRTH DAY

IN ATLANTA, AND URGE OUR CITIZENS TO FAMILIARIZE THEMSELVES WITH THE GOALS OF NAPSAC.

IN WITNESS WHEREOF I HAVE HEREUNTO SET MY HAND AND CAUSED THE SEAL OF THE CITY OF ATLANTA TO BE AFFIXED.

MAYNARD JACKSON
MAYOR

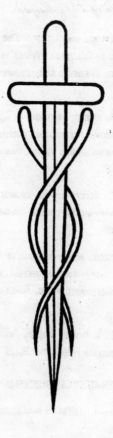

# Government Regulation

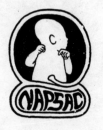

# CHAPTER TWO

## HOW DOCTORS USE GOVERNMENT TO MAINTAIN A MONOPOLY AND WHAT CONSUMERS CAN DO ABOUT IT

### By Ann Gray

The most striking characteristic of maternity care in the U.S. today is the medical monopoly which controls it. This article will discuss the government's role in helping to establish and maintain the medical monopoly, some aspects of the government which particularly affect maternity care, and what we ourselves can do to influence the government in the interests of women and children. Historically, the concerns of women and children have been underrepresented in the government, and have had few advocates, while men, and especially male physicians, have been well represented indeed. Hence, governmental actions affecting maternity care have tended to serve primarily the interests of physicians rather than those of women and children. Sometime these interests coincide, but other times physicians' interests appear to run more to maintaining their monopoly position and concurrent high fees.

The American Medical Association (AMA) was founded in 1847, and immediately learned how to use government to its advantage. Thus organized medicine has had over 100 years of experience in dealing with the government. One of the main goals of the AMA from the beginning was to increase doctors' fees by controlling the number of physicians and eliminating competing healers. The following information is from an unpublished paper by Ronald Hamowy at the University of Alberta. The paper is entitled "The Early Development of Medical Licensing Laws in the United States, 1875-1900."

### Use of Licensure to Maintain Power

There were two key reasons for occupational licensure: first, to ensure the qualifications of those practicing the healing arts, and second, to limit the entry of new doctors into the profession. The AMA accomplished this by having states pass laws requiring that a doctor must have attended an accredited medical school, passed a medical examining board, and been licensed by the state in which he or she would practice. At the same time, the AMA reduced the number of medical schools by raising the standards for training, and further cut down on the number of graduates by increasing the length and cost of medical training. From the beginning, the AMA used the government to help in its effort.

Ann Gray is editor of the Federal Monitor, a national newsletter concerning government involvement in family health care; she is former southern Regional Director, ICEA, and Director, District IV, NAPSAC.

Acknowledgment: This article is based on a presentation at a seminar, "Issues in Childbearing," Nov. 2-4, 1978, Issaqua, WA, sponsored by Resource & Development Services for Childbirth Educators, (RADS), 1100 23rd Ave. East, Seattle, WA 98112.

I do not wish to give the impression that the licensure laws and medical practice acts resulted in poor quality physicians. On the contrary, we have excellent doctors in our country, and undoubtedly the licensing laws eliminated some quacks. The problem is that our physicians are rather like Cadillacs — very expensive, and not enough to go around. And in many cases we do not have the option of picking a less expensive doctor or another sort of health professional. There are many occasions when we would like to be able to choose a Volkswagen instead of a Cadillac.

The AMA was very successful in introducing occupational licensure. Recognizing that it would be much easier to have licensing legislation passed if physicians were serving in state and federal offices, the AMA urged its members to run for office, which they did. Soon physicians were well represented at all levels of government. States started to pass licensing laws in the latter part of the 19th century, and by 1901 all the states and territories except for Alaska and Oklahoma had instituted medical examining boards.

The following census data statistics show how well the AMA succeeded in reducing the number of physicians relative to the population. In 1850 there were 176 physicians for every 100,000 people. By 1900 there were only 157 physicians for every 100,000 people, and in 1957 there were 132 for every 100,000 people. The number of medical schools in the country fell dramatically also, from 160 in 1900 to a low of 76 in 1930. By 1957 the number had crept back up to 82. In the past three years, 81,000 students have unsuccessfully applied for admission to medical schools in the United States.

The other part of the task was the elimination of competing healers. In the 19th century the main competition to physicians was from Eclectics, who relied on botanical and herbal remedies, and from homeopaths, who used minute doses of medications and the recuperative powers of nature. Orthodox medicine in those years relied heavily on bloodletting, blistering, and large doses of medicines. The AMA continuously denounced the eclectics and homeopaths as quacks in its literature, and sought broadly worded medical practice acts in each state to restrict competing professions. The AMA tried to extend the definition of medical practice to include "all those who desire to treat the sick for compensation," a definition which, if strictly interpreted, could be used to bring under the control of law the spiritual healers like the Christian Scientists, and drugless practitioners like chiropractors. All the states eventually passed medical practice acts; however, they vary from state to state as to how broad a definition they use. The constitutionality of medical practice acts has been consistently upheld by the courts ever since the 1889 U.S. Supreme Court case Dent v. West Virginia.

Today we are seeing the aftermath of the licensing laws and medical practice acts, as midwives — both nurse-midwives and lay midwives — struggle to be allowed to practice their professions. While the licensing efforts of the physicians in the 19th century were aimed to control entry into the profession and to limit competition, the midwives today are simply trying to establish their right to practice their profession within the law. The medical establishment is offering fierce resistance all along the line, but they have been unable to eliminate midwives and the demand for them continues to grow. Consumers can be optimistic about mobilizing and passing midwifery legislation today. The following are a few examples of the struggles over midwifery legislation in the states going on today:

1. In California, AB 1896, a bill originally known as the Midwifery Practice Act, was finally passed in a watered-down form. While the original bill called for the development and regulation of midwives under a Midwifery Examining Committee as independent health care providers for women in normal childbirth, the final version simply makes it possible for any government agency involved in health or education to apply to sponsor a pilot project for training innovative health care personnel. The Department of Consumer Affairs in California is expected to apply to sponsor a midwifery training pilot project.

2. In New Jersey, the Board of Medical Examiners has been trying to regulate nurse-midwives out of business by placing so many restrictions on them that they can not function. A successful letter-writing campaign by nurse-midwives and parents' groups staved off the first set of proposed regulations. A common statement by New Jersey physicians has been that they favor nurse-midwives in principle, but nurse-midwives are really unnecessary in New Jersey because there are physicians available to provide all the obstetrical care. Clearly the New Jersey physicians are more concerned about the competition than about the public welfare.

The objectionable regulations which they are expected to propose show just as clear an economic concern. To look at one example, the Board of Medical Examiners in New Jersey would like nurse-midwives to be restricted to caring for women throughout pregnancy and the postpartum check-up, but not for subsequent gynecologic care. Note that the Board is not saying CNM's are unable to perform routine gynecologic care at the time of the postpartum check, they are qualified to provide such care later as well.

3. Also in California, at the same time that AB 1896 was struggling its way through the California Senate, an unlicensed midwife, Marianne Doshi, was indicted on charges of practicing medicine without a license and murder, in connection with the death of a baby whose home birth she attended in June, 1978. In October of 1978 Marianne Doshi was cleared of both charges. In setting aside the indictment, the judge commented that he thought people probably have the right, under our constitution, to choose alternatives to "what the California Medical Association (CMA), or the AMA, or the medical profession wants to provide as far as the birth of children goes." He further commented that he hoped "that the medical profession has enough maturity. . .to say that there are alternative ways" to what they want to provide. In a 1976 case, Bowland v. Municipal Court, in which another unlicensed midwife was acquitted, the judge ruled that childbirth was not a disease but rather "a normal physiological function of women," and hence that "attending a woman in childbirth is not the practice of medicine under California law." This ruling could have gone the other way if California had had a very broadly worded medical practice act which included "treatment of any physical condition" as practicing medicine.

4. In Illinois, 11 women who wish to be licensed as midwives have a class action suit in progress which seeks to overturn an Illinois statute which discontinued the issuance of midwifery licenses in 1965. Their suit was dismissed before full hearings, and they appealed the dismissal. A Circuit Court of Appeal ruled in June 1978 that the women may have the right to practice their profession, and ordered the case returned to federal district court for full hearings. The state of Illinois has now appealed the reversal of the dismissal to the U.S. Supreme Court.

5. At the November, 1978 meeting of Resource and Development Services

(RADS), Representative A.A. Adams told about the midwifery licensing bill he
would be sponsoring for Washington state. Washington residents favoring this
legislation should take steps to help it pass and to influence the wording so it will
have the provisions you want. Ask to be on Rep. Adams mailing list for communications concerning this legislation. Call his office to learn when the
hearing he mentioned will be held. Plan to attend the hearing in large numbers,
and make arrangements in advance to testify on the bill if you wish to. Send
data on midwifery and home birth to your own state representative and
senator, and urge them to support the bill. Form an ad hoc committee to
coordinate the support effort, or become involved with the Washington State
Midwifery Council, which has been analyzing and reporting on the bill in its
publications.

These are the sorts of activity concerning licensure which are going on in
many of our states. If you wish to see nurse-midwives or lay midwives licensed
in your state, you need to be aware of the current situation. In some cases there
is an old granny midwifery law still on the books, yet no one has been licensed
for many years because of refusal to do so by physicians in control of such
midwife licensing procedures. I understand that was the situation in
Washington state, and a midwife did force the state to test her and license her
under the old law. If there is such a law, then there may be legislation proposed
to strike it from the books, as has happened in several states recently.

On the federal level, nurse-midwives have been seeking third party reimbursement. Again it is an uphill fight. In 1978 at least two such bills died in U.S.
Senate committees. One was S. 618, a bill to amend the CHAMPUS program so
that the services of a licensed registered nurse (and hence a nurse-midwife)
could be provided under the program without a requirement that such services
be specified by a physician. Another was S. 1702, a bill to amend the Social
Security Act to provide for inclusion of services rendered by a certified nurse-
midwife under the medicare and medicaid programs. Both bills failed.

### The Role of the FDA in Assisting Doctors

So far I have discussed occupational licensure, and its effects on maternity
care, and the courts' role in backing it up. Next I would like to discuss the Food
and Drug Administration (FDA) and its influence.

Some of you may have been following the FDA's progress in restricting the
use of oxytocic drug products for the elective induction of labor. Doris Haire,
the President of the American Foundation for Maternal and Child Health, has
been working for over a year to alert the FDA to the widespread use of elective
induction of labor and its possible hazards. The FDA's Obstetrics and
Gynecology Advisory Committee (now known as the Fertility and Maternal
Health Drugs Advisory Committee) heard testimony over a period of several
months from Lewis Mehl, Estelle Cohen (the mother of a brain-damaged child
in the Bronx), Sheila Kitzinger, Lewis Sullivan of San Francisco, representing
the American Society for Psychoprophylaxis in Obstetrics, and several others,
and finally has issued revised package labels for oxytocic drug products. The
new labels have a box near the top with the following words: "IMPORTANT
NOTICE. (Name of drug) is indicated for the medical rather than the elective
induction of labor. Available data and information are inadequate to define the
benefits to risks considerations in the use of the drug product for elective induction. Elective induction of labor is defined as the initiation of labor for
convenience in an individual with a term pregnancy who is free of medical

indications." These revised labels were mailed to the pharmaceutical manufacturing companies on August 28th, 1978 and they were to have 60 days to put them into use.

This was an important victory for the interests of women and children, but one must not forget the historic role of the FDA in assisting the medical monopoly. One of the last remaining forms of competition to physicians is self-treatment, and the FDA has been the tool for controlling this trend by naming certain drugs as prescription drugs, available only with a physician's approval. Again it is important to remember who has the most influence at the FDA. The Obstetrics and Gynecology Advisory Committee was composed entirely of obstetrician-gynecologists. It did not have a single consumer member or even a pediatrician. After it had been repeatedly suggested that representatives of both be added, the renamed Fertility and Maternal Health Drugs Advisory Committee is now appointing a pediatrician and a consumer member.

Another positive step the FDA has taken in recent years is to require patient package inserts for estrogens. Patient package inserts are labels to explain in layperson's language the directions for use, including purposes or indications for the drug, the proper method of administration, precautions, and significant side effects and adverse reactions that may result. The reaction of the pharmaceutical manufacturing association has been to challenge in several federal courts the FDA's authority to require such labels. The one court that has reviewed the matter so far has upheld the FDA's authority to require patient labeling of prescription drugs. It was a Delaware case in October of 1977.

Generally, any action to make more information available to the patient can be construed as being in her interest. The Drug Regulation Reform Act of 1978 called for patient package inserts for all new drugs, as well as a complete revamping of the mechanism by which new drugs come on to the market. The bill did not pass this year, but is likely to be reintroduced next year in substantially similar form. The fate and specifics of this bill are additional examples of the strong influence of the medical monopoly. Many physicians testified before House and Senate health subcommittees on the evils of patient labels, which they asserted would destroy physician-patient relationships. The act did contain a proviso that the prescribing physician could decide to withhold the insert from a particular patient, unless the FDA ruled that the insert may never be withheld for that particular drug.

I attended some of the hearings on the drug bill, and it was interesting to see that some of the legislators were confused about the potential effects of patient labels. They were concerned that patient labels which mention possible adverse reactions to a drug may make the FDA liable to suit if that reaction should occur. While this may seem to be a confused line of reasoning, I did see Representative Tim Lee Carter, a physician member of the House Subcommittee on Health and the Environment, question witness after witness along these lines. Rep. Carter asked many witnesses whether they did not think that the FDA could be held liable if, for instance, Health Education and Welfare Secretary Califano were to contract leukemia from taking the drug Butazolidin in the event that a patient package insert included with the drug were to list leukemia as a possible adverse effect of the drug. Clearly our Congressmen are not familiar with George Annas's work showing a lower instance of malpractice suits when more information was available to the patient. (See The Rights of Hospital Patients, by George Annas, $1.50 in paperback).

Later I learned why Rep. Carter was so interested in Butazolidin. At another time Doris Haire was testifying before the same subcommittee on the merits of patient package inserts, and Rep. Carter questioned her. He wanted to know of what use a patient package insert would be when even the physician package label does not list all possible adverse effects. He noted that the physician label for Butazolidin did not list leukemia as a possible adverse effect. Ms. Haire did not wish to contradict Rep. Carter, but volunteered that she did have a copy of the physician label for Butazolidin with her, and perhaps he would like to look at it, since she believed it did mention leukemia. The label was passed up to Rep. Carter, and the questioning continued on another line. After a short time Rep. Carter broke in and said he wished to apologize to Ms. Haire. Not only did the package insert list leukemia as a possible adverse effect of Butazolidin, but it noted that leukemia could occur even after only a brief period of treatment with the drug. Ms. Haire heard later that Rep. Carter's own son had contracted leukemia.

To come back to the Drug Regulation Reform Act of 1978, another aspect which consumers found highly objectionable was a reduction of the penalties for noncompliance by the pharmaceutical manufacturing companies from criminal penalties, as are now imposed, to civil penalties. It was noted that the drug companies have such high profits that civil penalties, or fines, are hardly a deterrent at all, while criminal penalties, which involve jail sentences, are more effective. Note that Secretary Califano was very anxious to have the drug bill pass, and in private life he is a lawyer whose firm has one of the large pharmaceutical manufacturing companies as a client.

To relate the drug bill to obstetrics, it is important to notice that patient package inserts would be required only for new drugs, while the great majority of obstetric drugs have been on the market for years. When the bill is reintroduced in 1979, consumers should ask that the obstetric drugs also have required patient package inserts, and, furthermore, that a new drug's safety for childbearing women be established before the drug is approved for that use.

### Bills You May Wish to Promote for your own State

Before leaving the subject of patient information, I would like to mention three good bills which you may wish to try to have introduced in your own state. The first is a New York state bill passed in 1978 which concerns drug information to be furnished to expectant mothers. It states, "The physician or nurse-midwife in attendance at the birth of a child shall inform the expectant mother, in advance of the birth, of the drugs that such physician or nurse-midwife expects to employ during pregnancy and of the obstetrical and other drugs that such physician or nurse-midwife expects to employ at birth and of the possible effects of such drugs on the child and mother." The other two are a New Jersey bill on the release of patient records, and a Massachusetts one on release of a patient's hospital records. The full text of each appears in Volume I Number 3 of The Federal Monitor, a newsletter on current legislative activities, $8 for annual subscription, 50¢ per single issue, address: Federal Monitor, Drawer Q, McLean, VA 22101.

Doris Haire has some suggestions for having legislation passed in your state. Try to have it introduced by a legislator from the majority party, and one who represents a large urban area rather than a rural one. Take advantage of election years, since a legislator who is up for re-election will be more eager to please. Provide the legislator with copies of sample bills from other states, so that the job of drafting one for your state will be made easier.

### The Department of HEW
Another area of the government which affects maternity care is the Department of Health, Education and Welfare (HEW), through its programs designed to improve the outcome of pregnancy for women at risk. I am thinking of the extension of the Special Supplemental Food Program for Women, Infants and Children, known as the WIC program, and Secretary Califano's new program for pregnant adolescents. Both passed the House and the Senate in October 1978. The WIC program was incorporated into S. 3085,      The Child Nutrition Amendments Act, which includes the School Lunch Program. S. 3085 was delivered to the President on October 30th and signed   into law on Nov. 10th. The sections of the bill concerning WIC provide for increased appropriations over previous years. These funds are used to provide nutritious supplementary food to pregnant women, infants, and children under five, who are at risk due to low income. The appropriations authorized are $550 million for Fiscal Year 1979, and $800 million for Fiscal Year 1980, as compared to $440 million in 1978. The large increase is justified on the grounds that one third of the counties in the United States still have not set up WIC programs because of uncertain funding in the past.

Apparently, the nutritious foods given under the WIC program help the recipients to establish good eating habits, and studies by the Center for Disease Control in Atlanta indicate that WIC is having a significant impact in improving the outcome of pregnancy.

Another program under HEW is the Adolescent Health, Services and Pregnancy Prevention and Care Act of 1978. This act was added as an amendment to S. 2474, the Health Services Extensions Act, which also passed the Congress and awaits the President's signature. The parts concerned with adolescent pregnancy establish a program to develop networks of community-based services to prevent initial and repeat pregnancies among adolescents, to provide care to pregnant adolescents, and to help adolescents become productive independent contributors to family and community life. None of the funds authorized for the program may be used to pay for abortions, although an adolescent may be counselled or referred for an abortion if she so requests. S. 2474 was signed into law on November 10th, 1978.

In evaluating programs like these, it is important to note that whenever government programs are set up, it becomes compulsory for all of us to support them through our taxes, so we should look at them carefully. The WIC program and the one for pregnant adolescents are primarily for services, as opposed to programs for research. HEW's research branch most directly concerned with maternity care is probably the National Institute of Child Health and Human Development (NICHD). The purpose of NICHD is to conduct and support research and training relating to maternal and child health, and human development, including the special health problems and requirements of mothers and children and the processes of human growth and development, including prenatal development. The Institute periodically identifies areas in which it feels research is needed, and calls for grant applications in those areas. The applications received are then evaluated and the awards made. You can request to be on the mailing list for the NIH Guide to Grants and Contracts by writing to the National Institutes of Health, Bethesda, MD 20014. Ask for a form called "Request of Inclusion on Mailing List."

In 1978 I attended an NICHD grants committee meeting with Doris Haire. The committee members were physicians, mainly obstetrician-gynecologists and pediatricians, with NICHD staff persons in attendance also. The first hour of the grants meetings are usually open to the public under the Sunshine Act, while the later parts of the meetings during which specific grant applications are discussed are closed to the public. It is apparently quite rare for observers to attend the open parts of the grants committee meetings, for we were greeted with considerable curiosity and asked several times to be sure we had signed in. After listening to a discussion of how the best research results seemed to be coming from the medium sized institutions, as opposed to very large ones or individual researchers, the chairperson asked if either of the guests wished to comment or ask any questions. Ms. Haire accepted the invitation to comment, and said that she was concerned that if they were to decide to give almost all their grants to medium sized institutions, then individual researchers without the financial support of an institution would be left out. She mentioned Lewis Mehl's research comparing home and hospital births to give an example of a solitary researcher who merited NICHD's support. One obstetrician on the committee interrupted to say bluntly that he was familiar with Mehl's work and thought it was very poor. Ms. Haire replied politely that the Center for Disease Control had reviewed Dr. Mehl's study to which he was referring and found the methodology admirable. Ms. Haire went on to say she felt there was a great need for research on the effects of obstetrical medications on learning, and one of the staff members noted they had never received an application on that subject.

At the break several NICHD staff members came up to Ms. Haire and me to introduce themselves and offer their assistance if any individuals or organizations with which we were associated wished to apply for grants. This is an area in which our childbirth groups and others may wish to become active. Note that the NICHD is concerned with grants for research, however, and not services. As Ms. Haire and I were leaving, an NICHD staff member came out into the hall to compliment Ms. Haire on standing up to the committee member's questioning so calmly and effectively, and on being such a well-informed consumer.

## Congress and National Health Planning

There are two other areas I would like to touch on before closing. These are the Senate subcommittee hearing on obstetrics which was held in April, 1978 at the instigation of Doris Haire, and the issue of national health planning. On April 17th Senator Edward Kennedy presided over a Senate health subcommittee hearing into obstetrics. Senators Kennedy, Javits and Schweiker heard testimony regarding the safety of ultrasound, the relationship between fetal monitoring and cesarean rates, the use of drugs during pregnancy and labor, and the incidence of elective induction of labor. Three separate panels testified before the subcommittee. The first was FDA Commissioner Donald Kennedy and two of his staff members. The second panel consisted of Dr. Roberto Caldeyro-Barcia, Doris Haire, Dr. Albert Haverkamp, and Dr. Ronald Rindfuss. The final panel included Drs. Ervin Nichols, Richard Paul and George Ryan, representing the American College of Obstetricians and Gynecologists (ACOG), and Dr. Leonard Smith, an obstetrician in private practice. The ACOG showed its political astuteness once again in choosing Dr. Smith, since he practices in Hyannisport, Massachusetts, where the Kennedy family spend their summers.

During the hearing Senator Kennedy pointed out the discrepancy between the

ACOG's policy statement on ultrasound and the views of FDA Commissioner Kennedy. The ACOG policy statement says that "presently there is no evidence to suggest that ultrasound is deleterious to the fetus; therefore external monitoring is safe." Commissioner Kennedy, on the other hand, stated that "the risks (of ultrasound) are unknown, and because there is reason to suggest that there might be some risks, a cautious physician would want to be reasonably well assured that there was some benefit to the procedure" for a particular patient.

Commenting on fetal monitoring, Senator Kennedy stated, "As in many areas of medicine, the development of obstetrical technology far outstrips our capacity to assess its appropriate value. As a result, common practice is established before appropriate practice can be defined." To address the latter problem, Kennedy had introduced legislation (S. 2466) to create the National Institutes of Health Care Research, which would be a separate institute to support research designed to evaluate the appropriate use of technology.

The outcome of this hearing was that Senator Kennedy's legislation for a health care research institute did pass, but in an amended form. Instead of a separate institute, there will be simply an Office of Medical Technology within HEW. In addition, the FDA and HEW are continuing their consideration of the issues raised at the hearing, and the FDA is studying the safety of diagnostic ultrasound. A limited number of copies of the hearing record are available from the Subcommittee ou Health and Scientific Research, U.S. Senate, Washington, DC 20510.

To move on to health planning, I will not go into much detail because other articles in this volume discuss the network of Health Systems Agencies which have been set up to plan future hospital facilities for each area around the country. When the National Health Planning Guidelines were first published in proposed rulemaking form in September of 1977, they called for the closing of obstetric units with fewer than 2000 births per year, unless they were in sparsely populated areas with no other obstetrical services. In December, 1977, Muriel Sugarman of the International Childbirth Education Association, David Stewart of the National Association of Parents and Professionals for Safe Alternatives in Childbirth (NAPSAC), Doris Haire and I met with the authors of the guidelines and substantiated that HEW had no properly controlled data which justified using a births-per-year criterion for closing obstetric units. That fall and winter HEW received over 55,000 letters protesting the guidelines' plans to close these small obstetric units. As a result of the outcry the guidelines were loosened somewhat, but the impact remains the same. This is clearly a case in which we can not ignore the government, because it is taking actions which will affect us, whether we participate or not.

Although the local Health Systems Agencies are required by law to have a majority of consumer members, the medical professionals tend to dominate the planning process. The medical monopoly has lost no time in sending its suggested model for maternity care, a pamphlet entitled "Toward Improving the Outcome of Pregnancy," to every Health Systems Agency in the country. In the ACOG model of regionalization, the emphasis is on technology and high risk care, rather than on screening, preventative care, community involvement, and use of alternative settings and birth attendants. Some childbirth and women's organizations are mobilizing and preparing alternative models to send to the Health Systems Agencies. As Norma Swenson of the Boston Women's Health Collective said at the NAPSAC conference in Atlanta in May of

1978, "Our government does not recognize it as a conflict of interest that the most highly paid group of physicians is also the most influential in planning maternity care."

It is important for each of us to see that there are some consumers on our local Health Systems Agencies' boards who will have family-centered maternity care in mind. While the elimination of multiple small obstetrical units may appear to be likely to cut costs, what is more likely is that all women would be treated at greater cost and with more technology at the larger centers, while the consumer of maternity care would lose the option of picking a hospital which offers the care she wants. Birth and the Family Journal, Vol. 4, No.4, 1977, has an excellent article on regionalization. We can expect to achieve results by working on the level of our local Health Systems Agencies. One example of childbirth consumers influencing their Health Systems Agency is the grant awarded earlier this fall to a project being cosponsored by a Western Massachusetts Health Systems Agency and an area childbirth group. The project, entitled "Berkshire Birth: Rights and Ritual," concerns a study of alternative birth settings which the Health Systems Agency is undertaking in response to the growing enthusiasm for home births in Berkshire County. The grant comes from the Massachusetts Foundation for the Humanities and Public Policy, which supports public education projects which bring the learning of the humanities to bear on current controversial issues for the benefit of the citizens of Massachusetts.

### Summary

In summary, it is important to remember in dealing with the government that the government is far more apt to have the best interests of physicians and drug manufacturing companies in mind, rather than those of women and children. So, we need to look every gift horse in the mouth. Evaluate proposed legislation to see whether it serves to limit entry into the medical practice field, or whether it gives groups other than physicians an opportunity to practice their professions. Look at proposed programs to see whether they are oriented toward patient information, toward health, toward prevention, screening, nutrition, consumer participation, and the use of alternative care providers and settings. Or do they emphasize technology, high risk care, specialists, and lack of consumer choice. Is there a non-government alternative? Will the program tend to be self-perpetuating and inflationary, heavy on the bureaucracy that administers it and light on the services provided? Will there be any assessment of the effectiveness, and any way to terminate the program if it is found lacking? Above all, do not ignore the government's actions which relate to maternity care, because the government is continuously taking steps which affect women and children, and not necessarily favorably. Remember, we can influence the government, and we have more chance of success today than ever before.

Want to Contact a Particular Author?
All of their Addresses are on Page 281

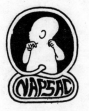

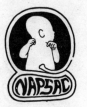

## CHAPTER THREE

### HOW GOVERNMENT GUIDELINES ORIGINATE:
An Investigation of How a National Standard was set
for minimum size of OB  Services

#### Ms. Robbi Pfeufer

#### Foreword
Since the investigation reported below was undertaken, there have been revisions due to pressure from the public of the obstetrical guidelines which are the subject of this paper. For example, the standard for large city hospitals was reduced from 2,000 to 1,500 deliveries per year. The revised guidelines can be found in:

Federal Register, Friday, 20 January 1978, Part V. Department of Health, Education and Welfare. Health Resources Administration. National Guidelines for Health Planning. Vol. 43, No. 14, 3060-1.

I decided to leave the article as is, for its value, if there is value to be found, lies in describing a piece of the process by which government policy comes into being as seen from a consumer's optic.

#### Introduction
Large decorated initials frequently illustrated the texts of medieval illuminated manuscripts. These lively images often seem to assume an independent life on the page. Forms turn, bend, densely interlace, producing and reproducing elaborations. Contained by a schema, this activity takes place within a totality, suggesting, along with inclusion, exclusion.

#### The Case of a Minimum Size Guideline
Early in October 1977, word came to the Ad Hoc Committee on Maternity and Newborn Care attached to the Area IV Health Systems Agency (HSA) (1), that a national guideline had appeared in the Federal Register recommending a minimum size criterion for obstetrical services. The news had not come through the HSA paid staff, there to provide technical assistance to the publicly elected HSA volunteer members. It had come through sources in the childbirth movement, a loosely-knit, although national, interest group.

On hearing of the guidelines, the Ad Hoc Committee, which I belong to, immediately called the HSA staff for copies. Soon after, I opened the Federal Register of 23 September 1977 (2) and there, in six point type, but illuminating the section like a large medieval decorated initial, was a minimum size criterion for obstetrical services of 2,000 deliveries (for Standard Metropolitan Statistical Areas (SMSA) with populations of 100,000 or more).

This quantitative standard, 2,000, encapsulated a totality of discourse and activity which we had watched come into being, first as an informal consumer committee, later as an HSA planning committee. From the beginnings of

---

Ms. Robbi Pfeufer is a childbirth educator, member of HSA, Sub-Area Council, IV, a candidate for MA and MPH degrees, Boston University, and author of several articles on Regionalization.

regionalized planning for maternity and newborn care (3), the process seemed to take on a life of its own. Like the medieval example, one or two essential design elements initiated endless elaborations at a rate which appeared to outstrip conscious intention. However, the framework within which this repetition took place remained exclusionary. Despite repeated efforts to enter the schema (4), most recently through election to the HSA, our committee remained for the most part operationally outside of it. Finally, catching us by surprise, a highly reduced summary image, which the number 2,000 is, of an entire pattern of obstetrical practice appeared as a proposed standard at the national level.

### The Purpose of this Study

The purpose of this paper was to find out what empirical data supported the figure 2,000, through interviews and a literature review. The study is by no means conclusive or even inclusive. It merely is intended to disclose information and issues and to make certain observations.

This preliminary search gave me academic rather than activist access to the schema, the latter having been, as I mentioned earlier, nearly impossible. Following this turn I came to find out more about how the number reached the Federal Register and why it was there, than to discover the firm empirical ground it rested upon.

To begin with, I would like to briefly describe the main elements of the proposed maternity care model which the guideline number summarizes. Then I would like to discuss the alternative model which is made up of those elements excluded from the schema. The alternative model begins from a shared premise — the need for a regionalized network of maternity and newborn care services. It assumes, however, an almost symmetrically dissimilar form from the other plan. Where one recommends centralized services, the other recommends decentralized services; where one is a high-risk model of care, the other is a low-risk model of care; and so on.

### The "High Risk" Model of Regionalization

The "basic text" of the regionalization concept, "Toward Improving the Outcome of Pregnancy, Recommendations for the Regional Development of Maternal and Perinatal Services," was written by the Committee on Perinatal Health, made up of representatives from the American College of Obstetricians and Gynecologists (ACOG), the American Medical Association (AMA), the American Academy of Pediatrics (AAP), and the American Academy of Family Practice (AAFP). Funded by the National Foundation March of Dimes (MOD), the project began work in 1972, issued a final draft which was used immediately, and published a monograph in 1976.

The document outlines a national plan to lower costs and improve quality of obstetrical care, intended, as the report states, as recommendations and goals rather than as directives. The Committee recommends the centralization of obstetrical units. Remaining services would be organized into a coordinated network for consultation, education, and transfer of patients, serving a population-based area. To justify their continued existence, obstetrical units would be expected to satisy certain standards and criteria. These would include annual volume of deliveries (2,000 suggested) and a relatively medically intensive baseline capability for all units. Different levels of care would be allowed between, for instance, teaching hospitals and community hospitals.

The argument for a medically intensive baseline of care rests on another number which, along with the 2,000 figure, needs careful study, but only can be noted here. The current assertion in obstetrics is that one-third to one-half of all complications cannot be predicted before labor begins (5). The alternative model, on the other hand, relies upon the statistic quoted world-wide (6) that approximately 80-90 percent of all women can give birth without complications. Planning strategies based on these two sets of statistics obviously would be and are quite different.

Justification for the high-risk model of care, formalized as planning recommendations in the Committee on Perinatal Health monograph, proliferated rapidly even before the Committee issued its final draft (7). Nevertheless, several nagging doubts remained, expressed in the literature. First, were the declines in mortality and morbidity over the last decade or so due to numerous advances in perinatal and neonatal medicine, including regionalized programs? Or were the improved rates due to the decline in the birth rate, the availability of abortion and birth control, and improved interconceptional spacing? — all of which took place during the same time period (8). Furthermore, despite slight improvements nationally, the U.S. infant mortality rate, a sensitive indicator of the health of a society, continued to compare unfavorably with other developed countries of the world (9). Secondly, did the adverse effects of various invasive diagnostic procedures and manipulations of the normal process of labor outweigh the benefits (10)? What were the long-term effects of these new practices and procedures (11).?

Despite these unresolved questions (known mainly to the medical profession), the approach outlined in the monograph appealed to health planners and policy makers. It seemed to reflect the prevailing spirit of cost containment and regional planning and happily too, filled a planning gap. Comprehensive Health Planning Agencies (12) and later Health Systems Agencies incorporated features into their own plans (13). State health departments across the country provided support and assistance for local implementation of the Committee recommendations (14).

In Massachusetts, for example, the State Department of Public Health (DPH), with funds provided by the U.S. Department of Health, Education and Welfare, the Tri-State Regional Medical Program, and Blue Cross of Massachusetts, Inc., collaborated on a statewide study of regionalization of maternity and newborn care. This comprehensive report (15) included proposed standards and criteria for all obstetrical services based on the recommendations of the Committee on Perinatal Health. Fortunately, before these regulations were completed, the newly formed Health Systems Agency intervened to block further work on the regulations until alternative models were explored and until DPH included broader representation in its planning efforts. Furthermore, DPH was reminded of its responsibility to work with the HSAs (16). Other forces outside the HSA such as vigorous opposition from community obstetricians undoubtedly contributed to the temporary halt in state regulatory planning for obstetrics.

Not too long after, similar standards, particularly the ubiquitous size criterion, this time for 1,500 deliveries, appeared at the national level in a bill proposing maternal and child national health insurance. Under this bill, only services operating at 1,500 annual volume would qualify for reimbursement (17).

Then the figure sprang up as a proposed national guideline for obstetrical services under PL 93-641. Potentially, this last development was the most important because regional HSAs were required by law to incorporate the guidelines set by HEW into their Health Systems Plans. Thus, efforts at state and local levels, some through HSAs, some not, to restructure or at least to modify existing patterns of obstetrical care might be curtailed severely.

### The "Low Risk" Model of Regionalization

The low-risk model for maternity and newborn care begins at a symmetrically opposite point from the Committee on Perinatal Health plan (18). It assumes that most childbearing women will have normal, uncomplicated labors and deliveries. It proposes, therefore, that the baseline for obstetrical care should be set at a low-risk level of care including: decentralized, non-institutional services located in communities (although maintaining links with a high-risk center); use of midwives as the primary care-giver; standardized, rigorous prenatal screening and supervision of pregnant women; and the like. Furthermore, this approach would seek to reduce the high-risk population (10-20 percent of women) rather than expanding capacities to handle a stable population of high-risk cases. Noting the apparent equation between high-risk and low-income, proponents of this model suggest attacking the problem at the level of primary prevention — nutrition supplementation, nutrition and childbirth education, education for parenthood, improved access to care, continuity and comprehensibility of care — rather than reserving resources for end-stage remedies. In the low-risk view, the U.S. infant mortality rate's poor ranking internationally demonstrates the need to re-examine maternity care practices in this country immediately as one possible causal variable. Patterns of care in countries with best ranking infant mortality rates should be studied for the possible application of their methods to our own system. Advocates of a low-risk model express much concern over the relative risk attached to molding normal childbirth to fit into a high-risk model of care (19).

Theoretically, each of these proposed systems, high-risk and low-risk, should be given equal weight by guideline makers, since proponents of each approach have gathered a substantial body of supportive evidence. Also, theoretically, either approach should lose persuasive force if scientific fact contradicted its assumptions. But the dominance of the medical model which our committee witnessed at the state level reproduced itself at the national level, empirical facts or no empirical facts. Political reality — who can tug hardest at the sleeve of government — rather than scientific reality seems to be the decisive factor. But to return to the original question: What empirical evidence is there to support an annual volume of 2,000 deliveries for most hospitals?

### On the Absence of Science in Policy Making

The literary sources I turned to, some of which I referred to earlier, did not shed light on the efficacy of the proposed quantitative standard. By the literature's own account, evidence for an ideal minimum size criterion tends to be unsystematically derived and contradictory (21). The most illuminating, although unexpectedly bald information, came from my conversations with half a dozen people (22), four directly or indirectly involved in the development of the guidelines, a consumer activist, and a medical economist.

Responses to the question, "Is there empirical data to support the number 2,000?" included the following: "No, it was put out for comment to test the waters." "Frankly, we started high to bargain down." "There was a great variation in recommendation; we took a middle figure." "Economic data is not uniform enough to prove economies of scale." "Mortality studies by size of hospital do not control for variables; they are poor studies." "There is a changing view of risk by what your economic requirements are." "Frankly, there hasn't been a lot of justification for the figure." "Clinically, the size of hospital only indicated improved mortality and morbidity for very tiny babies (1-2 percent of the population)." "No, we don't support it ourselves" (ACOG). "An approximated break even point for Level II service." "An ACOG study showed that the larger the hospital and the more closely associated with a medical institution, the higher the infant mortality rate (23). When I told this to HEW, they said they had a study which showed that when you control for the greater number of high risk cases at the large hospitals, infant mortality is shown to be lower there than at smaller hospitals. So someone went over to HEW to pick up a copy of this study, and they were told no such study existed."

I never expected the weight of scientific evidence to be so slight nor if so, to be acknowledged so candidly and universally. My next impulse was to say, "Why you are all nothing but a pack of cards!" After the frustrated efforts of our committee to enter the dialogue over the last three years, this would have been gratifying to me, but would not help at all. The figure 2,000 remained and remained to be dismantled, and if, as I soon learned, it was to be dismantled, how would a new standard be assembled? Potentially the same problems of process would recur. But problems to whom? Our problems, trying to enter the forum of policy making, were not shared by everyone else who had a stake in these guidelines. The common denominator though did turn out to be that everyone had problems with the figure 2,000. Even legal problems about compliance with due process. But not to get ahead of the story.

Once I discovered the absence of empirical evidence, I decided to find out how these guidelines came into being at the national level, for most definitely they were there, although not yet cast in bronze. This sleuthing effort found me deeper inside the medieval initial than ever. Apparently as well as there being no way in, there also was no way out. The few elements which created the high-risk model, its many elaborations at the state level, and the extensive literature supporting advances in perinatal and neonatal medicine were the main discourse consulted by HEW. But exactly how did the guidelines reach the Federal Register, and exactly why were they there?

### How General Legislation Turns Into Detailed Regulation

The Federal Register of 23 September 1977 (24) begins with the following supplementary information: "Section 1501 of the Public Health Service Act as amended by the National Health Planning and Resource Development Act of 1974 (PL 93-641) requires the secretary of HEW to issue, by regulations, guidelines concerning national health planning policy."

The introduction explains, among other things, that these guidelines are to include "National health planning goals, which, to the maximum extent practicable, shall be expressed in quantitative terms." The introduction further states that although PL 93-641 recognizes that cost, access, and quality of care all were urgent issues, these guidelines would address only short-term cost containment measures in the institutional sector, in order to help planning agencies with this task immediately. Thus these proposed guidelines refer only to resource standards within specific categories of health services, those which have been shown to be the most inflationary, namely, acute care. Additional guidelines, it was stated, will pertain to problems of access and quality, will take up ambulatory and long-term care issues, and will come out at a later time.

HSAs, the supplementary information continued, must comply in their Health Systems Plans with these guidelines within a year after promulgation and will be required to meet these resource standards within five years or less if possible. Certain exceptions to the standards are allowed.

Broadly speaking, national guidelines canalize the authority of regional HSAs so that regional decision-making flows within certain policy boundaries. To achieve this, guideline-makers specify the legislative intent of a Congressional act such as PL 93-641 in greater detail than is found in the act itself, which tends to be very broad in scope and general in language. Because they give further shape to the spirit of the law, these guidelines are very important. Administrative agencies, to whom Congress gives discretionary power to create guidelines, also are very important. For they not only have been delegated very broad powers, but they also have considerable latitude in carrying them out — who they consult with, how they make their decisions and based on what evidence, and how much public process they permit in creating guidelines.

Charged with the purpose delegated to them by PL 93-641, department staff within the Health Resources Administration, an arm of HEW, set about developing guidelines three or four years ago. These were scheduled to be completed a year and a half ago. Altogether, guidelines were needed for 16 areas of health services, an undertaking which cost one million dollars.

The initial step involved soliciting competitive bids for a contract to survey the state of the art and to publish these findings in a monograph, one for each of the 16 areas, each contracted independently. Contracts were awarded to bidders based on how well the project was done, whether it met the requirements, previous work done by the firm, the bid, and staffing capabilities. A consulting firm (there was some hedging over which it was) was chosen to produce the obstetrics monograph for HEW. In-house staff then took this document, added to it their own independent literature search and review of original documents, "talked to some people," and drew up a draft of the guidelines about a year ago. An advisory panel also was involved. Finally, the draft was circulated to various groups for comment at that time.

A bibliography, derived from all 16 monographs, was compiled and is available for inspection at Health Resources Administration Office of Planning, Evaluation, and Legislation in Hyattsville, Maryland. Each member of the National Advisory Council, the federal HSA planning body, has a copy of this bibliography. The Massachusetts member of the NAC has a copy of it (25).

Due to the change in administration, the guidelines were very overdue and when, in late June 1977, Julius Richmond, M.D., became Assistant Secretary of HEW, pressure was brought to bear to get the guidelines issued for comment. They were pulled together in a matter of weeks, "under great pressure," an HEW spokesperson emphasized more than once. The Congress, in general, and Senator Kennedy and Congressman Rogers (26), in particular, were impatient to see them in print immediately.

The next part of the story recounts the issuance of the guidelines and perhaps best can be introduced by a prophetic quote from the Federal Register supplementary information (27). "The state of the art of establishing specific quantitative resource standards is still in its infancy." As the next events show, it is a high-risk infancy at that.

On 23 September 1977, the proposed guidelines appeared in the Federal Register. At that time, no notice was given of any hearing which might pertain to them, only a date by which responses must be submitted (22 November, later extended to 9 December, the date of the next NAC meeting). As it happened, 23 September was itself the day of an NAC meeting. According to due process requirements, the NAC must approve proposed guidelines before they are issued. This was unlikely to have happened in the appropriate sequence, thus constituting an infringement of due process. When asked about this, one HEW spokesperson said, "It's Congress's fault for putting too much pressure on."

In response to the proposed resource standards, 25,000 written testimonies were submitted. About 80 percent of these came from consumers objecting to the closure of community hospitals, probably prompted by their obstetricians or gynecologists, since most consumers do not read the Federal Register, regularly or irregularly. The ACOG submitted a 10-page, single-spaced letter critiquing the obstetrical guidelines (28). They stated that it might not be permissible legally for HEW to impose federal standards, that the guidelines interfered with local and regional planning, and that the imposition of the size criterion would be medically and economically disastrous.

On 21 October 1977, a public hearing on the guidelines was announced in the Federal Register, only 18 days before the hearing was held. This hasty notice constituted another likely infringement of due process. At least 30 days must elapse between notification of a hearing and the day it is held. Certain groups were invited to send representatives, such as ACOG. But to the knowledge of the Area IV HSA, to take only one obvious example, no invitation was received by them. This undoubtedly was true for other such planning bodies, although it would seem logical to solicit their testimony at the hearing. Consumer representatives who had testified at the hearing on the bill for Maternal and Child National Health Insurance, another obvious, easily visible source of invitees, were not approached. A written summary of the 8 November hearing is available (29).

While those testifying all agreed on the need for regional systems, no one approved the size criterion. Apparently, a spectrum of objections was raised. The guideline's inflexibility, impracticality, potential infringement of states' rights, local planning agencies' rights, hospital rights, and perhaps above all, the rights of the medical profession to set its own standards were mentioned. On this last point, George Ryan, M.D., M.P.H., F.A.C.O.G., one of the main authors of the regionalization monograph, reportedly stated, "I support the figure but not its application." One witness objected to what he saw as a step toward socialistic and communistic medicine.

Responding to pressure from Congressmen, who were responding to pressure from constituents, Secretary of HEW, Joseph Califano, wrote a letter on 30 November (30) to Senator Kennedy and Congressman Rogers and "all members of Congress," calling for a reconsideration of the proposed guidelines. He said in his letter we "recognize that the current proposed standards for obstetrical units may be too strict. We intend to review this standard carefully and to revise it appropriately to take into account the objections that have been raised."

To our knowledge, a second public hearing was not called, although this would seem to be the appropriate step. Instead, at its 9 December meeting, the National Advisory Council delegated the revision of the guidelines to three men, Julius Richmond, M.D., Hale Champion, and a Dr. Foley, a member of the NAC

(31). They were asked to come up with revisions in one week's time. (Apparently a newsletter publication called the Health Finance Newsletter carries an excellent summary of the whole history of these guidelines, including perhaps most importantly, a clear presentation of the key figures involved. As the member of our maternity committee, herself an M.D., said on returning from Washington, "It's like Greek to find out who's who.")

The visit of the childbirth movement representatives to Washington was, as expected, inconclusive. A small group met with HEW representatives (who had changed the appointment hour three times in the previous week) on 5 December. Later they held a press conference and at the end of the day met with Roger's assistant, Robert Crane. He is reported to have said, "We're not happy about these guidelines ourselves." They gave copious amounts of materials to the various government representatives, which were costly to xerox, and picked up certain documents — a copy of Califano's letter, the testimony of the 8 November hearing, and some others.

But no precise mechanism was established to ensure an equal voice, or even any voice, in the reworking of the guidelines. Concern is strong that the schema will close over again, the inner elaborations set into motion as before, resulting in final guidelines not substantially different from the ones now under attack. Furthermore, these final guidelines could then be said to reflect a broad consensus, including contributions from the childbirth movement. This assertion would be minimally accurate, if that.

HEW representatives explained to our emissaries that Parts II and III of the guidelines will be issued in January and March respectively. While the present proposed guidelines address the most inflationary sectors of the health care system, these also are among the most powerful sectors politically. Thus, issues of access, quality, and ambulatory care will have to be fit into designs built around the acute care sector, which hardly will provide much room for innovation and genuine restructuring (and cost containment).

For example, if, as ACOG says in its written testimony (32), the 2,000 figure is too high (A survey of SMSAs showed an average of only 1,470 annual deliveries at larger units), large units will be forced to compete for patients with out-of-hospital facilities. Indeed, the latter type of service is likely to be strongly opposed come March. If guidelines for these deinstitutionalized services will not be proposed until the spring, which is the current plan, it almost presupposes the unlikelihood of their coming into being at all.

Final guidelines will have a powerful impact upon regional HSAs as the summary information in the Federal Register described (33). In order to receive continued funding, HSAs must comply with the guidelines in their Health Systems Plan. State health departments, already enthusiastic about the regionalization plan, would be likely to revise their regulations for hospital services to conform to the Health Systems Plan in their state. While Califano's letter says that the federal government has no right to close hospitals down, in effect this is what very well could happen. Philosophically, promulgating guidelines piecemeal seems foolish. (Politically, for those who stand to gain by this approach, it may make a lot of sense.) It contradicts the process by which regional HSAs have been asked to formulate their Health Systems Plans. Certainly a piecemeal approach is not likely to promote, let alone exemplify, integrated health planning. And yet the HEW guidelines are expected to be the binding agent which will smooth out lumps and inconsistencies in the health care system nationally.

If the story breaks off here it is because it is unfinished and because the future storyline is unclear to us. What the best next step for us to take may only be the next best step, since the best step is one which we are powerless to make. We would like to help revise the guidelines. We would have liked to help write the monograph.

But this is, of course, a fantasy. No more fantastic, though, than the strange shape obstetrical care has taken over the last decade in the United States. This pattern of care continues to warp in ways predictable and unpredictable patterns of family beginnings (34), a distortion which began in earnest when childbirth was moved to the hospital.

At the heart (35) of the current system of practice is a system of belief intertwined with such practical considerations as economic gain, career opportunity, and the like — all of which the number 2,000 mutely or not so mutely expresses. It is this system of belief and pragmatics which has created an impermeable schema on the outside and a rich inner culture on the inside where elements proliferate rapidly. To take just one example, neonatal and perinatal technology proliferates so quickly that techniques become obsolete before they can be evaluated through clinical trials (36).

This solipsistic totality, while resisting intrusion from any outside elements which truly seek to alter it, has demonstrated a remarkable capacity to absorb and transform certain modifications of present obstetrical practice. These incorporations include birth rooms inside hospitals, Leboyer deliveries, and family-centered cesarean births, to name a few. So long as the essential structure remains intact, these concessions are allowed.

### Conclusion

If there is one conclusion I can come to with reasonable confidence at the end of this inquiry, it is that, whatever else it may be, the stuff the schema is made up of is not objective scientific fact.

The "whatever else it may be" deserves close analysis, because the totality I keep coming back to to describe with variations on an image is compelling indeed, as all politically powerful things are. But, without question, the elements I have only hinted at here can be analyzed. It would be very useful to systematically demystify this reality in order to better work upon it, around it, and in spite of it. Unravelling how guidelines get written is a small contribution in this direction.

This piece of research raised serious questions in my mind about who had or perhaps more importantly, who had not been included directly or indirectly in a public process (at least nominally public) to create public policy.

Whatever the contest of forces outside the realm of public policy making (which is inequitable enough), our contention is that inside the domain of public policy a public process must be followed. This process would take into account that the available discourse found in the literature is biased, that consumer views are not represented, that physicians' views may carry great weight but are not broadly representative either of health care providers or of the overall population of the United States.

Policy makers have a duty to reach out to those groups not present in the discourse, who most likely work on volunteer time, who have neither xerox machines nor WATS lines at their disposal. The brief study I made revealed a relatively harried group of policy makers in Washington who did not seem able, even had they wanted to, to exercise this kind of initiative. In the absence of such efforts, the dominant view on any policy matter, which is not necessarily the view most broadly representative, can slip easily enough into the realm of public policy.

For the moment, the HSAs at the regional level show promise of supporting broad representation in policy planning. How these regional efforts will fare over time, how, for instance, executive planning will integrate with regional HSAs' health systems planning, remains to be seen.

## References

1. (1974) National Health Planning and Resources Development Act (PL 93-641); 93rd Congress, 2nd session, approved 4 January 1975. Created under this law, HSAs are regional health planning bodies. They are non-profit corporations with Boards of Directors. Members are made up of providers and consumers, with a consumer majority. Among other responsibilities, HSAs must develop Health Systems Plans for their areas, taking into account issues such as cost containment, access to care, and quality of care.
2. (1977) Federal Register, Part II, Department of Health, Education and Welfare, Health Resources Administration, National Guidelines for Health Planning, Advance Notice of Proposed Rulemaking, Vol. 42, No. 185, 23 September, 48502-48505.
3. Regionalization of obstetrical services is a separate planning effort from regionalization of neonatal intensive care. The latter system developed in the late 1960s and primarily involves education, consultation, and transfer of sick neonates to neonatal intensive care units (NICUs), rather than a reorganization of hospital units.
4. (1975) Ad Hoc Committee on Maternity and Newborn Care, HSA IV, draft report: The Proposed Plan for Regionalization of Maternity and Newborn Care in Massachusetts, Preliminary Analysis and Recommendations (Luce, Norsigian, Pfeufer, Swenson, Sugarman); A. Lynch (1977), The Crucial Role of Consumers in Planning Maternal Health Care, Library Bulletin 333 (June-July).
5. C. Donahue et al. (1977), The Closure of Maternity Services in Massachusetts, Obs. Gyn. 50 (3): 280-284.
6. P. Dunn (1976), Obstetric delivery today: For better or for worse? Lancet 10 (April): 790-793.
7. (1974) Modern Perinatal Medicine, ed. I. Gluck. Chicago: Year Book Medical Publishers, Inc.
8. (1974) Clinics in Perinatology. Philadelphia: W.B. Saunders Co., September 1:1, March 1:2.
9. J.M. Schneider (1977), Infant mortality and morbidity statistics — 1975, Perinatal Press 1 (No. 3, April: 1. Summary figures for 1975: U.S. IMR 16.1:1000. The U.S. continues to rank about 15th compared to other developed countries.
10. R.L. Schwarz et al. (1974), Conservative management of labor, Recent Progress in Obstetrics and Gynecology, Proc. VII, Congr. Int'l. Obstetrics and Gynecology, ed. L.S. Persianinov et al. Prague: Avicenum Checos Medical Press, 105-126; A. Haverkamp et al. (1976), The evaluation of continuous electronic fetal heart rate monitoring in high-risk pregnancy, Am. J. Obs. Gyn. 125 (3): 310-320.

11. H. Frost and M. Stratmeyer (1977), In-vivo effects of diagnostic ultra-sound, Lancet 7 (May):999.
12. (1974) Report on Hospital-Based Maternity Services in Health Planning Regions III, V, and VI, draft, prepared by the Planning and Standards Committee of the Health Planning Council for Greater Boston.
13. (1977) The Health Systems Plan for Massachusetts HSA IV, Draft Volumes 1 and 2, Health Planning Council for Greater Boston, Inc.
14. A. Pettigrew (1974), The role of the state department of health in regionalized perinatal care, Regionalization of Perinatal Care, Report of the Sixty-Sixth Conference on Pediatric Research, Ross Laboratories.
15. (1977) Massachusetts Maternity and Newborn Regionalization Project, Regionalization of Maternity and Newborn Care in Massachusetts, Final Report, 1 August 1974 — 30 September 1976.
16. (1977) HSA IV Board of Directors recommendation, 8 February.
17. (1976) Maternal and Child Health Care Act, HR14822, 94th Congress, 2nd session.
18. D. Stewart (1977), An Optimal Maternity Plan, paper given at 105th Annual Meeting of the American Public Health Association, Washington, D.C., 23-31 October, 2:00-5:00 p.m. (67 references).
19. D. Haire (1976), The Cultural Warping of Childbirth, Monograph of the International Childbirth Education Association, revised edition.
20. (1976) ACOG establishes Washington branch, ACOG Newsletter 20 (No. 9, September).
21. L. Kirsch (1976), Letter to Program Director, Office of Health Planning Facilities Development, Massachusetts Department of Public Health, 12 May; A. Fleck (1977), Hospital sizes and outcomes of pregnancy, Office of the Assistant Commissioner for Child Health, New York State Department of Public Health, 23 February; Project Report; Committee on Perinatal Health.
22. Marian Troyer, Program Analyst, Office of Health Policy Research and Statistics, Department of Health, Education and Welfare, Washington, D.C.; Laurell Shannon, Office of Planning, Evaluation, and Legislation, Health Resources Administration, Hyattsville, Maryland; Elaine Locke, Executive Assistant to Ervin E. Nichols, M.D., Director, Practice Activities, American College of Obstetricians and Gynecologists; Charles Donahue, J.R., M.A., Boston University Center for Health Planning; Lawrence J. Kirsch, M.A., Principal Associate, Center for Community Health and Medical Care, Harvard University Medical School; Doris Haire, D.M.S., President, American Foundation for Maternal and Child Health, Inc.
23. (1970) National Study of Maternity Care: Survey of Obstetric Practice and Associated Services in Hospitals in the United States, Committee on Maternal Health of the American College of Obstetricians and Gynecologists.
24. Federal Register, 48502.
25. Philip Caper, M.D., University of Massachusetts Medical Center, Worcester.
26. Senator Edward Kennedy, D.-Mass., Chair of the Health and Scientific Research Subcommittee of the Human Resources Standing Committee (Senate); Congressman Paul Rogers, D.-Fla., Chair of the Interstate and Foreign Commerce Committee, Head of Health and the Environment Subcommittee (House).
27. Federal Register, 48503.

28. (1977) Official response of the American College of Obstetricians and Gynecologists to the health planning guidelines, 21 November.
29. I haven't seen this summary yet.
30. I haven't seen this letter yet.
31. Julius Richmond, M.D., Assistant Secretary for Health, HEW; Hale Champion, Acting Secretary, HEW; Dr. Foley, NAC.
32. ACOG official response, 5.
33. Federal Register, 48502-3.
34. D. Haire; M. Klaus and J. Kennell (1976), Maternal-Infant Bonding, St. Louis: C.V. Mosby; M. Sugarman (1977), Perinatal influences on maternal-infant attachment, Amer. J. Orthopsychiat. 47 (No. 3); 407-421.
35. N. Devitt (1977), The transition from home to hospital birth in the United States, 1930-1960, Birth and the Family Journal 4 (No. 46, Summer).
36. Modern Perinatal Medicine.

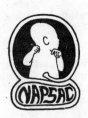

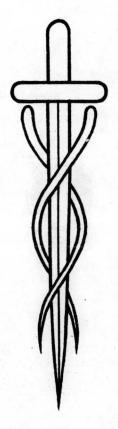

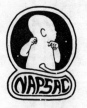

# CHAPTER FOUR

## HEALTH CARE PLANNING — WHO IS IN CONTROL?

### Diony Young

The question of who is in control of regional health planning is absolutely vital if the present system is going to work for the benefit of all of us who use health care services. But before I answer it, I need to describe briefly what is happening in health planning in the United States today and how we got there.

Since World War II various federal health planning bodies were created to try to solve the problems of rising costs, maldistribution of services, and quality of care. These bodies included the Regional Medical Program (RMP), the Comprehensive Health Planning (CHP) program, and the Hill-Burton hospital construction program. In these programs consumers had token or no participation. The power was in the hands of physicians and other providers, who failed in their attempts to reduce costs to prevent overexpansion of hospitals, to eliminate duplication of services, and to provide adequate primary care where it was needed. Decision making was largely secret, hospitals were fearful of sharing services or developing cooperative programs, and little accountability to the public existed. Health planning was essentially political game playing and empire building — with consumers carrying the increasing cost. Complex, large, and self-serving institutions provided health care, and "serving the sick," which was the original stated purpose, was replaced by "self-protection of vested interests." This is still a problem today (10).

In 1974, the Health Planning and Resources Development Act was passed to try to solve the problems of the past. This legislation assimilated the RMP, CHP, and Hill-Burton programs into one planning agency, the Health Systems Agency (HSA), over 200 of which are now planning health care throughout the country. The legislation provided new tools to work with. The question is, will the HSAs, with their mandated consumer majorities be able to use these tools? Before answering that question, we need to know how this new legislation functions.

Table 1 outlines the organization and major functions. The geographic areas which the HSAs represent will be the keystone in the reorganized system.

The law states that the purposes of HSAs are:
1. To improve the health of residents
2. To increase accessibility, acceptability, continuity, and quality of services
3. To restrain increases in health care costs
4. To prevent unnecessary duplication of services

Table 2 shows the composition of an HSA. All business meetings of the HSA and its committees and councils must be open to the public and announced well in advance, and all records and data are available to the public on request. Decisions require a quorum (not less than one half the membership). Public

---

Diony Young is an editor of medical books for C.V. Mosby Company, HSA Board Director, member of Regional Hospital Council, Board member ICEA, and author of ICEA pamphlet, "Bonding — How Parents Become Attached to Their Baby."

| Public Law 93-641 (1974) | |
|---|---|
| **NATIONAL HEALTH PLANNING & RESOURCES DEVELOPMENT ACT** | |
| Organization & Major Functions | |
| **NATIONAL** | |
| Secretary of Health, Education & Welfare (HEW) | Nat'l Council on Health Policy & Devl'mt (NCHPD) |
| 1. Designates & approves Health Systems Agencies.<br>2. Issues national guidelines for health planning.<br>3. Provides priorities for health planning goals. | 1. Advises, consults with, and makes recommendations to Secretary of HEW about National guidelines for health facilities, services and manpower. |
| **STATE** | |
| Statewide Health Coordinating Council (SHCC) | State Health Planning & Devel'mt Agency (SHPDA) |
| 1. Annually reviews & coordinates HSA's plans.<br>2. Prepares state health plan.<br>3. Reviews HSA budgets.<br>4. Approves/disapproves state plans and applications for certain federal funds.<br>5. Advises the SHPDA. | 1. Conducts state health planning activities.<br>2. Integrates health plans of HSA's into preliminary state health plan.<br>3. Reviews appropriateness of all institutional state health services every 5 years. |
| **REGIONAL** | |
| Health Systems Agency (HSA) | |
| 1. Assembles & analyzes health data about the population.<br>2. Establishes, implements & annually updates Health Systems Plan (HSP), which is long-range, as well as the Annual Implementation Plan (AIP), which is for one year.<br>3. Reviews & approves/disapproves applications for federal funds for health programs or state certification to provide services.<br>4. Coordinates activities with Professional Standards Review Organizations (PSRO's).<br>5. Recommends priorities for modernizing, constructing, & converting health care facilities. | |
| **LOCAL** | |
| Subarea Council (SAC) | |
| 1. Makes recommendations about local issues to the HSA.<br>2. Coordinates local planning efforts.<br>3. Participates in development of HSP & AIP. | |

**Table 1.** ORGANIZATION & FUNCTION OF THE 1974 National Health Planning & Resources Development Act.

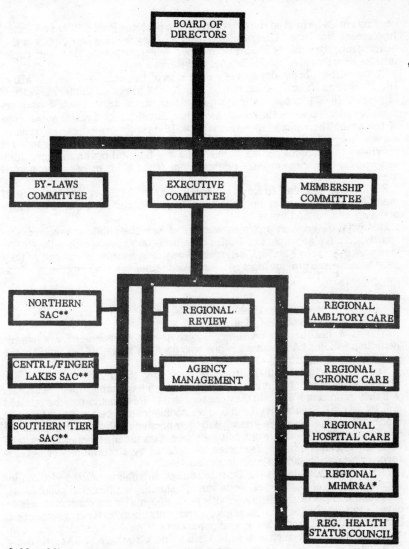

* Mental Health, Mental Retardation & Alcoholism

** Subarea Council (SAC); Other councils within each subarea are formed to undertake specific program areas (such as hospital care) or specific tasks (such as project review or membership).

Table 2. EXAMPLE OF THE COMPOSITION OF AN HSA (Health Systems Agency). Above Example is from Upstate New York.

hearings must be held on the proposed Health Systems Plan (HSP) and annual Implementation Plan (AIP), prepared each year by the HSA, and notice of that hearing must be published in the newspaper. When the plan is approved, copies must be distributed to public libraries in the area.

The governing body, depending on the size of the area, will be a Board of Directors or an Executive Committee, which must have a consumer majority of 51 percent to 60 percent, comprising residents of the area. These consumers must broadly represent the social, economic, linguistic, and racial populations of the area. The remaining percentage will be direct providers (physicians, nurses, hospital administrators, government health agencies, etc.) or indirect providers (physician's spouse, banker who is a hospital health insurer, childbirth educator whose earnings represent one tenth of his or her gross annual income).

Each HSA has a staff to carry out the policies of the governing board. Staff members should number no more than 25 and should be experts in health planning and related areas.

This brief description indicates where and how the public is involved. Obviously, to have an impact on health care decision making, either they must take part in an active and self-determined way as consumer members, or they must monitor and provide input as consumer or other community groups.

## Problems for Consumers
**Membership and representation.**

Who is a health care consumer? Perhaps for purposes here a simple definition will do: "A consumer is one who does not make his-her living in the health service industry." (17)

Now, we are faced with many other questions, the answers to which are critical to the issue of HSA control. Who will be the consumer members? Who will they represent? Who will they not represent? How should they be selected and by whom? Should they be the more sophisticated, better educated, and more affluent members of a group? Will their opinions reflect the group opinion or personal bias? These are difficult questions. Consumer representatives have been elected, appointed, self-selected, designated by a community or government organization, and often self-perpetuated.

The federal mandate says that consumer members must be "broadly representative of the social, economic, linguistic, and racial populations, geographic areas of the health service area, and major purchasers of health care." But in Dallas, for example, representatives of local government, businesses, banks, and other major purchasers of health care took over consumer seats (3). In such cases, in Dallas and elsewhere, HSAs are being challenged in the courts on the nature of their consumer representatives and how they are selected (3).

Several studies have showed that HSAs generally have governing Boards and Executive Committees which underrepresent women, minority groups, low-income groups, and the elderly (8,12). A significant number of HSAs included consumers who had direct or indirect ties to health providers and who were not "broadly representative" of the population in their area (11). Health provider membership is heavily weighted in favor of physicians and hospital administrators (12).

**Consumer bias.**

In any community there will be a variety of groups — young and old, black and white, sick and well, well-to-do and poor, urban and rural, and so on. Obviously, each consumer will enter the HSA with certain interests, biases, and motivation. Each person's focus will be essentially a narrow one and protective of his or her interests.

If we look at who is not represented on HSAs (e.g., economically disadvantaged persons, women, and the elderly), can we be sure that someone will address their special needs? Can I, a white, middle-class, college-educated, 39-year-old woman from a rural community whose special interest is maternal and child health, obtain sufficient feedback from the larger community to speak for all women, all ages, all socioeconomic groups?

There are, of course, consumers who think and vote like providers (and even a few providers who think and vote like consumers!) Also, during the learning process consumers may change or realign attitudes, beliefs, advocacy positions, and roles so that they no longer represent the views of their group but become provider oriented. Social relationships between providers and consumers may change, affecting consumer voting behavior.

Some consumers may distrust or feel victimized by all providers, and may be motivated to "get back" at the providers or the establishment, perhaps demanding more and new services instead of improved use of old ones. Others may want personal power and prestige (1).

Individual consumers will have different goals — the banker may view cost containment and closure of obstetrical units as an essential long-term goal, whereas a childbearing woman may focus on the need to retain obstetrical units that respond to family needs or on the necessity of establishing a free-standing maternity center. Consumers may identify different problems for priority and become frustrated when cost containment, for example, is constantly given higher priority than improving the health status of the citizens.

**Patterns of attendance and participation.**

Many consumers will have more difficulty than providers in attending meetings, especially in the daytime, and obviously "without the requirement of a quorum that is at least 50 percent consumers, consumer control of an HSA and its activities could be seriously jeopardized." (15) Low-income or elderly consumers may have transportation problems in getting to meetings, and without appropriate reimbursement, some members simply will not be able to attend. Low attendance is especially pronounced among consumers, and usually they are not a working majority, despite their mandated majority (6).

Once at the meeting, some consumers, for reasons of intimidation or lack of knowledge, may not actively participate, which in turn will lead to boredom and frustration, a high drop-out rate, and turnover. Participation must not simply mean a voicing of needs and concerns in an advisory capacity, however; it must mean a sharing in decision making. Thus, "There is a critical difference between going through the ritual of participation and having the power to affect the outcome of the process." (5)

**Lack of consumer organization.**

Provider groups are powerful, well organized, and amply funded to represent the best interests of the medical profession and hospitals. Consumers are not, and their input in decision making is fragmentary and seldom unified in what constitutes the best for the community, unless somehow they can get together and coordinate their views.

### Lack of information.

Consumer members are greatly handicapped initially by lack of knowledge of health matters. Thus they are learning during their tenure, making errors, not voicing concerns, not understanding, and often not participating until their term is about to expire. Providers, of course, come to meetings with their specialized fund of knowledge and a degree of sophistication that consumers usually do not have (15). To participate in an informed way, consumers must do much preparation, for which often there is little time available before decisions must be made to meet deadlines. Consumers are thus placed at a great disadvantage and may not assert themselves if in unfamiliar territory, and thus they can lose control because of the "providers-must-know" syndrome (15).

### Provider resistance to lay involvement.

Because of differing expectations, territories, and roles, problems and friction often occur when providers and consumers face each other. Conflict may arise over "territorial rights" — health professionals claiming the medical care aspects and consumers claiming the social, political, racial, financial, and humanistic aspects. Problems may occur when territories overlap, and neither group may be willing to yield.

Many providers have difficulty giving up their traditional authority in health care decision making and resist sharing it with consumers. It must be remembered that providers did not invite consumers into the health planning arena — politicians did (17). In addition, HSAs with their consumer majority, represent a definite threat to the independence, prestige, and jobs of health care providers (1). It has also been pointed out that some providers cannot separate the role of the consumer-patient from that of consumer-citizen (14).

### Passive consumer acceptance of provider expertise.

The physician-patient relationship is traditionally one of passivity and dependency, in which the consumer seldom questions the expertise and judgment of the physician. In the HSA arena the consumer is thrust into a different role and expected to shed the dependency role of the patient-client and become an assertive consumer. Many are unable to make this role transition, and too often at meetings I have seen them sit silently, meeting after meeting, and gradually drop out altogether.

### Staff pressures.

The effectiveness of consumer members partly depends on how they are viewed and respected by health planning staff. If consumers are not taken seriously by the staff, their impact can be diminished. Subtle "subversion" of consumers by staff can occur, and strong staff persons, in nurturing consumer members, can develop a dependency relationship (16). Consumers must be aware of how manipulation and pressures from staff on key issues can influence the way they vote.

### Political maneuverings.

A tremendous amount of political game playing goes on in HSAs, and it takes a while to catch on. One physician has described the participants in the HSA as "movers" — largely consumers and third parties whose chief goals are to save money and improve accessibility and quality of care — and "statics" — largely providers and bureaucrats who want to maintain the status quo (1). Strategies and counterstrategies, he believes, "can be expected to reach new heights of development and finesse as the HSAs gain continuing experience, not only in rational planning but in developing the fine art of political confrontation." (1)

In such a complex hierarchy of councils, there are many points in the system where specific interests can mobilize support, have access, and checkmate earlier actions and decisions. In my experience the consumers have not attained the political know-how and organization to use HSAs to their advantage.

**Task forces.**

Although a consumer majority is mandated at all levels of the working body, task forces are advisory and, depending on each HSA attitude, can have a largely provider composition. This is especially critical in the area of maternity and newborn care.

HSAs have designated or will be designating levels of perinatal services for all hospitals in the region. In the Finger Lakes HSA, New York, the Perinatal Services Task Force was one of the earliest to be appointed. Designation of perinatal services was top priority in 1976. The task force was appointed quietly by staff (possibly with provider input) and held its first meeting before many consumers were aware of its existence. Its makeup was 8 physicians, 3 nurses, 1 hospital administrator, and 5 consumers, 2 of whom dropped out early and were not replaced. Consumer representatives had little chance to influence the guidelines, which were adopted virtually unchanged by the Executive Committee.

Loud and efficiently orchestrated outcry from physicians, hospitals, and the public accompanied the designation of levels — several community hospitals objected to being designated Level I (hospitals providing low-cost, normal obstetrical care). They wanted to be Level II (more costly, specialized care), and obstetricians publicly spoke about the horrors of being "reduced to the role of a midwife."

Compromises were negotiated with the HSA, whereby level designations would be dropped, new labels given, and agreements reached between units representing different levels of care — regional, subarea, or community.

Provider domination of task forces is a critical influence on decision making at all HSA levels. Thus consumers may vote on proposals which have had little original consumer input.

### Solutions for Consumers

I have emphasized the problems consumers face in HSAs because they must know the realities involved in HSA participation if they are going to make them work the way they should — in the community's interests.

A recent publication by the Health Research Group describes how HSAs should operate: "Consumers should not be advising planners or providers; planners and providers should be advising and informing consumers, who finally decide what the health system should look like" (2). Providers are equipped to be the medical and technical consultants of health care and services, but this does not necessarily mean that they fully understand how the consumer perceives health care problems or how best to solve them (15).

Consumers and providers bring different skills and values into the health planning field. HSAs will only work effectively for the public when the providers and consumers combine their skills, listen to each other, and develop a constructive basis for joint planning. This cannot occur when one group surrenders its rights to the other group. How, then, can one go about making the consumer role in HSAs more effective and more viable than it is at present?

When considering the functioning of HSAs, one can examine the strategies consumer members of HSAs can use and the strategies that consumer and other groups in the community can use.

## Strategies for HSA Consumer Members

**1. Accept membership only if you are willing to spend the necessary time and energy required.**

Because consumers have the disadvantage of lack of health care knowledge, the preparation and education required for active participation at meetings is considerable. Effectiveness depends on asking questions, listening carefully, and challenging assertively, when necessary — but careful advance preparation is needed. Try also to determine earlier how other consumer members feel on the issue in question. Above all, do not allow yourself to be intimidated, and if you do not understand medical and health planning jargon, ask for explanations.

Suggestions for preliminary preparation for HSA participation and advice about meetings is given in "A Handbook for Consumer Participation in Health Care Planning."(9)

**2. Familiarize yourself with parliamentary and political strategies.**

Again, to participate effectively, you have to know procedures for introducing amendments, points of order, tabling, voting procedures, and so on to slow down proceedings or control critical votes. Assistance from a sympathetic staff member in these strategies can help, but "Robert's Rules of Order" (13) or a similar guide is necessary.

Many strategies can be used at meetings, some of which need practice, but the art of bargaining, negotiating, compromising (when necessary), and maintaining a calm and friendly demeanor (at least on the outside) can be helpful. Remember that an adversary on one issue can become an ally on another. Other political strategies in HSAs (albeit somewhat tongue in cheek!) are described by Berg (1).

**3. Investigate consumer and provider representation.**

This can be done initially by requesting from staff or the Membership and Nominating Committee a complete analysis of consumer membership — by family income, sex, race or ethnic group, occupation, and residence. Make sure consumers do not have a conflict of interest that ties them with providers.

Providers can be categorized according to specialty, institution representation, and financial interest. They should reflect a broad range of different health professions, but membership may be heavily loaded with hospital and nursing home administrators, physicians, and hospital trustees. Recruitment of providers who are sympathetic to the consumer viewpoint, such as childbirth and health educators, dieticians, nurse-midwives, family practitioners, community health nurses, social services representatives, etc., will help compensate for the provider imbalance (12).

When you can see who are underrepresented among consumers and providers, insist on immediate active recruitment to obtain equitable representation. A provider rotation system should be established to increase or decrease certain types of providers.

Determine the regularity of turnover of membership on the Board and Executive Committee. Look into the protocols for selection of membership. Does the Board reelect itself? It has been suggested that HSA Boards should be "chosen in a manner similar to that of the school boards."(12) This would enable greater public accountability — something that is largely lacking.

Attendance requirements should be strictly enforced, and members missing three consecutive meetings or more than 50 percent of meetings annually should be replaced. Consumer members must be encouraged to attend to avoid domination by providers. In addition, a requirement that a designated percentage of consumers be present at Board or Executive Committee meetings before a quorum is declared will ensure more effective consumer control. This should be written into the bylaws (12).

**4. Establish an orientation and ongoing training program for consumers and providers, separately and together.**

This is essential for active and effective consumer participation from the beginning. A joint program for consumers and providers should include the organization's history, structure, bylaws, goals, objectives, policies, funding, timetables, and how it is integrated into the federal and state political and legislative structure.

A separate consumer training program is crucial and should contain the following:

(a) Assertiveness and communication techniques

(b) Information about social and health needs and problems of the area

(c) Techniques, procedures, and rules of meetings

(d) Description of region's health care delivery system, listing consumer groups, hospitals, HMOs, clinics, medical societies, nursing homes, etc.

(e) Funding and reimbursement of health facilities and services; insurance programs

(f) Role, rights, and responsibilities of a consumer in HSA

(g) Skills in group participation; skills in working with providers

(h) Orientation manual that includes glossary of health care jargon and abbreviations

It is believed that training will increase consumers' confidence in their role, increase consumers' abilities to work together, and increase their knowledge and planning skills (11). But questions arise as to which forms of training are effective (5).

**5. Educate the public about HSAs.**

HSAs are not well known, and therefore extensive public education is necessary to explain their purposes and work and how this can affect the health of individuals and the community (12).

Publicity for meetings and for issues of special interest and importance to the community must be provided in local news media. Insist that all meetings are truly open to the public and press.

**6. Study the law under which HSAs were created and bylaws and procedures for your HSA.**

This will enable consumers to be much better equipped to question and monitor HSA operation. Factors such as conflict of interest specifications and secret or open voting procedures can become critical issues in important votes. If bylaws do not seem to function in the public interest, suggest amendments.

**7. Question task force selection and insist on a consumer majority for every task force.**

Consumers can lose effective control of an HSA if task forces are provider dominated and consumers vote on proposals that have not had both consumer and provider input. This may change, however, since the Department of HEW has recently proposed new rules for HSAs whereby advisory groups, such as task forces, would be required to have a consumer majority (18). Insist that the entire membership be advised before a task force is to be selected so that interested persons can indicate their desire to serve on it.

**8. Question reimbursement of consumer members for travel, meals, parking, etc.**

With consumer members who live considerable distances from meeting places or are not financially well-off, "transportation and other related costs must be borne by the agency." (12)

**9. Get to know consumer and other community groups and leaders in your area.**

This will enable consumers to represent their community more responsibly and effectively.

Not only will such groups inform you about community concerns and needs, but they can be valuable allies at public hearings and applying pressure for changes in health plans. At the same time, you can keep such groups informed about HSA activities, priorities, etc. Members with concerns in maternity and newborn health care can mobilize support from sympathetic community groups for innovations in maternity care or on regionalization issues.

**10. Familiarize yourself with consumer-patient rights.**

Consumers are usually sensitive to the needs of consumers, but this is not enough. They must become informed about what a consumer's human and legal rights are within the health care system, including such matters as informed consent, advocacy and ombudsman services, equal rights of minorities, provision of language alternatives in educational material, and humanistic, emotional, and social aspects of health care.

**11. Maintain constant communication with at least one HSA staff person.**

It is very important to find a sympathetic staff person — someone you can trust and who will keep you informed — to help you work in the community's interests. There is no question that provider members such as medical societies and hospital associations will cultivate inside sources of information from HSA staff to further their particular interests (2). Behind-the-scenes action can usurp your effectiveness, so take some lessons in tactics from others.

### Strategies for the Community —
### Particularly in Relation to Perinatal Services

Most regional plans for perinatal care follow a medical model and comprise crisis-oriented policies. They generally fail to address the emotional and social needs of healthy childbearing families; they limit choices; and they separate family members in high-risk situations. Emphasis on a comprehensive maternal and child health care plan throughout pregnancy, birth, and postpartum is generally lacking.

**1. Find out everything possible about how HSAs function and fit into federal and state health planning.**

Use this information to plan your strategies.

**2. Endeavor to be appointed to HSAs.**

Fill out resumes so that they will be on file and will be considered when vacancies occur on the Board and on other councils. Make yourself visible and keep in touch with HSA activities. Inquire regularly about the status of regionalization of perinatal care and ask to be considered for membership when relevant task forces are going to be appointed. Make efforts to have key persons appointed to HSAs whose influence can be used both as a positive or constructive force or as a negative or obstructive force.

**3. Study the Health Systems Plan (long range) and Annual Implementation Plan (one year) as it applies to perinatal care.**

See what services they fail to provide for childbearing families — what the deficiencies are. Analyze the location of the maternal population in relation to available services and determine who is-is not being served. Then, develop a model of perinatal care that meets all the needs of families in the community or region. If perinatal guidelines have been adopted, again determine what they fail to provide and mount a campaign to get them changed.

**4. Make sure your group is on the mailing list for notices of meetings, agendas, information, minutes, and newsletters of the HSA.**

**5. Find out the schedule for preliminary meetings and public hearings on the HSP and AIP.**

Request a preliminary draft of these plans. Make a statement from your group on the deficiencies in perinatal services and present your alternative model (orally and written). Use reporters and the press to disseminate your views (2) It is well to be aware that HSA public hearings may be more ritualistic than substantive, so be sure to follow up to determine if your testimony was acted upon. If it was not, determine why not. Don't give up! HSA staff who are sympathetic to your views may be able to advise on strategy.

**6. Make use of the fact that you are in a buyer's market.**

In the market of maternity and newborn services, there is a highly significant variable — that of the birth rate. When that rate is declining, hospitals want to improve their services to attract clients; thus the consumer-client is in a position to demand, to negotiate, and to initiate alternative models of maternity and newborn care.

**7. If you are dissatisfied with your HSA's responsiveness to the needs of consumers, do something about it.**

Initial constructive criticism can be directed to the HSA Board. If there is no action, complain to the HSA Board, the Governor, the Statewide Health Coordinating Council (SHCC), your Congressperson(s), the Department of Health, Education, and Welfare, and the Public Citizen's Health Research Group, Suite 708, 2000 P Street, N.W., Washington, D.C. 20036.

Establish a local health or childbirth action group.

### The Future

In the past, consumer participation in health planning has demonstrated little actual results (7). It is too early to tell how effective HSAs will be in saving money, but a recent survey by "Health Manpower and Planning Reports" of 68 HSAs in 30 states "believes that modest inroads are being made against a voracious American appetite for heavy health-care expenditure." (4)

As to who is in control of health planning, however, it is clear that in most cases the balance of power in HSAs is with the providers. Active public involvement both inside and outside HSAs is needed to weight that balance in favor of consumers. It has already been done in different parts of the country by establishing consumer health coalitions and action groups to put pressure on HSAs by requiring them (sometimes by court action) to fulfill the mandates of the Health Planning and Resources Development Act. Consumers must work to make this legislation accountable to the public, to us all.

What about maternity and newborn care? It is time for childbirth and consumer groups to plan and mobilize their resources and move in on the HSAs with an alternative model of comprehensive maternity and newborn care, with the aim of having it incorporated into the Health Systems Plan (16). Innovation must be a part of health planning. We cannot allow family-oriented maternity centers to be wiped out by regionalization. It has been recommended that the focus for normal birth, including family planning, parenting education, and prenatal care, should be removed from the expensive, high-risk perinatal centers (16). Increased availability of nurse-midwives and direct reimbursement of their services must be emphasized. Health professionals within a community have an ethical and moral responsibility to provide care for all childbearing women, regardless of the birth environment, and childbirth and consumer groups must actively develop ways of meeting their needs. Consumer and childbirth groups must be informed and up-to-date on federal and state maternal and child health legislation and must start initiating legislation that relates to the emotional and social needs of childbearing families. We must not merely wait for things to change, we must change them ourselves.

## References

1. Berg, R.L.: "Movers" and "statics" refine political strategies in HSAs, Hospital Progress 56:64, 1977.
2. Bogue, T., and Wolfe, S.A.: Trimming the fat off health care costs: a consumer's guide to taking over health planning, Washington, D.C., 1976, Health Research Group.
3. Consumer issues around HSAs: the Dallas experience, Health Law Project Library Bulletin No. 333, June-July, 1977, Health Law Project, Philadelphia.
4. Financially strapped HSAs save money despite slow pace of health planning, News Sheet, Finger Lakes Health Systems Agency, p. 2, Feb., 1978.
5. Galiher, C., Needleman, J., and Rolfe, A.: Consumer participation, HSMHA Health Reports 86:99, Feb. 1971.
6. Greer, A.L.: Training Board members for health planning agencies: a review of the literature, Public Health Reports 91:56, Jan.-Feb., 1976.
7. Hochbaum, G.M.: Consumer participation in health planning, American Journal of Public Health 59:1698, 1970.
8. HSAs have few women, minorities, The Nation's Health, p. 9, April, 1978.
9. Judd, L.R., and McEwen, R.J.: A handbook for consumer participation in health care planning, Chicago, 1977, The Blue Cross Association.
10. National Symposium on Patients' Rights in Health Care, Washington, D.C., May 17-18, 1976, U.S. Department of Health, Education and Welfare.
11. Parker, A.W.: The consumer as policy maker — issues of training, American Journal of Public Health 60:2139, 1970.
12. Placebo or cure? State and local health planning agencies in the South, Atlanta, 1977, Southern Regional Council.
13. Robert, H.M.: Robert's rules of order, New York, 1967, Pyramid Books.
14. Salber, E.J.: Consumer participation in neighborhood health centers, New England Journal of Medicine 283:515, 1970.
15. Sypniewski, B.P.: Do consumers really control an HSA? Health Law Reports Library Bulletin No. 332, May, 1977, Health Law Project, Philadelphia.
16. Tannen, L.N., and Sparer, E.V.: Consumer issues around HSAs: HSAs as an arena for consumer struggles — as illustrated by maternity care needs, Health Law Reports Library Bulletin No. 337, Nov., 1977, Health Law Project, Philadelphia.
17. Varricchio, L.: The consumers in health planning: their emergence and dilemmas of participation, Dec. 6, 1976 (unpublished manuscript).
18. Federal Register, Part II, May 26, 1978.

Puzzled By An Unfamiliar Abbreviation
Such As "HMO", "AIP", or "RMP"?
See Glossary on Page 284.

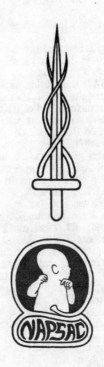

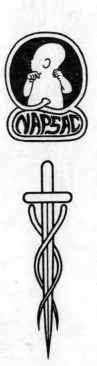

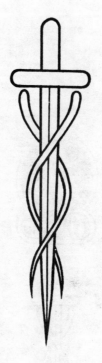

# Perinatal Regionalization

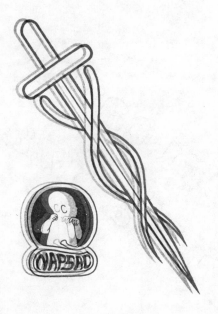

## CHAPTER FIVE

### PERINATAL REGIONAL PLANNING
### WHAT IT IS, AND WHY DOCTORS RECOMMEND IT
### George M. Ryan Jr., M.D., M.P.H.

Regional planning is neither new nor unique to perinatal health services. Certainly everyone is familiar with the regional programs established some years ago for the management of heart disease, stroke and cancer. We also remember the concept as applied to the battlefield with battalion aid stations, regimental hospitals and M.A.S.H. units, and larger general hospitals to serve a specific region or military force. Other models exist in Canada, the United Kingdom, the United States, and the Commonwealth of Puerto Rico. The purpose of all such programs is to marshal the resources of a region to provide all the expertise needed for all patients within the region to be served.

Why do doctors support it? Because they believe that regional planning of perinatal services will improve the quality of care available to patients and will result in the prevention of much of the deaths and injury suffered in the past.

Let's look at the actual concept and the reasons for this belief in greater detail.

It is easy to understand that patients fall into three general categories. First is the uncomplicated normal patient, the second is the patient with some threatening complications which should ordinarily be handled in a good maternity unit, and thirdly there are the patients who have extraordinary needs for services and facilities which are not usually available. Out of this three-leveled concept grew the recognition that patients in this country are even now being served by hospitals capable of handling Level I, Level II, or Level III problems, but no attempt is at present being made to plan for the rational triage of patients to appropriate units. With careful examination of the categories of patients, it becomes clear that the so called "normal patient" is an entirely retrospective diagnosis that can only be made after mother and infant are discharged home in good health. The fact is, many patients unexpectedly develop complications during labor, delivery, or their postpartum course; hence every patient is a potential type II or complicated patient (1). Therefore, those hospitals not able to manage most of the unexpected complications unnecessarily endanger the mother and her infant.

We believe that any obstetrical unit charged with the responsibility for the safety of mother and infant should be able to manage unexpected complications in an optimal manner. As a result, those hospitals not able to handle these complications should only function when there is no practical alternative such as in cases of geographic isolation. We also feel that every patient should have reasonable access to an intensive care unit in the event she needs it either for

George M. Ryan, Jr., M.D., M.P.H. is a professor of obstetrics and gynecology and community health, University of Tennessee, Center for the Health Sciences; secretary of the ACOG, author or coauthor of more than 20 technical papers in obstetrics and gynecology, including the original blueprint for regionalization entitled "Toward Improving the Outcome of Pregnancy."

predictable or for unexpected complications. Out of these basic thoughts grew the concept of defining the capability of hospitals as Level I (those capable of performing only normal perinatal care), Level II (those also able to manage most unexpected complications), and Level III (those also offering intensive care to that small portion of the population needing it).

In order to add flesh to the bare bones concepts, the Committee on Perinatal Health was established, representing major professional organizations and seeking input from a broad cross section of interested groups. The document "Toward Improving the Outcome of Pregnancy" (2) was published which in essence reiterated the concepts I have presented and proposed guidelines to be used in the establishment of services and personnel for the various facilities as well as guidelines for the interrelationship of the facilities.

The principles of triage of high risk patients to appropriate facilities, establishment of those facilities where none exist, and educational programs to teach people how to use the system are all based on actual programs and not just on theoretical concepts. The results of a variety of programs involving the various principles have been made available. They represent a variety of settings and approaches, but all would indicate that they have contributed to an improvement in the pregnancy outcome. In Wisconsin (3) in the late 1960's a retrospective analysis of fetal and neonatal deaths in 35 hospitals was undertaken. The data showed that half of the fetal deaths and two-thirds of the neonatal deaths in the state could be classified as preventable, meaning that if the patients had received optimal care by current standards that this sort of improvement in perinatal mortality could have been achieved. Half of the preventable deaths were judged to have been avoidable at the local level while the other half could have been avoided only by care in a regional Level III facility. As a result of this information, ongoing educational programs and site visits were initiated to improve care at the local levels, and by 1973, nine neonatal intensive care units were established. The first perinatal center providing both high risk maternity and perinatal services was established in 1971.

Since institution of the statewide program of neonatal intensive care centers and transport of the sick newborn, the neonatal mortality has decreased from approximately 10 deaths per 1,000 to 6 deaths per 1,000 live births, a 40 percent reduction.

In Wisconsin's south central region, the site of the first center to offer maternal high risk care, fetal deaths per 1,000 births decreased from 9 to 7 in the first year of the center's operation. In addition, an increasing number of maternal transfers for fetal indications was noted. This program demonstrates the effectiveness of identification, education, consultation, transportation, and both maternal and perinatal intensive care.

In 1960 the statewide infant mortality rate in Arizona ranked 45th in the 50 states (4). In addition 43 percent of the severely retarded children in the Arizona Childrens Colony were judged to have acquired their condition during the perinatal period. Arizona began in 1962 to define its problems and institute a program suitable for the sparse population density in that southwestern state.

A broadly representative Maternal and Child Health Committee first mounted a demonstration project in which two major maternal and perinatal units in Phoenix were selected as newborn intensive care centers. Sick newborns were transported from rural areas to these centers under the direct responsibility of the neonatologist at the center. After three years the mortality rate was halved for infants in the project with birth weights of 1000-2500 grams.

Because of these encouraging results, the State Health Department requested and received funding by the State Legislature to convert the demonstration project to a statewide program. Eventually four maternal and perinatal centers were established and coordinated transport provided. Between 1966 and 1972 the decline in infant and neonatal mortality in Arizona was more rapid than the national trend. Between 1960 and 1972 the infant mortality ranking improved from 45th to 11th nationally, while neonatal mortality improved from 35th to 3rd. This program involved joint participation of the practicing community and the State Health Department and demonstrated the potential benefits of neonatal transport and intensive care.

In Canada the Quebec Perinatal Committee began collecting perinatal data in 1967 and has continued up to the present. The initial report in 1967 showed a perinatal mortality of 22.1 per 1,000 for infants weighing more than 1,000 grams (5). The committee studied the effects of neonatal intensive care and referral of the sick newborn on perinatal mortality within the Province. Hospitals were thus classified as non-referring, referring, and intramural neonatal intensive care hospitals. The perinatal mortality rate per 1,000 live births in each of these was respectively 19.0, 16.9, and 14.7. This was widely interpreted as demonstrating the benefits of transport of the sick newborn and the even greater benefit of delivery of the sick newborn in a facility with a neonatal intensive care unit.

In 1970 a universal health care system was established in Quebec. Under this program maternity and perinatal care is paid for by the government. Government agencies are responsible for health planning and financial management. "Regrouping" of obstetrical services was begun, embodying the same concepts we term "consolidation." It was determined that maternity services with less than 2,000 deliveries per year were economically inefficient and that the perinatal mortality rates in hospitals with less than 1,000 deliveries per year were 30 percent greater than in larger hospitals. The long term goal was established of providing a system of maternity services with intramural fetal and neonatal intensive care units wherever geographically possible. Short term goals included continuing development of intramural high risk centers, increased training of appropriate personnel, and increased utilization of referral to existing intensive care services. Results of this program have been impressive (6).

From 1967 to 1973 the perinatal mortality for infants weighing more than 1,000 grams fell from 22.1 to 14.4 per 1,000, a fall of 35 percent (perinatal mortality includes stillbirths and neonatal deaths during the first seven days). The prematurity rate remained unchanged from 1967 to 1973. Therefore, the reduced perinatal mortality rate is believed to be due to the improved care of mother, fetus, and newborn under the new system. While the 1967 report of the Quebec Perinatal Committee stressed the importance of neonatal intensive care, the 1973 policy statement indicated the advantages of maternal and fetal intensive care for those at risk. Programs involving recognition of risk factors during the prenatal period, precise management of prenatal conditions hazardous to the fetus, and intensive monitoring during labor and delivery produced still another increment of improvement over neonatal intensive care alone. When added to neonatal intensive care, maternal and perinatal intensive care produced a further reduction in perinatal mortality from 15.2 to 11.6 per 1,000 (6). Stillbirths on these services were 28 percent below the Quebec average and signs of neonatal asphyxia were 40 percent below the Quebec average. Evidence of an asphyxic injury was reduced 40 percent to 85 percent in comparison with the five years prior to institution of maternal and perinatal intensive care.

The Quebec programs included elimination of unneeded maternity units, consolidation of remaining units, establishment of appropriate facilities, creation of a transport system, and the development of short and long term regional planning under government auspices.

Massachusetts is a state with large urban and rural areas. After the Massachusetts Medical Society study in 1967 and 1968 (7) concluded that one-third of the state's perinatal deaths were preventable, the Massachusetts Department of Public Health sought to improve the standards of care by issuing new licensing regulations for newborn services and for obstetrical services. These included requirements for 24 hour blood bank services and 24 hour staffing of nurseries by registered nurses as well as the designation of seven intensive care nurseries as transfer nurseries and the requirement that each maternity unit in the state furnish the health department with their plans for management and possible transfer of sick newborns.

One of the interesting developments in Massachusetts has been the dramatic reduction in the number of maternity services. There were 120 maternity units in 1960 and only 65 by 1975. A recent study of the causes and process of closing of maternity services in Massachusetts as well as the subsequent impact on the hospital as a whole certainly did not indicate they were closed in most part, because of any regional planning activity (8). Instead, the analysis indicated that a hospital closing its maternity service typically had less than 150 beds, had less than a 15 bed maternity unit, and delivered less than 500 babies per year. The occupancy rate averaged less than 45 percent on the maternity service, and the hospital was losing money in this endeavor. The primary factor in most closings was economic. Other considerations included the concern for quality of care, vacant maternity beds while more medical surgical beds were desired, and staffing problems such as the retirement of physicians. In spite of the commonly expressed fears of the impact of closure of maternity services, the study indicated that most hospitals undergoing this process noted financial improvement in their overall operation, that there was no evidence that access to maternity services was limited, other hospital services were not adversely affected, and most nursing staff and other hospital employees continued their employment. Thus it was concluded that much of the opposition to closing of many small units was based on fear and not fact.

A recent survey was conducted of the effects of regional planning programs on the patterns of practice of the obstetricians in Massachusetts (9). Of those physicians involved in hospital closures, three quarters were originally at Level I units with the remaining 23 percent at Level II and Level III units. After the closures, the percentages were reversed with some 27 percent at Level I units and the remainder in Level II and III units. These are significant changes and would indicate that the consolidation of services by elimination of small units has improved the accessibility of better resources for needed care for the patients of these physicians. The fact that the obstetricians are utilizing their new found access is indicated by the fact that 20 percent of the obstetricians transferred maternity patients to other hospitals where they had practice privileges and they transferred about one mother per month. The reasons for these transfers related in over half the cases to prematurity and diabetes and were done more for the benefit of the fetus and newborn than because of risk to the mother. I believe this is clear evidence that the basic concept of triage of high risk patients is gaining acceptance among the practicing physicians.

While a substantial minority of the responding obstetricians felt threatened by planning for regionalized perinatal care, these fears evolved mostly from the possibility of closure of one of "their hospitals." Most felt that regional planning could reduce perinatal mortality and improve access to care, but only about one-third thought it was an effective method to curb the high cost of care.

The introduction of a consideration of cost into this discussion brings me to the next segment, - the response of government. The low occupancy rates of many maternity units and the excess numbers of beds as required for the needs of the population, as calculated by many formulas, as well as the soaring cost of operation of the intensive care units makes obstetrics a tempting target for cost containment governmental planning. A nationwide survey of state maternal and child health departments in 1974 revealed active operating perinatal regional planning programs in 28 states, and all but four states estimated that they would have program implementation by 1977 (10). The Health Planning and Resources Development Act of 1974 established a federally mandated program for planning, mediated through state and local agencies, while the federal government was to establish and fund this program. The concept was that planning and program development would be carried on locally subject to approval by state and federal review. In addition, it is clear that many people responsible for health planning at all levels of government embrace the principles embodied in the report of the National Perinatal Committee entitled "Toward Improving the Outcome of Pregnancy." In fact, the 18 states with the highest perinatal mortality were identified and $400,000 made available last year to each of those state departments of health for the promotion of regional planning of perinatal care and these programs are known as projects "to improve the outcome of pregnancy."

With all of this warmth of mutual effort toward common goals, HEW dropped a bomb-shell with its announcement in the federal regulations of Sept. 23, 1977 of the proposed rules for national guidelines for health planning. It was clear that these were meant to be cost control measures, were to be completed in five years, and furthermore, the guidelines for pediatric and obstetric services were totally different, therefore preventing any sort of mutual planning. The obstetric services guidelines demanded at least 2,000 deliveries in an obstetrical unit located in a standard metropolitan statistical area with a population of 100,000 or more. In addition, at least 500 deliveries would be necessary in any obstetrical unit outside these SMAs. The only exception to these numerical demands was if travel time to the unit exceeded 45 minutes under normal driving conditions for 10 percent or more of the population.

A second requirement was that there should be an average annual occupancy rate of at least 75 percent in each obstetrical unit. A brief review of the situation in various states and areas of the country revealed that the implementation of these guidelines would be economically and medically disastrous. Iowa for instance had over 90 maternity units and none of them delivered 2,000 babies a year. At the public hearings, the American College of Obstetricians and Gynecologists, the National Foundation, The American Hospital Association, and many others appeared and emphasized (1) that closures or consolidation of services that are not planned in conjunction with the creation of needed Level II and III units have the potential for creating serious deficiencies in the quality of care in some areas. (2) Due to the short five year period for implementation and the large number of hospitals involved, the political reality is that the impact would have been tremendous and the public furor unprecendented. (3) The fact that these proposed national guidelines usurped the planning authority of local HSAs was pointed out as well as (4) the fact that a complete set of guidelines was contained in the document "Toward Improving the Outcome of Pregnancy."

As a result, and to my pleasant surprise, new guidelines have now been drafted that include the requirement that neonatal services should be planned on a regional basis with continuing linkages with obstetrical services. Level II and III units are still listed as needing 1,500 births annually, and an average occupancy rate of 75 percent, but the Level I unit is not included in these requirements and there is no mention of standard metropolitan statistical areas. The emphasis on the linkage between neonatal and obstetrical services and the extensive quoting in the discussion of the basic tenets of "Toward Improving the Outcome of Pregnancy" indicate a recognition of the need for a system of care.

With this rewriting of the proposed guidelines, it would appear that we can return to the basic principles as outlined in "Toward Improving the Outcome of Pregnancy" which stressed that these are simply guidelines and represent goals to be worked toward over the next decade, not to be precipitously demanded.

And what of the public response? In general, the public has been apathetic. Occasional spurts of interest have been elicited by impending closure of maternity services, but generally we have done a poor job of public education to motivate the public to demand the kind of improved care envisioned by regional planning. Active opposition has been expressed by spokesmen presumably representing the viewpoints of the International Childbirth Education Association and NAPSAC.

Such viewpoints were expressed by Madeline H. Shearer in a recent issue of the magazine she edits, "Birth and The Family Journal" (11). She expresses the opinion that the Level I, II, and III recommendations were made to solve many of the problems of the urban obstetrical hospital. "By closing down small hospital maternity units more women must use the remaining hospitals." "By setting high risk standards of obstetrical care in the Level II and III hospital, including a 20 - 25 percent cesarean rate, more can be charged for births." Also, "obstetrical residency programs can retain the interest of new medical graduates, since there are increased opportunities for surgery and research." Such malicious statements do not represent the truth and are only a few of the distortions and inaccuracies in the article.

It is stated that no consumer groups or community groups back the principles of regionalization, conveniently ignoring the fact that the National Foundation of the March of Dimes is one of the largest consumer organizations in the country. Ms. Shearer keeps asking "Where will uncomplicated patients have normal childbirth if all that is available is intensive care?" The fact that the guidelines indicate that uncomplicated obstetrics will be carried out at all levels and that the purpose of the guidelines is to make more complex care immediately accessible to the patient who needs it is never mentioned. She also states that "obstetrical intensive care is being recommended for all women and all the remaining hospitals" and "this system has no provision of hospital services for normal birth" and she persists in referring to both Level II and III hospitals as providing only intensive care when the most superficial reading of the document indicates this is not so. In fact, Level II does not provide "intensive care." She also indicates her support for a transport service and transfer of infants to intensive care units while at the same time decrying the definition of services and personnel needed at those transport facilities, which is what the I, II, III, classification attempts to do.

I am in complete agreement with those who would improve the childbearing experience within the hospital setting. Proposals for regional planning of perinatal services in no way interfere with these goals. We should rightfully be concerned about the humanistic considerations raised by earnest patients, and in our rush to provide the best care possible to each group of patients, we must not fail to provide a gratifying emotional experience for the whole family. However, if we are to offset the distortions of information presented by the adherents of the "good old days" philosophy, we must take every opportunity to provide correct and responsible information to the public. My appearance at a NAPSAC conference is clear evidence of the depth of commitment to that responsibility.

In summary, I have presented the basic reasons for and the concepts of regional planning for perinatal health services, the results of programs embodying these concepts, a brief mention of the impact on physicians and their hospitals, government activities in the field, and a comment on consumer viewpoints. We are witnessing the early developments in a series of changes which will have far reaching impact on perinatal care in this country. Some have, and will, accuse us of irrationality in our support of the concepts of regional planning. I would respond by a quote from George Bernard Shaw who said, "A rational man will change his beliefs to conform to the world around him while an irrational man will try to change the world to conform to his beliefs. Therefore, all progress is made by irrational men."

The title of this presentation is "What is regional planning and why do doctors support it." I have given you two statements in the beginning of this presentation which I sincerely believe. I invite you to join me in that belief. They are, first, that regional planning for the delivery of perinatal health services is an attempt to improve the quality of medical care and improve access to it by the population. Secondly, doctors support it because a preponderence of evidence would indicate that the adoption of regional planning for perinatal services will benefit mothers and infants.

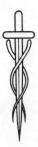

### References

1. Hobel, C.J., Hyvarinen, M.A., Okada, D.M., et al: Prenatal and intrapartum high risk screening. Am. J. Obstet. Gynecol. 117:1-9, 1973.
2. Report of the Committee on Perinatal Health: Toward improving the outcome of pregnancy. The National Foundation March of Dimes, 1976.
3. Schneider, J.M., Graven, S.N.: Regionalized obstetrical and gynecological care in Wisconsin. Contemp. Ob.-Gyn. 3:35-47, 1974.
4. Meyer, H.B.P.: Transportation of high risk infants in Arizona, in: Regionalization of Perinatal Care, Report of the Sixty-sixth Ross Conference on Pediatric Research, Ross Laboratories (unpublished).
5. Carrier, C., Doray, B., Stern, L., et al: Effect of neonatal intensive care on mortality rates in the Province of Quebec. Pediatr. Res. 6:408, 1971 (Abstr.).
6. Policy Statement of the Quebec Perinatal Committee: Perinatal Intensive Care After Integration of Obstetrical Services in Quebec. Quebec, Ministry of Social Affairs, 1973.
7. Committee on Perinatal Welfare of the Massachusetts Medical Society: Report on perinatal and infant mortality in Massachusetts. 1967 and 1968. (1971 unpublished).
8. Donahue, C.L., Pettigrew, A.H., Young, K., et al: Closure of maternity services in Massachusetts. Obstet. Gynecol. 50:280-284, 1977.
9. Ryan, G.M., Fielden, J.: The impact of regionalization programs on patterns of perinatal care. (in press).
10. Berger, D.S., Gillings, D.B., Siegel, E.: The evaluation of regionalized perinatal health programs. Am. J. Obstet. Gynecol. 125:924-932, 1976.
11. Shearer, M.H.: The effects of regionalization of perinatal care on hospital services for normal childbirth. Birth and the Family Journal 4:139 (Winter) 1977.

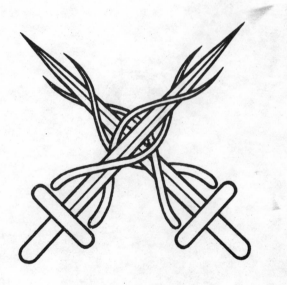

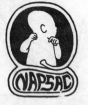

# CHAPTER SIX

## REGIONALIZATION: A MODEL OF
## PLANNED NEGLECT FOR PRIMARY CARE

### Judy Norsigian

It has taken us a couple of years to really pinpoint what it is that is so inappropriate about the plan for regionalizing maternity and newborn care. At first, we thought we just needed a different model for regionalization, one that emphasized prevention more and provided for childbearing options both in and out of the hospital. But recently we realized that regionalization, which refers primarily to avoiding the unnecessary duplication of expensive technology, expensive personnel, and hospital facilities, just cannot be used as the descriptive umbrella term for all of maternity and newborn care. Moreover, the term "maternity and newborn care" is itself inappropriate, as this refers primarily to in-hospital care. What we want to be talking about is maternal and child health care, and about options for childbearing women and families that do not assume the hospital as the main or only focus. What should never be forgotten is the fact that most maternal care is primary care. As many critics of hospital maternity care have said, "Why is it that we have emphasized hospital-based maternity care, increasingly in university medical centers which are tertiary care institutions, when 80-90 percent of all maternity care is, in fact, primary care?" With this in mind we must ask, "Are regionalization of maternity and newborn care plans designed for the greater good of the greater number?" We think not.

With this perspective it makes sense to talk first about a "system" of maternal and child health care that is community-based and prevention-oriented. Certainly, within such a system arrangements will have to be made for both predictable and unpredictable high-risk situations. But we are not talking about applying a high-risk model of care to low-risk childbearing women (for example, having a fetal monitor for every childbearing woman). We are talking about things like the following:

1. A preventive approach highlighted by an emphasis on prenatal nutrition, effective prenatal screening, and community-based outreach programs, designed to reach as many pregnant and likely-to-become pregnant women as possible.

2. A system with built-in consumer control, such that parents, in collaboration with consumer health education groups, professionals, and other health workers, make the key decisions about their childbearing experiences. Professional dominance, now the reality in most health and medical care settings, remains a formidable obstacle to greater parent responsibility and control. This is one area where we need more effectively to be organizing for change.

Judy Norsigian is a member of the Board of Directors, HSA, IV, MA, Board Member, National Women's Health Network, Administrative coordinator for the Boston Women's Health Book collective, and co-author of the book, "Our Bodies, Ourselves."

3. A system with appropriate hospital back-up services for those childbearing women who choose to give birth in out-of-hospital settings and find at some point that they require medical intervention in a hospital setting.

That being a sketch of how things ought to be, the fact is that we must begin with what we've got. We are now confronted with a variety of regionalization plans, some already being implemented, that we need to scrutinize carefully. We need to develop thorough critiques of these plans, to pose alternatives that better meet the needs of childbearing families, and to begin the kind of community organizing that will establish wide-spread support for alternatives. Hopefully, as more childbearing families and non-professionals speak out and organize themselves, increasing numbers of sympathetic professionals and healthcare workers will have the courage and support to do the same themselves.

If we find, as most of us will, that we are not able to change the model to begin with, we can at least work towards improving what plans exist.

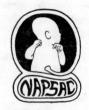

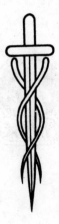

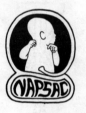

# CHAPTER SEVEN

## THE POLITICS OF REGIONALIZATION

### Norma Swenson, MPH

Regionalization has been presented to us as a life-and-death medical necessity, and as rational planning for the distribution of scarce resources. But maternity care is mainly a political process, and Regionalization of maternity and newborn care is primarily a social policy. It is nothing more or less than a national childbirth policy for every single family giving birth in the United States.

Unfortunately, most of us don't know very much about how policy gets made in this country. Furthermore, when we hear discussions about legislative processes or health systems planning, we usually get bored or tune out. We do this partly because these activities take us so far away from the mothers, babies and families we are concerned about; and partly because in general so many of us feel powerless and removed from control over the forces which are shaping our lives.

Increasingly we no longer have a choice about whether to educate ourselves about these issues or to organize politically. Health planning is here to stay. If we don't learn soon how to act as special interest groups able to influence the legislative regulatory and health planning processes, and at all levels, we will eventually have no choices left at all.

We, as childbearing parents, are a small and shrinking number. We are a minority. We are transients who visit the system once or twice and then leave. As a result we have organized, if at all, around the individual experience, for survival, for the short-term. But the old strategies we have developed—using consumer power in the competitive market place of hospitals and doctors, using the legal system for recognition of our constitutional and civil rights, or educating ourselves to more effectively negotiate the system by superior preparation—somehow all of these aren't working very well anymore. We need to know why. One reason is that professionals, largely physicians, do organize themselves politically, for the long-term and for control over the childbirth setting as their workplace. The contest between parents and professionals is, at the moment, a totally unequal contest.

Most of us aren't aware that organized obstetrics and gynecology has moved into health planning and government influence-peddling in a major way over the last few years. We should realize that there is nothing illegal about this activity. Our government does not recognize it as a conflict of interest that the group which makes the largest income of all—practicing physicians—from the care of women should also be the group having the major influence on women's health policy, particularly maternity care.

The ACOG, for example, has a gorgeous Washington, D.C., office, with two

Norma Swenson, MPH, is former president, ICEA, co-author of books, "Our Bodies, Ourselves," and "Citizen Evaluation of Community Health Services," and many other publications on women's health and maternity care. She is an alternate member, MA-SHCC, HSA, IV.

paid lobbyists--a man and a woman--and the services of two board-certified obstetrician-gynecologists. One or another of them is present at every public hearing and many private meetings to advise federal government regulators and planners about women's health and maternity care. Only rarely are consumers present to testify on their own behalf. The ACOG has publicly stated that it expects to be regarded as a spokesMAN for women's health, and the primary care physician for all women. The specialty is seeking federal government recognition and government funding for this designation. ACOG's current headquarters is in Chicago, but to more effectively influence federal policies to their own ends, they are now contemplating the moving of all their offices to Washington D.C.

ACOG has also begun plans to move into the media in a big way, by organizing dramatized TV shows about childbirth. Soon, we will be hearing paid public service announcements about why we should implement the Regionalization plan.

How did all this come about, and where does the money come from for all these activities? Why did Regionalization, in particular, get launched, and how has it come to have so much influence? There are several key points we'd like to make.

I am indebted to Dr. George Ryan for my first glimpse of how the idea of Regionalization of Maternity and Newborn services came about. George was a year ahead of me at Harvard School of Public Health and it has always been a source of amazement to me that the curriculum might have changed so much in just one year. Somehow he and I managed to learn completely different things there. What George learned was that Comprehensive Health Planning was a provider's dream, hospital-focused and easily controlled by physicians and private sources of funding. The advantages to providers of such private and voluntary planning over public or government planning were obvious. George's planning group basically secured HEW's blessing to create a national plan for the "rationalizing" of obstetric services. This is not the place to discuss health planning and whether it works for anyone, if at all. But what I learned at school of public health and working in Comprehensive Health Planning at HEW in Boston was that our government was giving lip-service at least to the idea that consumers were intended to be involved in health planning, and furthermore, that they should have a majority voice.

The document, "Toward Improving the Outcome of Pregnancy," sponsored by the March of Dimes and co-authored by George Ryan, deserves careful study and I urge everyone who is not familiar with it to obtain a copy. It has become the basic guiding model for Regionalization. I would like to point out several important features of its origin, and the group that planned it.

The Committee on Perinatal Health which prepared the document was composed entirely of physicians representing physician organizations: The American Academy of Family Physicians (AAFP), the American Academy of Pediatrics (AAP), the ACOG and the AMA. Not only were all of these committee members men, but all were board-certified specialists in academic medicine. Most were past or present officers in their own specialty groups, that is, in their own guilds or unions. As far as I know, all of them were also white men. The Task Forces themselves were all composed of men and physicians with the same kinds of backgrounds, and a significant number of them were obstetricians, representing the AMA committees, while also being part of the ACOG. It seems scandalous that no national nursing groups were invited into the planning and decision-making at that level, not the American College of Nurse-Midwives (ACNM) or even ACOG's own nursing group (NAACOG). But it is even more outrageous that no consumers or consumer organizations were invited at this level, not even as tokens or consultants, and not even from the National Foundation of the March of Dimes. (Of the 34 people on the combined Task Force and Consultant roster, only seven people were women, largely nurses, but all as consultants only. All but three of the men were physicians.) Furthermore, there were no mental health professionals at all. One does not have to be a feminist or a politician to recognize whose interests would be served by a planning group like this. Let's look closely at the results. What exactly are the benefits to physicians and hospitals? I have described all of this in the Appendix to our book "Our Bodies, Ourselves," which I will summarize briefly here:

(1) The plan guarantees to teaching hospitals that their needs will come first. The survival and perpetuation of the university hospital complex is the first goal of modern medicine. This model guarantees that the academic group in obstetrics would control the entire system of professional obstetric and perinatal practice from the top, setting standards for everyone down to the smallest unit and most obscure physician delivering babies. It guarantees an unlimited supply of teaching material and an unlimited supply of money to pay for expensive personnel and equipment. The system also perpetuates specialty medicine, by placing it out of reach of any other standards but its own, that is, the standards set by obstetrician-gynecologists.

(2) The plan is designed to protect the individual physicians as much as possible from being accountable either to their own patients, to consumers in general, or to the hospital or the state, for the quality of pre-natal care and supervision. This model of regionalization requires no standards of screening or practice which must be met by the physician involved before the delivery. Protection of incompetence is offered by building in a guarantee that any carelessness or mismanagement of pregnancy will be rescued at the time of delivery–and by the full armamentarium of the hospital if necessary.

In this same plan, these physicians advise Level I hospitals to build in a "strong component of preventive services," since these patients can't get easy access to high risk care. Why not stress this same component at Level II and Level III hospitals? Why not make rigorous screening and standards binding on every physician granted privileges at every hospital? If physicians were required to screen rigorously in every setting, most hospitals wouldn't need such an expensive unit. In fact, they wouldn't have to have so many doctors. In fact, they wouldn't have to have hospitals at all. As the Maternity Center Association in New York has shown, you don't need a hospital or a doctor for a normal birth.

But this is not the question. The question for us is, why is the self-interest of this small group of physicians being allowed to serve as childbirth policy for our whole nation? And how does it affect us? What are we going to do about it?

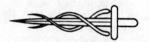

For a copy of the pamphlet mentioned on previous
pages the original publication that outlines the concept
of regionalization of perinatal services, write to:

NAT'L FOUNDATION OF THE MARCH OF DIMES
1275 Mamaroneck Avenue
White Plains, New York    10605

Ask for:

Toward Improving The Outcome of Pregnancy
by George Ryan & Others

# The National Foundation

# March of Dimes

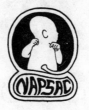

# CHAPTER EIGHT

## A MOTHER'S RESPONSE TO REGIONALIZATION
## THE HEART OF THE MATTER

### Judith Dickson Luce

Birth is an experience that cannot be separated from women giving birth, from the person born, or from the families in which these births take place, anymore than death can be separated from the dying person. But in this society we try desperately to do both and also to separate the dying and birthing person from all of the rest of us. To birthing and to dying we bring our histories, our relationships, our rituals and the deepest values and hopes that give meaning to our lives. Perhaps what is most wrong with medical plans like "Regionalization" is that they enforce the separations I have just described and in no way address the more central needs and values that women and men bring to their birth experiences. These are needs and values that relate to intimacy, sexuality, the quality and style of family life and community, and our deepest beliefs about birth, life and death.

One of the problems we face in trying to respond to Regionalization plans is that we can begin to perceive ourselves as part of the health care team and forget who we are: birthing women and men, mothers and fathers. In a sense we are not able to approach birth on our own terms, with our own language. The topic has been defined in another tongue and too easily we find ourselves reacting, criticizing, counter-proposing, but on their terms: medical ones that so narrow our experience of birth. (We begin to speak in terms of "good outcomes," "optimum experiences," and "levels of risk.") And in turn we see the professionalization and medicalization of roles and relationships that rightfully belong to mothers, ·fathers, siblings and friends. We must keep reminding ourselves that for 95 percent of women birth is not a "medical event" — there are few if any medical dimensions to that experience. And even when complications do exist the medical dimension must be kept in perspective. Life-supporting procedures cannot be allowed to impinge upon or replace values and experiences that are equally life-sustaining.

The medium is the message and I believe there is a symbolic dimension to all this planning that cannot be ignored. The message of Regionalization, a high risk model of care for every woman, is that women's bodies don't work. By definition, to be a woman has come to mean to be "high risk." By describing and categorizing a woman "high risk" or even potentially "high risk" we cement fear to a process that most women are already alienated from (and fear creates problems in childbirth). Being afraid of natural bodily processes and dependent on men and machines damages women in birth as forceps, drugs and meddling hands damage newborns. And fear and the experience of failure keeps women distant from each other. The message, most often not spoken but heard even in the silence, becomes: "my body did not work for me and yours might not either." So we are bound together in a circle of fear rather than strength.

Judith Dickson Luce is a member of Birth Day, member of ICEA Task Force on Regionalization, a birth attendant, woman and mother of three.

Many of us are familiar with the poster: "I am a woman giving birth to myself." For too many of us this process of becoming, every bit as real as the physical birth of a child, is aborted or ends in miscarriage. We can't let this continue to happen.

Historically it has been impossible to talk about birth without talking about midwives — wise women, healers, enablers of women, protectors of the process of birth. The midwife was the bridge builder between women and families. She taught women about their bodies, about birth and the ways in which the richness of the culture would be transmitted to their children. I do not glorify an idyllic image of the past. I am certain that knowledge was limited but as limited as it may have been it was not alienating. Today we need bridges between us — as women and as families.

My vision of the future is that every woman who labors and births will be capable of helping one other woman birth — be it sister, friend or daughter; that a woman who knows and trusts her body and lets it work will share the memory of that knowledge with other women; that women and men who have taken responsibility for their birthing will help others do the same. I see women learning birth from their mothers and sisters not from professionals. I see "prenatal care" — "primary care" being just that: the care we give ourselves and our unborn children, the care we give to and receive from those most primary in our lives.

We can create our own rituals of birthing that are rich, that nourish us and bind us together and that say something about who we are and who we want to become. This is what birth is about. In doing this women will be able to say "birth is ours;" families will be able to say: "birth is ours."

I have given birth three times. My third child, Damara, was born at home three and a half years ago. I believe her birth, the way I gave birth to her, the way our family gave birth, was not just a wonderful, personally fulfilling experience, but one whose roots went deep, connecting me to women who have given birth before me, binding me closer to all women, to all birthing families.

So, I share with you the account I wrote of her birth:

### Damara's Birth

Our decision to have a home birth was both simple and very complex. It was simple in that from the very beginning of this pregnancy it never entered our heads that this baby would be born anywhere but in our own home. It was complex in that the decision to do this represented personally a stage of growth and awareness of many issues, social, philosophical, political and even religious. These were related to my sense of being a woman, being in touch with and responsible for my own body. It had to do with Tom's and my sense of family, of the naturalness of life, of birth, of sexuality. We were learning slowly and somewhat painfully but gladly a sense of the seasons of things. We wanted our children to learn these things naturally from the early years of their lives. Being part of Damara's birth in our own home with our friends we felt was a way of doing this. We wanted to have a real choice about how we gave birth, where and with whom. We wanted to shape and create the environment our child would be born into. We wanted her birth to be a celebration. We wanted her to be born in a happy, colorful, yet peaceful place. I wanted music for labor and people to support me and celebrate with us. Mostly we didn't want the rhythm of our family life disrupted by separation from each other or from Jonathan and Peter.

We also had developed strong feelings about what technology poorly used and institutions which become ends in themselves can do to depersonalize, dehumanize and in many ways take from us the most basic and for some of us the peak experiences of life, like birth — and death. They become so removed from us that we don't even experience them. I had felt painful ruptures in the births of my other two children and had been able to reflect on what happened and why it shouldn't again. Most painful had been that initial 10 to 14 hours separation, routine in most hospitals. My best instincts told me that the initial contact and being together was critical and that separation was no less painful for the one being born. At home we knew there would be no separation. As it turned out it was those first few hours of skin-closeness and warmth that were most precious to me and to Tom.

In deciding to have a home birth we had to deal with the possibility that something could go wrong (as it could in the hospital, although we are led to believe otherwise), meaning we had to deal with death, the possibility of death. Our sense was that the quality of life is as important an issue as the fact of life; that how we birth is as important as birth.

Damara is our last biological child. We wanted to end with a bang by bringing all we were and knew to make her birth our very own experience that would be as rich as possible.

And it was: it was rich and it was uniquely ours. Most amazing had been how in touch with my body and its messages I had become. I knew the baby was coming. Awaking at midnight out of a deep sleep (my body had told me to go to bed at 8), finding myself in labor, my energies were totally directed. I knew the baby was coming and coming soon. The memory of her two and a half hour journey is filled with images, feelings, sounds. The long hot bath I took, the water soothing, relaxing, easing the intensity of the contractions. Peter, our two year old, resting his head on my lap as I labored sitting on the rug while Tom fixed the bed, vacuumed the rug (tried to — I protested, at this point a little lint wouldn't hurt anyone), and set up the stereo. And then the music, soft, beautiful in the background, totally concentrated out during contractions. It was September 25, 1974. The first cold night of the Fall. I will always remember hearing, "Try to remember — the kind of September when life was slow and oh, so mellow — when grass was green and grain so yellow." It seemed to come on just for me. The words, "Without a hurt the heart is hollow," spoke to my labor, the intensity of the very powerful thing happening within me. And there was the support I felt in between contractions from the people who were with me.

And there were the funny things. Christina, my friend, saying I did not look comfortable. My response being, "What did she expect, I wasn't and couldn't imagine being so until it was over." Her asking if I'd like a bigger clock to watch (I had become wedded to Tom's wrist watch); my answering emphatically, "No, if it were bigger it would take longer for the seconds to go by!" For me, time was of the essence; to experience completely the sensations of labor, knowing they only came a minute at a time. It was good being able to drink all I wanted when thirsty, a sharp contrast to my hospital labors. I had thought of everything. Even the three 35-cent lollipops from Brighams: one for Jonathan, one for Peter and one for me. Mine went untouched. There was the birth itself. The still excitement I felt in the room; Jonathan and Peter't intent gazing, my own excitement and eagerness to push and then the shock of the pain (those good old posterior presentations). I just pushed and pushed. I remember voices gently saying, "push, push, you can do it." It was like everyone was pushing with me. I remember the strength of Tom holding me, voices again: "It's a girl, it's a girl." There she was, quiet and still and so beautiful. She waited before she breathed. I can still hear Christina saying, "come on, little girl, breath for us." And she did. Our fingertips touched as she let out a little yell. All was quiet and peacefulness and so much welcoming. I felt all my energy had drained into her. The intensity of the feelings that followed in those hours, in the next few days were such that they overshadowed the events themselves. But I remember the wine, the music, the song, "Moments To Live By", Tom had practiced for months ahead of time. And there was Peter's request for "Old McDonald" that had to come first.

Everyone left as quickly and quietly as they came. It was 4 a.m. and we were left with Peter sleeping on the floor next to our bed. Jonathan was back in bed. Tom and I lay there with Damara between us, her skin touching both of ours. Tom slept, but I lay there and watched the changes that each moment brought — in her and in me. I was joyful and grateful. Through our window I watched the sun rise. Outside our room were beautiful wild yellow flowers silhouetted against the predawn sky. They turned yellow and then almost golden as they blew gloriously in the Autumn breeze. The sun rose and we rose. The day was such a celebration. Family and friends came and feasted on turkey and heard of Damara's birth as if there had never been another birth. The days that followed were a time of rest and reflecting on all that had happened. I thought of how Damara would someday share in her own birth in a way I never knew of mine, a birth that was hers and no one else's. There was hope that this would be a point where we could again touch as she moved one day into womanhood.

The second day was warm and sunny. Tom and I buried the placenta next to our house. We planted a yellow chrysanthemum over it to remind us always of the pain and joy that was Damara's birth, to remind us of the golden days of September, to remind us "without a hurt the heart is hollow", to remind us of the oneness of life and creation. Life is birth, but it is rebirth too. To remind us, for others, that birth is one of the moments we are given to live by, and it shouldn't be taken from anyone.

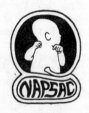

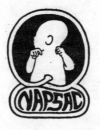

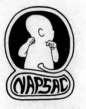

# CHAPTER NINE

## REGIONALIZATION OF MATERNITY AND NEWBORN CARE: FACTS, FANTASIES, FLAWS, AND FALLACIES

### Muriel Sugarman, M.D.

### Summary

Motivated by a concern for improving perinatal outcome, rationalizing care delivery, and containing costs, many regions in the nation are designing and implementing plans for regionalization of maternity and newborn services. This paper analyzes the origins, clinical biases, strengths and weaknesses of regionalization plans in general and suggests modifications designed to incorporate or enhance mental health and humanistic principles, cost-effectiveness analysis, consumer acceptability, and consonance with Federal health planning guidelines.

### Introduction

The concept of regionalization of health care services first originated in application to such major health care areas as coronary care, burns, and emergency medical services. The principal behind such regionalized planning was to be sure that cases had access to that institution with the appropriate capability to handle the level of seriousness of the patient's condition, without needless duplication of services.

The idea was that there would be many small, easily accessible, community-based institutions capable of caring for less serious cases, some larger institutions which could care for moderately severe cases, and one or two centers in each geographical region to which would be transferred the most serious cases — those which required the most sophisticated equipment and the most highly trained, specialized caregivers. Agreements among institutions would also assure continuity of care and sharing of up-to-date knowledge. Applied to major disease conditions, this appeared to be a logical, economical, effective, and beneficial way to distribute care.

In recent years this model came to be applied to maternity-newborn care. Yet birth is surely not a major disease condition. True, there are life-threatening, high-risk conditions in a small percentage of mothers and-or newborns (10 to 15 percent), but the prototype plan for regionalization of maternity-newborn care aims to apply to all births. It is therefore crucial that we look closely and critically at its origins and development.

Several years ago, representatives of the American Academy of Family Practice (AAFP), American Academy of Pediatrics(AAP), American College

Muriel Sugarman, M.D., is Assistant Child Psychiatrist, Beth Israel Hospital, Boston; Psychiatric Consultant at Boston Hospital for Women; former chairperson, ICEA Regionalization Committee; she is author of "Perinatal Influences on Maternal-Infant Attachment," in the Journal of Orthopsychiatry, and "Regionalization of Maternity and Newborn Care," Journal of Perinatology and Neonatology.

of Obstetricians and Gynecologists (ACOG), and the American Medical Association (AMA) formed a self-appointed national body known as the Committee on Perinatal Health. This Committee set up voluntary task forces to design a system of regional health planning for maternity-newborn care with the expressed goal of reducing rates of maternal, fetal, and neonatal mortality.

With administrative and financial assistance from the National Foundation— March of Dimes, the Committee on Perinatal Health published its recommendations in 1976. That document — "Toward Improving the Outcome of Pregnancy: Recommendations for the Regional Development of Maternal and Perinatal Health Services" (7) — sets forth guidelines for regional planning of perinatal services which are being incorporated into local health plans and regulations in many parts of the country as well as into national health planning guidelines, and have already begun to be widely circulated and adopted — sometimes through actual regulation or regional planning; in other instances, through private agreements among institutions.

Regional planning of maternity-newborn care — or regionalization — is a concept which is now clearly upon us and is rapidly gaining momentum throughout the country. This paper examines the reasons behind and the goals of regionalization, attempts to critically evaluate its weaknesses, and suggests modifications.

### Motivations for Regionalization

To go back to the origins of the concept of regionalization of maternity-newborn care, we must briefly look at four motivations: (1) statistical indicators of health status such as mortality rates; (2) therapeutic issues; (3) the deficiencies of the general health care system; and (4) economic and political issues.

Stated motivation number one behind the formation of the Committee on Perinatal Health was the objective of reducing mortality rates. Since 1970 the United States has ranked 11th to 15th among the developed nations of the world in infant mortality (38) — a statistical measure long considered to be an extremely important indicator of the health status of a population.

Although this embarassing showing has been explained away by criticisms of the methods of data collection and analysis of other countries, and by the greater physical and socioeconomic differences among segments of our population, etc., no one in the field of maternity and newborn care has been proud of these statistics or satisfied that we could not do better. The document published by the Committee on Perinatal Health states its aim to reduce mortality by four means: early detection of abnormality, higher quality of care, better access to scarce resources, and earlier dissemination of advanced technology. We will examine the efficacy of these methods more closely later.

Second, there is a therapeutic motive for regionalization — good quality obstetrical-newborn care is not easily available to large segments of the population because of maldistribution of services and personnel. Duplicating specialized technical services in poorly served areas would be costly; placing highly-trained personnel in underserved areas would not only be costly but would result in loss of technical skill for these personnel through lack of sufficient practice in areas where the number of high risk cases is small. Hence the alternative plan calls for transporting high risk mothers and newborns to centralized facilities which already have the expensive technical equipment and highly skilled personnel to render the most specialized care.

The third motivation for regional planning is the current state of the health care system in general. Rising costs, maldistribution of professional caregivers, duplication of equipment and services, too many hospital beds, unequal access to care, and lack of systematic planning have forced awareness of the critical need for careful, rational, and more cost-effective planning in all areas of health care.

Economic and political issues related to maternity-newborn health care are a fourth but very important motivation for regionalization. Almost all hospitals are today in difficult economic straits. Maternity units have not been a money-making part of general hospitals. Indeed, they have often been a financial liability. With falling birth rates and increasing reliance on sophisticated, expensive equipment, these problems have become more acute. Many maternity units are seriously overbedded and-or understaffed and under equipped by today's stringent standards, while current health care personnel and equipment costs and reimbursement methods provide no incentives for correction of these conditions.

With falling birth rates, there is increasing competition between teaching and community hospitals, between obstetricians and neonatologists and less highly specialized caregivers such as family practitioners and midwives, over the dwindling number of birthing families. Quite understandably, the large urban centers with highly specialized personnel and equipment claim to be the best places for birth for medical and safety reasons and wish to decrease the competition of other forms of care.

Basically, the prototype plan for regionalization — set forth in Toward Improving the Outcome of Pregnancy (7) — consists of closing or consolidating "underutilized" or "inadequate" maternity units; defining three basic levels of care for the remaining institutions; setting standards of care for each level of hospital; listing criteria for consultation, referral, or transfer among perinatal units at the three levels; and encouraging education by and input from the high risk perinatal specialists into all of maternity-newborn care.

The three levels of care are: Level I, uncomplicated or primary maternity-newborn care; Level II, moderate risk, secondary care; Level III, high risk, intensive, high technology tertiary care. The levels are defined by availability of special personnel, equipment, and services (laboratory, ultra-sound, bloodbank, etc.) but even a hospital with Level III status can and will care for low risk, normal patients. Minimum numbers of births per year will define which hospitals will close or merge. For example a minimum of 1000 - 2000 births per year is suggested for any maternity unit, and tertiary care units may well aim for 1400 to 3000 births per year.

If this plan is implemented, in many areas small, local, community hospital maternity-newborn services will close and in some areas moderate and high-risk care (Level II and Level III) will be housed in one institution.

Normal, healthy childbearing families will have little choice: Either hospital birth in Level II or Level III centers where care will be very technologically oriented, or out-of-hospital birth.

(There are a few areas of the country where Regionalization has not meant total reliance on Level II or III care. According to Madeleine Shearer of Birth and the Family Journal, Arizona, the Rocky Mountain States, Wisconsin, and North Carolina, use Level II and III care only for high risk women and have kept open their Level I institutions. This more sensible implementation needs further exploration.)

This plan has been presented as a set of guidelines — for redistributing scarce, costly resources; for centralizing the care of high risk mothers and infants; for liaison mechanisms to increase continuity of care and responsibility for a regional population; for education, teaching and sharing of new skills and knowledge; for reducing overbedding and — hopefully — costs. Yet there are many who have grave misgivings about the impact of implementing plans for regionalization of maternity and newborn care as they now stand. They feel an urgent need to raise questions, suggest changes, and contribute their input to any regional planning for current and for future maternity-newborn health care.

### Limited Orientation to Plan

The document that is the foundation for most regional or state regionalization plans — for all maternity-newborn care — Toward Improving the Outcome of Pregnancy — was almost totally conceived and produced by organized medicine. The task force members and many of their consultants were practicing or academic obstetricians, pediatricians, and family practitioners and members of their specialty societies. Not invited by this self-appointed group were consumers and consumer groups, representatives of national nurses' organizations including the American College of Nurse Midwives, rural health care providers, and mental health professionals. The document itself then is heavily oriented to treatment of disease, high risk care, crisis intervention; i.e., treating the already present problem at the end of pregnancy and in the perinatal period. In fact, this plan focuses almost entirely on tertiary care — that is the detection and care of the high-risk mother and newborn.

While prevention of mortality and morbidity was an avowed goal of the Committee on Perinatal Health, the guidelines do not spell out in detail any program of true prevention to begin early in pregnancy. The preventive focus of the guidelines consists only of early detection and identification of factors statistically associated with high risk conditions, e.g. maternal age, parity, previous history of need for special neonatal care, or detection of true medical disease such as diabetes, heart disease, etc. There is no emphasis on or plan for community outreach, for early involvement in prenatal care, improved prenatal nutrition, education for childbirth and parenting, alcoholism counselling, etc. which might decrease the numbers of high risk deliveries. As with so much of medical care in this country, the focus is on more, better, newer technological interventions to treat end-stage problems.

A corollary of this disease orientation is the heavy focus on technology and the neglect of health-oriented and humanistic issues. Nothing is said about informed consent, foreign language interpreters, support for families with complications of the birth process, prevention of maternal-infant separation, providing knowledge, support, and encouragement for breast feeding, etc. Although psychiatric problems are mentioned as high risk factors for screening purposes, the roster of consultants and required staff mentions only medical social workers — not psychiatrists, psychiatric social workers, or other mental health professionals. In planning for the closing of excess beds no mention is made of evaluating a given service or hospital not only as to its technological excellence and annual number of deliveries, but also as to its competence in giving family centered, humanistic care and its acceptability to patients.

A significant omission from the guidelines is planning for normal pregnancy and birth. Nowhere are there criteria for low risk pregnancy, labor, and birth. Nowhere are there guidelines for non-interventionist management of the normal birth process. Only brief mention is made of the use of midwives; almost no mention is made of prenatal care, delivery, and postnatal care by the family physician, nurse practitioner, etc. In point of fact, the care of the vast majority of healthy, normal women and their infants is largely ignored, while all resources and attention are on the high risk situations, which occur in a small minority of cases. (10 - 15 percent by the estimates of most obstetrical experts).

### Cost Effectiveness

We must also raise the whole complex question of the cost effectiveness of the proposed prototype plans for regionalization. Specialized high risk services are costly but effective in the situation where complications are either already present or highly likely to make an appearance. We realize that even all-out efforts to prevent such complications as low birth weight, prematurity, toxemia, fetal alcohol syndrome, etc. will not prevent all of these and other complications. No one quarrels with a need for tertiary care centers. But central to most plans for regionalization is the goal of closing down many small, less costly primary care maternity units (for example, in Massachusetts, the plan proposes to close all but one or two in the entire state (31, 371). This forces patients to go to Level II and III (secondary and tertiary care) units where even normal, uncomplicated birth will be more costly. Since the trend in maternity and newborn care already is toward greater and greater management and intervention (11, 18, 45), one can predict that in centers where equipment and personnel are available for more of the increasingly fashionable, technologically sophisticated, but costly diagnostic and therapeutic procedures, these procedures will be overused. This may be done for teaching, research, or practice purposes, through lack of good criteria for utilization, or for legal self-defense. Such over-utilization will of course drive costs up, not down, as well as increasing the number of iatrogenic complications of birth, since every one of these procedures carries with it seldom-mentioned risks and hazards.

Highly specialized maternity centers wish to admit uncomplicated cases because of the need for teaching material, the need for practice of skills, and problems of current third party medical care payment. Teaching and practice requirements could alternatively be dealt with by moving personnel to the teaching cases instead of the reverse. Reimbursement by insurance or state and federal payers is a thorny but crucial practical issue. Under current reimbursement plans where there is a flat daily rate-bed (per diem rate), all maternity cases subsidize the high risk cases, as in general hospitals, all low risk patients subsidized high risk care. This is because low intensity care costs less per day than the daily rate set and high intensity care costs more. Large numbers of low risk cases are needed to offset the cost of high risk treatment. The hospital, caught in an economic squeeze, has an irresistible incentive to overuse beds, prolong stays, and perform specialized procedures frequently to

Note: According to a recent study, risks of dying are three times greater with Cesarean delivery than with vaginal delivery. (PAS Reporter 14: Special issue 1976)

offset the costs of personnel and equipment (6). However, since pregnancy is not a disease, putting healthy childbearing women into such costly, disease-oriented environments is costly and unfair as well as demoralizing and unhealthy (2, 36). It is unhealthy because the likelihood of infection, of having a Cesarean section, and therefore of dying are greater; (see note) also, where low risk women and high risk women are cared for together, low risk women are more likely to get less attention when things get busy and staff are pressed for time. Attempts to replace this attention by machines create situations which are unarguably not always in the best interests of the healthy, childbearing family unit.

Another question to be raised is the requirement for a minimum number of births for a maternity unit to provide high quality care and to survive economically. Various figures have been named (7, 8, 14, 20, 21, 23, 34) — but at least 1000 to 2000 deliveries per year is the minimum cited as optional. Here it is not clear why these numbers are so important: Are they the numbers that provide the best quality care — both technological and humanistic — or are they merely arbitrary numbers needed for the hospital to "break even" financially? Neither may be the case. At least three public health experts have seriously questioned whether number of deliveries has really been proved to be an indicator of good outcome or economy of operation (15, 16, 25).

In all the concern over cutting costs by closing down under-utilized maternity units and increasing the number of births per year in more centralized facilities, too little attention has been paid to patient access. Closing community maternity centers would mean a great increase in travelling time, the burden of which would fall most heavily on those without automobiles, those living in areas without public transportation, mothers with other young children who must accompany them to prenatal visits, and those who are physically ill or handicapped. Such families, often those most in need of care, would have longer travel times for prenatal visits, for family visiting of either mother or newborn in the hospital, and for reaching the maternity unit during labor. One can predict a great increase in elective inductions, with all their complications and increased risks, for those women likely to develop complications whose homes are further than ever from the maternity unit.

### A Proposed Alternative Model

Guidelines for an alternative system of maternity-newborn care should take into account, among other factors, the following critical issues:

(1) cost containment

(2) risk and cost-benefit analysis (risks and costs vs benefits of care)

(3) financial fairness for patients and institutions through better reimbursement strategies

(4) prevention efforts throughout pregnancy, labor and delivery, and the postpartum period

(5) mental health, social, and humanistic issues

(6) consumer input and patient acceptability

(7) accessibility of care — (how long it takes to arrive at the maternity unit and how to get there)

(8) continuity of care — (follow-through and familiar caregivers)

(9) regional responsibility for a given population

(10) data collection and quality assessment

(11) health education and training

(12) long term followup

There is a need for a consistently broader and deeper focus, with greater diversity of input, to arrive at a truly rational regional plan for caregiving. As they now stand, plans for regionalization may create serious humanistic, mental health, social, and patient acceptability problems; may lead to cost increases rather than containment; and may not actually prevent or decrease morbidity and mortality.

One means of obtaining diversity of input is through the Health Systems Agencies created by PL 93-641. The National Health Planning and Resources Development Act of 1974 — which mandates statewide health plans drafted by local Health Systems Agencies and other Federally designated state agencies — provides for consumer and provider input, public hearings, and Federal approval, thus promoting much greater diversity in health planning. Another means would be for planning and regulatory bodies at the state and federal level to seek out consumer and consumer organization input, input from midwives, childbirth educators, etc. instead of only inviting input from the provider establishment.

The following plan deals with the prenatal, perinatal, and postpartum periods as a caregiving continuum. It is meant as a framework around which individual communities and families could set up a system with choices and alternatives yet still include sound health care principles. This represents an alternative prototype regionalized system for all maternity-newborn care.

## Proposed Prenatal Care System

Prenatal care which is acceptable, accessible, community-based, and prevention-oriented should be available to all pregnant women. In order to encourage pregnant women to be involved in care as early in pregnancy as possible, there should be a system of public education, patient transportation, and community outreach enlisting specially trained community workers. Each community should have a coordinated neighborhood based network of prenatal clinics, staffed mainly by midwives and-or nurse practitioners with assistance from community aides or advocates especially where language and other cultural barriers might prove a problem. These prenatal centers would also have access to physician backup. The clinics would offer comprehensive prenatal care including:

(1) abortion counselling where needed

(2) education about normal physical and psychological changes in pregnancy; signs of abnormality; how, when, and where to request assistance with problems

(3) childbirth preparation including normal anatomy and physiology of birth, benefits and risks of drugs and procedures, relaxation and breathing techniques, patients rights and responsibilities, etc.

(4) nutritional evaluation, education, and supplementation where necessary to maintain superior nutritional intake throughout pregnancy; education about the importance of avoiding drugs, alcohol, pesticides, solvents, smoking hazards, etc.

(5) emotional and factual preparation for parenting, child care, infant feeding (especially breastfeeding), etc.

(6) special support for pregnant adolescents

(7) careful screening and prompt referral to perinatal centers for further evaluation of patients with carefully defined medical, psychiatric, or obstetrical complications or risk factors; this must include a means of tran-

sportation, and continued community clinic support, followup, and responsibility.

(8) for pregnant women with complications requiring bedrest, there should be in place a mechanism for home care-home help to prevent unnecessary hospitalization and separation of family members.

Certain data are needed to evaluate the success of these programs. There need to be specific criteria for the low risk patient in order to designate a population which can receive cost-effective care safely where it is most accessible and acceptable. The effectiveness of outreach efforts and community-based prenatal care could be assessed by indicators such as:

(1) average prenatal week of first visit

(2) average number of appointments kept

(3) ratio of referral appointments kept to referrals made (how many patients referred and how many kept appointments and continued care)

(4) incidence of low birth weight, prematurity, metabolic toxemia

## Proposed Perinatal and Neonatal Care System

A rational, coordinated system for maternity-newborn care must take into account reduction of excess inpatient beds and duplication of services; the cost-benefit and risk-benefit ratios of using medical and technological intervention; the wishes of consumers for more flexibility of care; the economic, social, linguistic, cultural and psychological needs of childbearing families; and the financial and educational needs of institutions. Low and high risk care should be provided in different settings.

## Low Risk Perinatal Care

The majority of pregnant women are healthy, normal, low-risk individuals for whom birth should be a social, familial, and emotional event rather than an illness. There is ample evidence in this country and from other nations that this population, once identified, can receive adequate, safe care through far less costly and intrusive means than are currently in common practice in the United States (3, 17, 18, 30, 46). With careful screening and full information, families should be offered a spectrum of birth alternatives. These should include the following:

(1) For the many low risk women who will elect to deliver in hospitals or who require minimal obstetrical intervention best performed in a hospital (such as analgesia, local or conduction anesthesia, low forceps delivery, treatment of infection, observation because of bleeding, etc.) there is a need for a moderately reduced number of small to medium sized, community based, accessible hospitals whose focus is on the low-risk, normal birth experience. Such hospitals should put the greatest emphasis on safely humanizing and normalizing the birth experience for the entire family.

Rather than using arbitrary numerical standards to decrease the numbers of excess maternity hospital beds, broader criteria for allowing small, local hospitals to remain open should be devised to include the following:

(a) economical operation and low cost care

(b) community acceptability

(c) staff privileges for and delivery by family practitioners and midwives in uncomplicated cases

(d) a demonstrated commitment to avoidance of technological interventions such as induction of labor, intravenous pitocin, fetal monitoring, drugs and anesthesia, episiotomy, forceps delivery, cesarean section, etc.

(e) use of labor-delivery (birth) rooms and labor lounges designed with as little atmosphere of hospitalization and illness as possible

(f) presence of loved ones and friends during labor and delivery as elected by the birthing couple

(g) ad lib movement and position choice for the laboring and birthing woman

(h) no separation of mother, father, siblings, and newborn unless medically necessary by valid, specified criteria, and with parent consent

(i) encouragement of and support and education for breastfeeding; no use of formula or sugar water unless medically required for complications (not as routine)

(j) early discharge (6-24 hours) with home followup by visiting nurses or midwives for healthy mothers and infants

(k) nurses who care for the family as a unit with support for the developing parent-infant attachments if families remain longer in the hospital

(l) standardized, objective obstetrical record keeping

(m) consultation, referral, and transfer arrangements for families with complications (mother and newborn to be transferred together whenever not contraindicated for specific medical reasons)

(n) sympathetic, non-punitive, non-judgmental back-up hospital care for families who have planned out-of-hospital birth but required intervention best done in a hospital for complications

(o) maintenance, to the greatest degree possible, of the caregiving relationship between the birthing family and their out-of-hospital birth attendants if hospitalization is required as in (n); attendants to participate in caregiving in hospital

(p) strict attention to informed consent and patients' rights

(2) In-hospital maternity and newborn care — even with great attention to avoidance of unnecessary technological interventions and short stay practices — is costly and associated with illness. Out-of-hospital alternatives should also be available for carefully screened, healthy, low risk women who choose not to go to a hospital for birth. Out-of-hospital, low cost domiciliary birth centers — staffed by midwives with obstetrician backup and within short transport distance to a hospital — are well under way in several states with excellent results in terms of healthy outcome, cost control, and consumer acceptability (24, 30). Attempts have been made to duplicate this type of center within a hospital but, at present, this seems to result in a loss of economic benefits, flexibility, non-interventive management, and patient satisfaction. Those patients who want a truly home like setting for birth do not merely want a hospital birth room with home like decor.

(3) The other option, home birth with attendance by sensitive, well trained midwives or family physicians and backup by obstetricians and neonatologists in a nearby hospital, perhaps with the availability of a transport vehicle and team, is another viable birth alternative. Though generally opposed by the medical profession in this country, there is ample evidence that birth at home, in cases which have had meticulous prenatal care and have been carefully screened for serious risk factors, and have easy access to skilled backup services, can be safe and health-promoting (3, 12, 17, 19, 32, 46). Regardless of established medical opinion, there are informed, responsible families who will insist on home birth (19). The medical profession cannot ethically abandon these individuals, but must provide as great a margin of safety as possible through careful screening, education in dealing with emergencies, non-

judgmental assistance in the case of complications, and assistance with rapid transport to hospital if necessary.

In the matter of home birth, the medical profession is dealing with the beliefs and attitudes of a subculture just as it does when confronted with Jehovah's Witnesses or Christian Scientists who refuse blood transfusions and certain treatments or Native American or Oriental patients whose healing practices may be in conflict with Western medicine. Medical care, as practiced in other cultures and countries, is not by definition inferior to our system; indeed, many of the beliefs and practices of other societies may offer superior results, both medically and psychologically. A good example of this is the efficacy of acupuncture, long scorned by Western medicine as "quackery" now studied as a new medical technique. The medical system does not have to agree with the beliefs of the subculture; it cannot force an unwilling practitioner to care for patients under conditions he or she considers too risky; but it cannot prevent, ridicule, or interfere with — indeed should support — the provision by willing practitioners of the best medical care possible under circumstances chosen (as is his or her right) by the patient. (44)

I see the threat of use or actual use of professional and-or legal sanctions against those who would provide care at home births as a highly unethical tactic to attempt to prevent out-of-hospital birth. Midwives have been threatened with arrest, loss of any professional certification; physicians have been threatened with malpractice suits, loss of hospital privileges, and loss of licensure with the avowed purpose of rendering families unable to obtain attendants. When confronted with the argument that the inability to find experienced, well-trained attendants may merely render homebirth more hazardous, those same professionals state their purpose to be one of making home birth difficult and hazardous so that fewer families will choose it as an option. I can think of no more unethical and irrational a maneuver than deliberately barring access to good care for those who refuse to compliantly accept the terms of provider institutions and organizations.

### High Risk Perinatal Care - Tertiary Care

For the small percentage of pregnant women and-or their newborns, who will have complications during pregnancy, labor, delivery, or postpartum, centralized perinatal centers serving a large geographic area will be necessary. These centers must maintain specialized technological services, personnel, and resources which are scarce, costly, and which require frequent use and-or practice to maintain optimal skill and cost-effectiveness. Planning for such centers should include the following:

(1) Sophisticated prenatal screening and diagnostic capability, inpatient and outpatient, using carefully formulated and individualized high risk criteria, not blanket categories.

(2) Equipment and resources for preventing or handling complications of labor and delivery for those patients diagnosed as high risk prenatally and for those referred during labor or postpartum from out-of-hospital or primary care hospital settings.

(3) Transportation arrangements for both mothers and newborns, and facilities for joint transportation and care when either requires transfer to a perinatal center.

(4) Highly trained obstetrical and pediatric personnel skilled and experienced in the care of the high risk mother and infant.

(5) The families of high risk maternity or neonatal patients require much more social and psychological support because of the long term traumatic effects on family life of perinatal complications (4, 13, 22, 26, 27, 28). To minimize long term morbidity, perinatal centers need to have the service of specially trained nursing and mental health personnel who can offer emotional support, guidance, information, and preventive intervention to those especially needy families.

(6) Arrangements for continued follow-up involvement in the perinatal center (to the fullest possible extent) by the midwife, nurse practitioner, family practitioner, or clinic aide who have cared for the family during pregnancy, labor and-or delivery and on whose support the family members depend.

(7) Since cultural and language barriers between caregiving personnel and patients are likely to increase patient anxiety, barriers to communication of factual material for treatment and informed consent, the use of general anesthesia during labor and delivery, and the problems of parent support and education, perinatal centers should have available foreign language interpreters and-or community representatives to improve and assure communication with such families, many of whom are already at risk.

(8) Criteria for designation of a perinatal center should be determined according to specific population needs, cost-benefit issues, and need for adequate practice to maintain skills rather than arbitrary numerical criteria such as number of deliveries, number of beds, location, etc. for every center. Centers should be located in areas where high risk patients actually live, whenever possible.

(9) Innovation in rate setting criteria by third party insurers should provide for reimbursement of high risk centers according to actual cost by diagnostic category or procedures required rather than the unfair and inequitable assessment of all patients in a center for the costs of these expensive resources; this would counteract current incentives to treat large numbers of low risk women in high risk centers to balance off the costs of treating smaller numbers of very sick patients (6).

(10) Careful liaison arrangements among perinatal centers, primary care maternity hospital units, birth centers, and home birth attendants with respect to mutual exchange of clinical and theoretical information, continuity of care, responsibility for patients, transportation, and particularly rotation and exchange of trainees; the last would give the broadest base of clinical experience in maternity-newborn care to all trainees and personnel without requiring low risk women and their families to travel to tertiary care centers for birth. For example, physician and nursing trainees could get a valuable view of normal, non-interventive birth attendance from rotation through primary care maternity units and out-of-hospital birth centers.

The quality and effectiveness of this system should be assessed by collection and periodic determination of outcome indicators, including, but not limited to:

(1) Perinatal, intrapartum, maternal, and neonatal mortality using nationally and internationally accepted formulae.

(2) Perinatal morbidity of mother and neonate: Cesarean section, significant perineal or cervical laceration, hemorrhage, retained placenta, need for infant resuscitation, birth injury, etc.

(3) Postnatal maternal morbidity: Infection, prolonged stay, psychological disturbance or depression, etc.

(4) Neonatal morbidity: Respiratory problems, infections, jaundice, seizures, etc.

(5) Long term family morbidity: There is need for careful follow-up to determine the incidence of family problems such as post-partum maternal depression or psychosis, parental separation or divorce in the first year post-partum, child abuse or neglect, and parenting failure.

(6) Morbidity in early childhood: Problems in infant development which may be related to the events surrounding birth such as developmental or mental retardation, failure to thrive, cerebral palsy, learning disability, infantile autism, etc. should be detected and related to the prenatal and perinatal care and events.

### Proposed Postpartum System

At present there is a glaring absence of resources responsible for postpartum family care in the first weeks and months of life. During this time many young families do not have adequate external supports or previous preparation for the arduous task of caring for and relating to a helpless newborn. Moreover, there is ample evidence that the postpartum stay in the artificial environment of the hospital may delay or interfere with the development of attachment and the delicate equilibrium between parents, siblings, and infant (5, 39, 40, 42, 45). In order that parent-infant and sibling infant relationships may get off to as natural a start as possible, families for whom birth occurs away from home should be returned to their own environment as early as is medically possible. This early discharge has been successfully attempted in several settings (30, 33, 47). A vital cornerstone of such an innovation is the use of specially trained visiting or public health nurses or midwives making home visits in the first hours and days after birth. In this manner, the medical condition of mother and infant, the status of lactation, the psychological condition of mother, father, siblings, and their interaction with the neonate can be followed at first hand in the home in the crucial first days and weeks of life. Since most families do not seek out professional care before the first pediatric and postpartum checkup at six weeks, by which time problems of lactation failure, bonding disturbance, postpartum depression, marital and sexual difficulties, etc. are more difficult to reverse, this aftercare can be much less costly and more effective over the long run than later treatment of already entrenched problems.

Longer-term counselling and mutual support services should be available to families with infants. (A list of such services, both professional ones and non-professional self-help groups, should be given to all pregnant women and encouragement to make contact prenatally should be part of prenatal care). These would provide information on infant and child development, preventive health care, and parenting, especially in high risk situations where there are such complications as a handicapped or defective infant, or handicapped, adolescent, emotionally unstable, alcoholic or drug dependent parents. As has been demonstrated by several self-help organizations such as COPE (Coping with the Overall Pregnancy-Parenting Experience) and the Tufts Family Support Service in the Boston area, as well as many childbirth education groups, such intervention does not have to involve costly individual therapy with highly trained mental health professionals, but can be done in groups with less highly trained but sensitive and experienced nurses, social workers, paraprofessionals, or lay counsellors with supervision and backup when needed from psychiatrists and-or psychologists.

## Conclusion

The National Committee on Perinatal Health and groups in many areas of the United States which are working to regionalize maternity-newborn care are consciously motivated by the wish to bring higher quality of care to more pregnant women and their offspring — "Toward Improving the Outcome of Pregnancy." The product of their efforts addresses a number of technological, staffing, and planning issues but is limited in its scope: It is deficient in its approach to humanistic needs, prevention strategies, and utilization of less expensive, more cost-effective, less technologically sophisticated alternatives. To fill the gaps in present regionalization endeavors the suggestions of health planning bodies, consumer groups, third party insurers, mental health experts, and the public should be enlisted. To fail to do this, to insist that only actual providers of hospital services can plan maternity-newborn care, will be to go further down the bleak path of mistrust and antagonism which has become so evident in health care issues in this country today.

Many childbearing families, their organizations, and their advocates possess valuable and increasing knowledge of health care issues. They are not wedded to increasing acceptance and use of the newest, best, most intrusive technology in order to know every answer and control every situation. They have no legal or financial "axe to grind." They have a common sense perspective on humanistic issues of health care, access to care, acceptability of care, over-utilization of services, and economy of operation, areas in which many professionals have serious blind spots. This input has been ignored for too long by health planning bodies, Congressional committees, State and local health departments. Such deliberate policies of exclusion can only be overcome by relentless and vigilant consumer pressure and activism.

## References

1. ACOG News Bulletin, 1972: Rural nurse midwives in Appalachia reduce maternal death rate. Page 1, (May 4).
2. Ad Hoc Committee on Maternity and Newborn Care, Health Service Area IV, 1976: The Proposed Plan for Regionalization of Maternity and Newborn Care in Massachusetts. Preliminary Analysis and Recommendations. Unpublished draft.
3. ARMS, S., 1975: Immaculate Deception. Houghton Mifflin, Boston.
4. BENFIELD, D. ET AL, 1976: Grief response of parents after referral of the critically ill newborn to a regional center. New England J. Med. 294(18): 975-978.
5. BURNS, P. ET AL, 1972: Distress in feeding: short term effect of caretaker environment of the first ten days. J. Amer. Acad. Child Psychiat. 11:427-439.
6. CISNEROS, R.J., 1977: Illness is rewarding - can health be the same? Presented at a meeting of the Massachusetts Public Health Association, Boston, Massachusetts, April 21.
7. COMMITTEE ON PERINATAL HEALTH, 1976: Toward Improving the Outcome of Pregnancy: Recommendations for the Regional Development of Maternal and Perinatal Health Services. National Foundation - March of Dimes, White Plains, New York.
8. COMPREHENSIVE HEALTH PLANNING AGENCY OF SOUTHEASTERN WISCONSIN, INC., 1976: Guidelines for Perinatal Services. Milwaukee, Wisconsin, (February).

9. DEPARTMENT OF HEALTH, EDUCATION, AND WELFARE; Public Health Service, 1976: National Guidelines for Health Planning, (October). Issued under P.L. 93-641, National Health Planning and Resources Development Act of 1974.

10. DEPARTMENT OF HEALTH, EDUCATION AND WELFARE; Public Health Service; Bureau of Health Planning and Resources Development, 1977: Guidelines Concerning the Development of Health Systems Plans and Annual Implementation Plans. Issued under P.L. 93-641, National Health Planning and Resources Development Act of 1974, December 23.

11. DUNN, P., 1976: Obstetric delivery today: for better or for worse? Lancet (April 10): 790-793.

12. EPSTEIN, J. ET AL, 1976: A safe homebirth program that works. In: Safe Alternative in Childbirth; NAPSAC, Marble Hill, Mo.

13. FANAROFF, A. ET AL, 1970: Follow-up of low birth weight infants: the predictive value of maternal visiting patterns. Pediatrics 49: 288-290.

14. FINGER LAKES HEALTH SYSTEMS AGENCY, 1977: Guidelines for Perinatal Services. Rochester, New York, (March 22).

15. FLECK, A.C., 1977: Hospital Sizes and Outcomes of Pregnancy. Office of the Assistant Commissioner for Child Health, New York State Department of Public Health, (February 23).

16. GAUSE, R., 1977: Personal Communication.

17. HAIRE, D., 1970: Childbirth in the Netherlands: a contrast in care. ICEA News, (Nov.-Dec.).

18. HAIRE, D., 1976: The Cultural Warping of Childbirth. Monograph, 3rd edition, International Childbirth Education Association.

19. HAZELL, L., 1974: Birth Goes Home: An Ethnographic and ATTITUDINAL Study of 300 Couples Electing Home Birth in the San Francisco Bay Area. NAPSAC, Marble Hill, Mo.

20. HEALTH BOARD OF THE METROPOLITAN COUNCIL, 1977: Health Systems Plan for the Metropolitan Area. St. Paul, Minnesota, (Apr. 14).

21. HEALTH SYSTEMS AGENCY OF NEW YORK CITY; HSA Task Force on Restructuring Hospital Service Delivery System, 1976: Report on Maternity Services. New York City, (October 22).

22. HELFER, R. AND KEMPE, C., eds., 1968: The Battered Child. University of Chicago Press, Chicago.

23. INDIANA STATE BOARD OF HEALTH, 1976: Criteria and Standards and Guidelines for Areawide Planning of Perinatal Services in Indiana - Draft. Indianapolis, (December).

24. INTERNATIONAL CHILDBIRTH EDUCATION ASSOCIATION NEWSLETTER, 1975-76: Maternity care alternatives: The New Life Center. 14(4), Winter.

25. KIRSCH, L.J., 1976: Letter to Program Director, Office of Health Facilities Development, Massachusetts Department of Public Health, (May 12).

26. KLAUS, M. AND KENNELL, J., 1970: Mothers separated from their newborn infants. Pediat. Clin. North Amer., 17(4): 1015-1035.

27. KLAUS, M. AND KENNELL, J., 1976: Maternal-Infant Bonding. C.V. Mosby, St. Louis.

28. KLEIN, M. AND STERN, L., 1971: Low birth weight and the battered child syndrome. Amer. J. Dis. Child, 122: 15-18.

29. LEVY, B. ET AL, 1971: Reducing neonatal mortality rate with nurse-midwives. Amer. J. Obstet. Gynecol., 109(1):50-58.

30. LUBIC, R.W., 1977: Comprehensive Maternity Care as an Ambulatory Service – Maternity Center Association's Birth Alternative. J. New York State Nurses Association, Vol. 8, No. 4.

31. MASSACHUSETTS MATERNITY AND NEWBORN REGIONALIZATION PROJECT, 1976: Regionalization of Maternity and Newborn Care in Massachusetts: The Final Report, Condensed Version. (Address inquiries to: Ann Hallman Pettigrew, M.D., 5 Follen Street, Cambridge, Massachusetts 02138).

32. MEHL, L. 1976: Statistical outcome of homebirths in the U.S.: current status. In: Safe Alternatives in Childbirth, D. Stewart and L. Stewart, eds. NAPSAC, Marble Hill, Mo.

33. MEHL, L. ET AL, 1976: Outcomes of early discharge after normal birth. Birth and the Family Journal 3(3).

34. MINNESOTA STATE BOARD OF HEALTH, 1976: Guidelines for Development of Regional Perinatal Care in Minnesota. Minneapolis, Minnesota, (April).

35. NATIONAL HEALTH PLANNING AND RESOURCES DEVELOPMENT ACT OF 1974 (PL 93-641). 93rd Congress, 2nd session, Approved January 4, 1975.

36. PFEUFER, R., 1975: Communities, community hospitals, and regionalization of maternity care. Unpublished manuscript.

37. REGIONALIZATION OF MATERNITY AND NEWBORN CARE PROJECT, 1976: Perinatal Regulations, in conjunction with the Massachusetts Department of Public Health. Unpublished draft.

38. RYAN, G.M. ET AL, 1977: Regionalizing perinatal health services in Massachusetts. New England J. Med. 296(4): 228-230.

39. SANDER, L., 1969: Regulation and organization in the early infant-caretaker system. In: Brain and Early Behavior, R. Robinson, ed. Academic Press, London.

40. SANDER, L. ET AL, 1970: Early mother-infant interaction and 24-hour patterns of activity and sleep. J. Amer. Acad. Child Psychiat. 9: 103-123.

41. SANDER, L., 1975: Infant and caretaking environment: Investigation and conceptualization of adaptive behavior in a system of increasing complexity. In: Explorations in Child Psychiatry, E. Anthony, ed. Plenum Press, New York.

42. STECHLER, G., 1975: Perinatal psychiatry. Presented to seminar on Development of Infants and Parents, Boston. (From: Infant looking and fussing in response to visual stimuli over the first two months of life in different infant-caretaking systems. Presented to Society for Research in Child Development, January 28, 1973, Philadelphia).

43. SUGARMAN, M., 1976: Comments on the Draft of Perinatal Regulations of the Massachusetts Regionalization of Maternity and Newborn Care Project. Unpublished manuscript.

44. SUGARMAN, M., 1977: Testimony for the Public Hearing of the Massachusetts Board of Registration in Medicine, (March 30).

45. SUGARMAN, M., 1977: Perinatal influences on maternal-infant attachment. Amer. J. Orthopsychiat. 47(3): 407-421.

46. WARD, C. AND WARD, F., 1976: The Home Birth Book. Inscape Publishers, Washington, D.C.

47. YANOVER, M. ET AL, 1976: Perinatal care of low-risk mothers and infants: early discharge with home care. New England J. Med. 294(13): 702-705.

### A Fence or an Ambulance

"Twas a dangerous cliff, as they freely confessed,
Though to walk near its crest was so pleasant;
But over its terrible edge there had slipped
A duke and full many a peasant.
So the people said something would have to be done,
But their projects did not at all tally:
Some said, "Put a fence around the edge of the cliff,"
Some, "An ambulance down in the valley."
But the cry for the ambulance carried the day,
For it spread through the neighboring city;
A fence may be useful or not, it is true,
But each heart became brimful of pity
For those who slipped over the dangerous cliff:
And the dwellers in highway and alley
Gave pounds and pence not to put up a fence,
But an ambulance down in the valley.
"For the cliff is all right, if you're careful,"
they said, "And if folks even slip and are dropping,
It isn't the slipping that hurts them so much,
As the shock down below when they're stopping."
So day after day, as these mishaps occurred,
Quick forth would these rescuers sally
To pick up the victims who fell off the cliff,
With their ambulance down in the valley.
Then an old sage remarked: "It's a marvel to me
That people give far more attention
To repairing results than to stopping the cause,
When they'd much better aim at prevention.
Let us stop at its source all this mischief," cried he,
"Come, neighbors and friends, let us rally;
If the cliff we will fence we might also dispense
With the ambulance down in the valley."

                                        Joseph Malins

Copied from
Wildwood Sanitarium and Hospital brochure
Wildwood, GA

# ICEA

NOTE: The International Childbirth Education Association (ICEA) has a new publication entitled, Position Paper on Planning Comprehensive Maternal and Newborn Services for the Childbearing Year. It has adopted a position of favoring a maternity program that offers alternatives both within and outside of the hospital – including free-standing birth centers and home birth services under the direction of certified nurse-midwives or physicians. The publication is 15 pages long and quite thorough in its recommendations. If you would like copies of this excellent position paper to distribute to your local Health Department, hospital, or Health Systems Agency, write to: ICEA, P.O. Box 20852, Milwaukee, WI 53220.

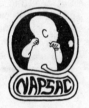

# CHAPTER TEN

## ANALYSIS & CRITIQUE OF A REGIONALIZATION PROPOSAL FOR MASSACHUSETTS WITH RECOMMENDATIONS FOR ALTERNATIVES

Susan M. Basham, M.S., Judith Dickson Luce, Judy Norsigian, Robbi Pfeufer, Muriel Sugarman, M.D., and Norma Swenson, M.P.H.

### Postscript May 1978

While this paper refers primarily to plans for regulations incorporating Regionalization of Maternity and Newborn services in Massachusetts, the model follows the national document (74) so closely that it serves as both a general critique of regionalization and a model for criticism of many state plans. New regulations in Massachusetts have yet to be promulgated, but the Health Systems plan does call for establishment of an out-of-hospital birth center in HSA IV.

### Abstract

This paper summarizes the intent of the current proposed revision of the Mass. D.P.H. maternity and newborn regulations, and analyzes data which supports and does not support their implementation. A re-conceptualization of maternity services follows, emphasizing provisions for a wide variety of low cost service delivery models for the majority of women. The report closes with an analysis of the Mass. Regionalization plan as an outmoded expression of health planning philosophy, a plan which ignores both consumer demand and consumer input in the planning process. A statement of consumer standards for optimum maternity care in the Commonwealth is included.

Susan M. Basham, M.A., is on the Board of Directors, HSA, IV, Massachusetts, Co-Director of Birth Day, and MBA candidate in Health Care, Boston University.

Judith Dickson Luce is a member of Birth Day, member of ICEA Task Force on Regionalization, a birth attendant, woman, and mother of three.

Judy Norsigian is on the Board of Directors, HSA, IV, Massachusetts, Board member, National Women's Health Network, and co-author of book, "Our Bodies, Ourselves."

Robbi Pfeufer is a member of HSA, IV, a childbirth educator, an MA and MPH candidate at Boston Univ., and author of several articles on Regionalization.

Muriel Sugarman, M.D., is former chair person of the ICEA Task Force on Regionalization, author of several articles on Regionalization and other topics, and a faculty member at Harvard University.

Norma Swenson, M.P.H., is former president of ICEA, Co-author of book, "Our Bodies, Ourselves," and alternate member of MA-SHCC, HSA, IV.

## Summary

The present proposed complete revision of hospital regulations for maternity and newborn services in the Commonwealth specifies planning for regionalization of specialized care and intensive care services for high risk mothers and infants, two to five percent of the population. Although not specified, these regulations and the regionalization plan also apply to low-risk mothers and infants, the majority of the childbearing population. In addition, the regulations indirectly affect all non-childbearing hospital users and health consumers in the Commonwealth, virtually the entire population. The regulations thus represent broad social policy as well as technical medical standards for all obstetric and newborn care.

Analysis of the regulations reveals that there are insufficient data to support either the cost-effectiveness or quality-effectiveness of the plan, as follows: (1) There is insufficient cost or quality information to justify the minimum size maternity unit criterion on which the planning is so largely based; (2) There is inadequate, inappropriate and outdated information on costs of implementing the entire regionalization plan, and the perinatal centers in particular; (3) the equity of imposing these implied costs on all taxpayers and consumers has not been addressed; (4) The conceptualization of a high-technology, crisis-intervention model of routine medical care, - on which the plan and the regulations are based - runs counter to fundamental considerations widely recognized to be optimum in the care of all pregnant women, e.g., primary care, preventive care, and outreach, ideally neighborhood based; (5) There is no mention of safeguards to ensure that informed consent is obtained for all procedures in all units; (6) The mental health and cultural needs of the high-risk group in particular and the childbearing population in general have not been addressed; (7) Consumer demand, as expressed by the choices of child-bearing women in Massachusetts and other states, and provider innovation, as demonstrated in a wide variety of settings by a range of personnel in many other states, is not acknowledged. Documentation in support of these 7 points is contained in the 75 references cited in the bibliography.

Recommendations which would provide for a wide variety of appropriately supervised, more cost-effective, community-based alternatives, geared for the majority of low-risk women, are included, allowing for the flexible utilization of existing hospital maternity units as desired.

The regionalization plan is placed in the context of the development of health planning philosophy generally, and critiqued for its failure to keep pace with current concepts. The process by which the regulations and the regionalization project in Massachusetts has been developed is chronicled, with particular reference to federally mandated consumer participation in health planning, and the history of citizen participation in the state regulatory process, noting the virtual absence of any but token consumer input during all phases of these processes. The report concludes with a statement of consumer standards for optimum maternity care for all women.

## I. Introduction

The Commonwealth of Massachusetts is now considering new Perinatal Regulations which would create a regionalized system of hospital, maternity and newborn services. These proposed regulations, if adopted, would be binding on all present and future maternity units, establishing certain standards for the operation of such units. The regulations include:

1. Minimum size for a maternity unit as determined by the number of deliveries annually at a fixed occupancy rate.

2. Capability for certain types of emergency care and for recognition and transfer of infants in need of special care.

3. Establishment of specialized regional perinatal centers for delivery of mothers at risk and for intensive care of newborns in difficulty.

4. Establishment of teaching and consultative linkages between existing units to enable all units to meet standards maintained by the regional perinatal centers.

The concept of regionalization of maternity and newborn hospital care, as described in the national report "Toward Improving the Outcome of Pregnancy" (74), has as its major goals:

1. The more effective reduction of infant and maternity morbidity and mortality.

2. The more efficient utilization of resources, to be achieved by concentrating expensive technology and specially trained personnel in regional perinatal centers serving a wide geographic area.

3. Savings in overall hospital costs by the planned reduction of maternity beds through consolidation of existing maternity units.

The Perinatal Regulations presently proposed deal with the implementation of these goals based on the following sources of data:

1. The above mentioned national report, "Towards Improving the Outcome of Pregnancy" (74), developed by a committee of physician planners.

2. A Massachusetts study of maternity facilities, their utilization patterns and their infant and maternal outcomes (22), co-sponsored by the DPH Division of Standards (funded by the Regional Medical Program) in conjunction with the former CHP "b" agency, the Health Planning Council of Greater Boston, now the designated HSA for Region IV.

3. Previously existing DPH regulations pertaining to obstetric and newborn facilities.

These proposed Perinatal Regulations, while focused primarily on the relatively small percentage of mothers and infants (currently 2-5 percent) who are in need of special care, also represent planning for all childbearing families, the vast majority of whom will be having normal, uncomplicated births. In addition, it also is assumed that these perinatal regulations are designed to ensure maximum cost savings and cost effectiveness in hospital facilities planning generally. Maternity units have consistently been among hospital units operating at great losses, which are then passed on and absorbed in the form of higher rates for the hospital as a whole. In this sense, the regionalization plan that would be implemented by these Perinatal Regulations is a policy which affects all citizens of the Commonwealth who use or might use hospitals for other types of care besides maternity care.

The data gathered in the Massachusetts study and the data supporting the national report, which has been the basis for the proposed Perinatal Regulations, show the need for the following:

1. Better capability in recognition and transfer of neonates in difficulty.

2. Better capability in treating these infants once their difficulty has been recognized. Also:

3. The cost savings in concentrating rather than duplicating expensive equipment and personnel required by perinatal centers is widely recognized.

4. Falling birth rates, as well as a surplus of maternity beds in general, clearly warrant the need for reduction in maternity beds and maternity units.

These aforementioned needs will be met by the proposed Perinatal Regulations, and it is generally accepted that they should be met. However, there is no data to support other features of the Regulations and there are other needs not addressed by the Regulations at all. Furthermore, the Regulations would implement a regionalization plan that was originally conceived under the earliest concepts of health planning (PL 89-749 - the CHP legislation), a plan that would not be fully consistent with certain HSA goals as mandated by PL-641. Therefore, it must be asked whether or not the regionalization of maternity and newborn care, as it would be implemented by these proposed Regulations, is the best way to achieve the stated goals. As a social policy, does it meet the requirements of far-reaching, broad-based community involvement?

## II. Limitations and Possible Consequences
### of the Proposed Perinatal Regulations

There has been little consideration of the limitations and possible consequences of the proposed Perinatal Regulations, especially in the following areas:

### A. Size Criterion

Amendments to the Standards and Criteria for Acute Care Beds in Massachusetts, discussed at the public hearing of May 3, 1976, suggest a minimum of 1000 deliveries per year for existing maternity units and of 1500 deliveries per year for new or expanding units. This standard is based upon the assumption that fewer, bigger maternity units will both improve quality of care and reduce costs. However, such an assumption does not appear to be well founded in light of the following:

1. Quality Considerations:

A. "The highest mortality rates (ed. note: in Mass.)are among the small percentage of infants — 7 to 8 percent — who weigh less than 2500 grams at birth. For these high-risk infants, particularly for the smallest ones (many of whom may be screened prenatally), there is indeed some evidence that bigger, more sophisticated maternity units do contribute to better outcomes." (15) "In terms of quality, at least as measured by neonatal mortality, the principle differences between big and small units show up in the outcomes of very small babies — the 2½ to 3 percent that weigh less than 2000 grams at birth — and in the records of the smallest units, those with fewer than 500 deliveries per year. Inasmuch as a large fraction of the prematures can be spotted early in pregnancy (and handled specially as high risk situations) one must question the qualitative impact of a 1000 - to - 1500 delivery minimum criterion." (15)

b. "For the large majority of full-term infants, however, the evidence of unit size: outcome relationship is far more difficult to see, except for the very smallest of the maternity units." (15)

2. Cost Considerations

a. "Unfortunately, few proper studies of the economics of hospital maternity units exist. Thus, in establishing public standards for the size and utilization of maternity units, the regulatory body needs to make a fresh inquiry into the relationship between cost — total and per unit — and different levels of activity. Moreover, inasmuch as the ratio of high-risk and-or complicated deliveries to the total of all deliveries will vary from hospital to hospital, it is important to adjust the cost figures to reflect differences in the work performed by the maternity units. (Adequate techniques exist for performing this type of adjustment)." (15)

b. "While there may be economies of scale over some range of maternity-unit activity, it is not at all clear where such economies of scale begin (if at all) and where they end. Correspondingly, there may or may not be diseconomies of scale; some units may be too large for efficient economic operation. This possibility does not seem to have been considered at all in terms of the Determination of Need regulatory framework. In the absence of any direct cost and case mix study of Massachusetts hospitals (of the type outlined above), the Comprehensive Health Planning A-B Task Force seems to rely heavily upon the findings of the Regionalization Task Force that: "A Minimum of 1000 deliveries per year would be necessary for the maternity service to meet all its costs with its own revenue." (15)

c. "If this conclusion is to be used as a basis for regulatory standard setting, it should be noted that it is somewhat misleading in two important respects: (a) it is not based upon any analysis of actual costs, but instead it uses a hypothetical estimate of the running costs of a so-called Level I maternity unit; it should be noted that only one Level I facility, on Martha's Vineyard, has been proposed for Massachusetts; and (b), it used an $800 average price figure as a basis for calculating a break even operating level. If the average price that is charged for a delivery is lower than its actual cost, i.e., if maternity services are priced at a subsidy level, then, by definition, more deliveries will be necessary to defray any fixed level of maternity costs. Hence, while there may be some valid social justification for subsidizing the price of maternity services, it is economic cost — rather than the subsidy price — that must be used to calculate the efficient scale of operations. In a similar vein, while the 1970 ACOG National Study of Maternity Care shows more intensive use of certain facilities (delivery rooms, labor rooms, etc.) in bigger units, the report is entirely silent in terms of the cost of more intensive operation." (15)

In another study, Fieck (54) of the N.Y. State Department of Health also showed that the size criterion was not a valid basis for maternity facilities planning.

B. Technological Impact

"It is frequently argued that new technologically sophisticated services are desirable, but they require a cadre of specialized personnel and a large pool of patients to prove feasible economically. Dr. George Ryan makes this point as follows:

It will be increasingly difficult for the smaller volume obstetric service to provide services, facilities, and personnel for application of the development I have outlined, not to mention future developments. Costs will be prohibitive, and the scarce, highly trained medical personnel will be unavailable in many instances. If, as predicted, the maternal high-risk center with intensive care delivery units becomes the expected standard for delivery of maternity care in hospitals, a legal element is introduced. When you speak of an expected standard, you imply a responsibility of institutions or physicians for unsatisfactory outcomes when the standards are not met (31).

Regulations which mandate a minimum size maternity unit are likely to have the indirect effect of encouraging the proliferation of sophisticated services. Whether this is or is not desirable depends upon the scientific evidence adduced on behalf of these technologies as well as upon the costs and benefits of alternative programs. Regulatory bodies should be aware that professional opinion divides on the issue of technology. There is, for example, a recent prospective, randomized study of electronic fetal monitoring that raises important questions about the benefits of some of the newest techniques and also points to the high incidence of cesarean section (3-fold rate increase) that is associated with this monitoring (12). Cesarean sections in turn, have maternal mortality rates significantly higher than normal deliveries, 80:100,000 vs. 27:100,000 in PAS hospitals. Furthermore, infection rates are also dramatically increased by monitoring, in both mother and baby. Many babies so infected contract meningitis as a result, and of this group, half die.

A recent retrospective study of approximately 17,000 women also challenged the efficacy of monitoring, especially for low-risk women (76). To summarize in the words of Dr. Raymond Neutra:

> A large fraction of women who deliver at term without any demonstrable risk factors (e.g., prematurity, breech presentation, etc.) have an average neonatal death risk of 1 in a 1000. Therefore, the maximum benefit which monitoring would provide in this group would be 1 life saved for every 1000 babies monitored. In order to do a randomized trial on this group, it would take over 100,000 monitored women and over 100,000 nonmonitored women to demonstrate such a benefit for low-risk women. (May 1978)

## C. Cost

"Another consequence of the proposed regulation which has not been fully recognized is the cost of developing a regionalized system. Apart from any capital costs which may flow from the consolidation or expansion of certain units, there are undoubtedly significant operating expenses that are entailed. The very process of coordination will require staffing support as well as transportation, education, and other backup systems. To our knowledge, no estimate of the additional costs implied by the proposed system have been made; thus, there is no real way of balancing the costs and benefits of the existing system against those proposed for the future."

## D. Equity

"Who will bear the financial burden of the additional costs imposed by the regulations? If the average cost per delivery increases as a consequence of these regulations, it may be passed on to users and non-users of maternity services alike. Hence, a decision at the DON level is really a decision concerning social costs and financing — and just like a tax, its incidence and overall impact should be clearly assessed." (15)

### E. Mental Health of the High Risk-Crisis Group

1. Personnel: The present plan omits mental health professionals from the health care team and from the committees which review hospital maternal and newborn services. This omission compromises the care of high-risk patients and families who may already be in a major or minor medical crisis and who, without consultation from mental health professionals may suffer further psychological consequences. In addition, this lack mirrors a shortcoming in health services well documented by the CHP agencies several years ago.

The present plan also neglects to provide foreign-speaking personnel on all service shifts, an oversight which, with the apparent equation between high-risk and low-income, and between low-income and non-English-speaking populations, most affects the high-risk group.

2. Procedures: The regulations do not minimize separation of family members during the course of hospitalization. For example, transfer of babies to a high-risk center does not include provisions for transfer of mothers, a situation which is most likely to affect the high-risk family, and which has known hazards, including possible long-term effects on the mental health of families.

### F. Informed Consent

Because of the risks attached to an increasing number of obstetrical medications and procedures (3,4,5,7,12,34,35,36,45,46,47,50,51,52,53,56,59,62,71) it is now more crucial than ever that childbearing women be able to provide their truly informed consent, that they have full knowledge of the positive and negative consequences of all medical interventions being proposed to them, as well as the estimated effects if there is no intervention. It is a serious omission that the Perinatal Regulations do not include specific mention of informed consent.

Informed consent is vital not only for health consumers but for providers as well. In a recent study of malpractice suits in California, it was found that most cases involved the complaint that a procedure was performed or medication given without the informed consent of the parturient woman (36). These findings do not support the frequent contention of many physicians that failure to perform certain medical practices would result in an increasing number of malpractice suits (though such malpractice suits do occur, they by no means represent the greatest proportion, as has been suggested).

### G. Primary-Preventive Features

Though it has been well documented that thorough prenatal care, including sound nutritional counseling (30) and the use of rigorous screening techniques (13,41) represents a highly effective approach to reducing maternal and infant mortality and morbidity, the proposed Perinatal Regulations (22,39) concentrate instead on crisis intervention. The adoption of such regulations only serves to further de-emphasize the fact that most maternity care is basically primary care. In the words of Dr. Phillip Lee, current director of the Health Policy Program at the University of California School of Medicine (San Francisco), while commenting on how a number of recent critics have been relating current problems in U.S. health care delivery more specifically to maternity care:

> Why is it that we have emphasized hospital-based maternity care, increasingly in university medical centers which are tertiary care institutions, when 80 - 90 percent of all maternity care is, in fact, primary

care? (from remarks made at the dedication ceremony for the Maternity Center Association Childbearing Center, New York, N.Y., Oct. 9, 1975).

As an example of effective prevention, we note that since a program of nutrition counseling was adopted in 1970 at Cambridge Hospital, there has been a 50 percent drop in the prematurity rate. (Prematurity and low birth weight are a major cause of infant mortality and morbidity).

The best examples of strong preventive approaches to maternity care are represented by many of the midwife-staffed birth centers (both free-standing and hospital-based) and the home birth programs with medical backup scattered around the country. Since all of these have reduced costs and since none have shown any increase in maternal and infant morbidity and mortality, in fact, several have reduced maternal and infant morbidity and mortality (32), it would seem appropriate to build into any regionalization plan mechanisms for the monitored growth and development of such options.

Moreover, it is well known that the population which shows the highest rates for neonatal and infant mortality is among that group which comes into delivery without any prenatal care whatsoever, and that these rates decline as prenatal care is received earlier and earlier in the pregnancy. Any proposed program which intends to improve the outcome of pregnancy cannot deal simply with the women who voluntarily present themselves for care. In order to improve the infant mortality rate in Massachusetts, as elsewhere, programs of outreach must be developed, so that those who are not presenting themselves for care, or are presenting themselves late, will be reached, involved, watched earlier and cared for. Such programs should include provisions for child care, transportation problems, language barriers, cultural differences and similar problems. Whenever possible, neighborhood prenatal care should be made available.

### H. Impact on Alternatives

For the majority of childbearing women the regulations make no real accomodation. Although the Regulations (22) assert "these systems (of perinatal care) provide an integrated and coordinated network of different levels of maternity and newborn care which are accessible to patients and appropriate to their needs," the Regulations do not bear out this assertion. Except for hospitals in geographically isolated areas the present plan does not put forth a developed model of low-risk care, thus restricting options for the bulk of the maternity population both within and among institutions.

Implied in the lack of a specific model for low-risk care is routinization of care based on the high-risk model, with the possible iatrogenic effects of needless medical intervention in a normal physiologic process. Provisions are lacking to keep families together. For example, there is routine separation of parents and infants for 24 hours following birth. There is no provision for early discharge, although this would represent a cost benefit (39,40,43,69).

"Regulatory bodies should consider the impact of these regulations on the development of nontraditional maternity units such as out-of-hospital birth centers, short stay units, and supervised home births. Surely, to the extent that (1) more high risk expectant mothers are identified during their pregnancies; (2) better prenatal care is extended to all mothers; and (3) the risk factors external to medical care itself (including socioeconomic factors) are improved, it should be possible to orient the childbirth process away from the medical model rather than increasingly towards it. Accordingly, it would be unfortunate to discourage or bar the development of more extensive out-of-hospital or lower-intensity services for low risk mothers by virtue of these regulations." (15)

## I. Consumer Demand

Increasingly, there is consumer demand for alternatives to hospital-based, physician-attended birth (32). In Massachusetts, since nurse-midwifery is legal only in facilities licensed by the Department of Public Health, and since there are no free-standing birth centers, parents have few options. If they do not wish to be in a hospital, then they must stay in the home. Currently, it is estimated that between 1 percent (Dr. George Ryan) and 3 percent (recent newspaper article) of Massachusetts births occur at home.

In other parts of the country, where options for out-of-hospital birth have been made available, parents have been seeking them out in increasing numbers (32,38,63). Currently, there are about five free-standing birth centers where delivery is attended primarily by nurse-midwives. They are found in places like Cliffside, N.J.; Albuquerque, N.M.; Raymondville, TX; Eugene, OR, and New York, N.Y. Some of these are booked up months in advance. For example, at Birth Center Lucinia, in Eugene, OR, where there are about 20 planned births per month (one nurse midwife and 2 nurses staff the center with obstetrical backup), the schedule is booked up through July 1977. In California, where there are a number of homebirth programs with hospital backup, it has been estimated by the State Department of Health that in some counties 15 percent of all births in 1975 occurred in the home. (Editor's note: as of October 1978, there are between 40 and 50 free standing birth centers in the U.S. and many others planned.)

Parents seek these alternatives to hospital birth not only for the type of care offered but also for economic reasons. At Birth Center Lucinia the total cost of all prenatal, intrapartum and postpartum care for both mother and baby is $550. This includes childbirth classes, nutrition counseling, prenatal exams, care during delivery (assuming no complications requiring hospitalization), and five postpartum visits which include all the immunization shots for the baby. Homecoming, a homebirth program in San Francisco, charges $450. for prenatal, intrapartum and postpartum care (this is midwifery-attended).

As new studies (8,23,24,32) further document the safety of these birth centers and homebirth programs with hospital backup, more parents seek such options. It is important that they be made available.

## III. Recommendations

In light of the foregoing documentation, we propose that no regulations be promulgated which close off options and alternatives for the service delivery models both more appropriate and more cost effective for the vast majority of low-risk childbearing parents. Therefore, we propose that:

1. The minimum size criterion be dropped.

2. That Massachusetts establish Level I hospitals, apart from the geographic isolation requirement, but otherwise in accordance with Level I criteria as specified in the national document, with appropriate linkages as specified in the Massachusetts proposed regulations. Such operation would specify rigid screening criteria for low risk women, and major utilization of nurse-midwives with physicians in consultant role on call. Technological capability would not be expanded beyond basic ER resources.

3. That Massachusetts hospitals which would like to maintain their maternity units be given the option of doing so, in conjunction with input from their local citizens, consumers, and service area clientele, and the Department of Public Health, according to two alternatives.

a. Operation as Level I Hospitals as above.

b. Operation as Pilot Project birth centers, with nurse-midwives providing basic care, including delivery, in consultation with physician on call, in accordance with standards established principles of geographic centering and the concentration rather than the duplication of specialized expensive, intensive care units, equipment and personnel. First conceived in conjunction with the Regional Medical Program (R.M.P.) Regionalization was based on certain assumptions, such as:

1. The nature of the illness being treated, e.g., heart disease, cancer, and stroke, represent an acute care crisis which implies the need for massive, emergency tertiary care for which no short-range preventive programs yet existed. Only specialists are presumed to be qualified to treat such conditions.

2. The population involved is primarily a population suffering a pathological condition of long-developed etiology which may be ameliorated by intensive care but which can rarely be completely cured.

Later in the development of health planning concepts the term Regionalization came to be applied more generally to programs of consolidation of beds and geographic centering of specialized units, largely under the impetus of academic-based specialty medicine. Intensive evaluation of all federal health planning programs during '73-'74 revealed a variety of serious shortcomings as well as important strengths. These can be summarized as follows:

1. Health planning represents an important mechanism for reducing capital expenditures, and therefore, overall health care costs, and should be strengthened.

2. The reorganization, limitation and consolidation of tertiary care facilities, while important, is only a first step in the overall development of health planning, particularly the development of area-wide long-range health plans which emphasize ambulatory-primary care preventive programs and health education.

3. Health planning bodies are, overall, probably less well equipped to carry out regulatory functions than legally constituted bodies traditionally are, (such as state departments of public health) and such functions represent a diversion of energy from the main planning efforts, which should include coordination with consumer and provider groups, and with other federal programs emphasizing cost containment and the reduction of tertiary care utilization, such as HMO, PSRO, etc., as well as the consolidation of RMP, Hill-Burton programs, etc.

While the philosophy of health planning has moved on from facilities planning, as reflected in the current HSA Act, PL 93-641, and in the Forward Plans for Health 76-81 and 77-82, published by HEW, many health planning proposals do not reflect this more advanced sophistication in concepts.

With this condensed summary of changes in health planning as background, the current proposed Regionalization Project in Massachusetts needs to be re-examined from these three points of view.

Changes such as: incorporation of primary-preventive services for a normal population; the systematic effort to reduce the number of high-risk cases; the effort to reduce the utilization of tertiary care facilities as much as possible, particularly by the non-pathological, low-risk population — all these are absent from the Massachusetts plan, clearly marking it as outdated from a progressive health planning point of view. Since pregnancy and childbirth have been established as 85-95 percent primary care (see discussion in earlier section), the total absence of primary care, prevention and outreach features in the mandated segments of the standards is noteworthy. While high-risk perinatal centers are naturally indispensable, so that as many viable infants as possible may be saved, it appears irresponsible not to require the attempt to prevent so many high risk births from occurring, to the maximum extent possible. Emphasis on prenatal screening and preventive services as a feasible approach to reducing high risk births is only emphasized in Level I units, as described in the national document, as follows:

> Since such patients (in geographically isolated areas) do not have ready access to a facility capable of delivering high-risk perinatal care, a strong component of preventive services and early detection of existing or potential problems must be stressed at the Level I unit. Therefore, those services must be a strong force in health education and in the development of interconceptional and antepartum services if the outcome of pregnancy is to be improved.

This language does not appear at all in the Massachusetts proposal, which only intends to allow one Level I unit, one on Martha's Vineyard, to exist. Why are these rigorous standards for prenatal screening and prevention not mandated in all Massachusetts hospitals as a way of reducing some percentage of the high-risk births?

By its failure to mandate screening and preventive services as required only in the Level I criteria in the national level document, by its failure to make prenatal care and outreach major features of its design, and by its failure to provide lower-cost personnel and lower-cost facilities for lower-risk patients, the present proposal both maximizes cost and fails to decrease risk.

In a period of shrinking resources we have to establish priorities and to make certain decisions about whether or not we will emphasize primary preventive measures or crisis medical intervention. Frequently, we cannot do both. For example, if we cannot have both a thorough program of nutrition as well as a fetal monitor for every childbearing woman, what do we do? The former, along with other kinds of preventive prenatal care, has been proven effective in improving pregnancy outcome for both mother and baby, especially among low-income women, who comprise the majority of high-risk women. The latter, which has been of some value in high-risk situations, has not been proven to be of significant value to low risk women, who comprise the great majority of pregnant women. In view of the above, it would be unwise to implement a program using fetal monitors for all low-risk cases, particularly if nutrition programs would suffer as a result.

### B. Regulatory Functions

As previously mentioned, the relationship between health planning and health regulation functions has been examined and questioned by many experts. In the case of Regionalization of Maternity Care, this question can be raised much more specifically, especially in Massachusetts. Lawrence Kirsch writes:

Regulations which pertain to capital development (such as DON) are poorly equipped to deal with the contingencies of program operation. Thus, the regulations, here, attempt to stimulate mergers, consolidations, and closures, and they do not concern themselves too much with subsequent events. How is the public interest served should the unit that ceases to function be far better than the one that receives the monopoly franchise in its service area, courtesy of the DON process? And what if one of the ripple effects of closure, merger or consolidation includes a retrenchment in existing prenatal-postnatal services?

Kirsch is clearly pointing here to two features of the Massachusetts situation: (1) the irrelevance of unit size to quality except where either the baby or the unit is very small; and (2) the importance of preventive and follow-up services for pregnancy outcome, which are not discussed in the Regulations. That the regulations are a poor vehicle to achieve consistent quality of a comprehensive nature seems clear.

## C. Health Planning Process

In light of majority consumer participation as a mandated special characteristic of health planning, and particularly in view of the even more systematic requirements under the new law, approval of the present Regionalization project would be unfortunate. The history of the Massachusetts Regionalization project in this respect is as follows:

Only one of the CHP "b" agencies was involved in the original study of Massachusetts maternity care, and that study only involved the utilization patterns in the "b" agency area. Even that co-sponsorship, however, was disapproved by the agency's consumers, and in the actual conduct of the study only the agency staff was involved, working with the DPH staff.

At the "A" agency level, a Committee on Standards and Guidelines, composed of both consumers and providers, did meet to discuss criteria for maternity and pediatric units in Massachusetts. However, their actual function, when finally carried out, became to approve criteria already established by a task force of "A" - "b" staff and DPH staff, thereby excluding consumer involvement once again. Even so, a number of crucial recommendations affecting these standards were introduced by consumers present at the "A" Standards Committee meetings, such as the vital importance of maintaining effective translators for women in labor. Although the body present accepted these recommendations, they never appeared in the final proposed regulations which emerged from the Task Force, indicating the one-way flow of information between these bodies.

Only two sets of public meetings have ever been held to discuss the Regionalization of Maternity Services in Massachusetts, one in 1972, the other in 1975. Both meetings, sponsored by the HPCGB, were poorly advertised (no notices appeared in any daily paper in the Boston area) and very poorly attended, especially by consumers or any other invited providers and hospital representatives routinely involved in the planning process. No consumer appeared on the platform as an official member of the program on either occasion. Consumer protests, voiced at both meetings by those who did learn of the meeting, were dismissed by providers from the platform. Written objections and commentary on behalf of the consumer, presented to subsequent DPH hearings on proposed amendments to the regulations (preparatory to introduction of the Regionalization regulations for Maternity Services), have not been acknowledged or incorporated into the present proposed regulations in any way.

It has been characteristic of the DPH regulatory process in this Commonwealth that input by the general public is deliberately delayed until the providers have given significant shape to the code, so that no major changes could be made through the public process. Indeed, it has been a source of pride to many members of the DPH staff over the years that this characteristic has been maintained. Yet the new role and authority of the DPH in implementing the health planning component of the overall health management process requires far greater responsiveness to consumer and citizen input than has been characteristic in the past.

One of the key questions for the Public Health Council in the future might be, "To what extent have consumers and citizens been involved in shaping the recommendations before us?" The present Regionalization Regulations, as proposed, will be promulgated in blatant disregard of consumer efforts to improve the quality of maternity care in the Commonwealth.

### References

1. American College of Obstetrics and Gynecology News Bulletin. Rural nurse midwives in Appalachia reduce maternal death rate. May 4, 1972.
2. Boston Association for Childbirth Education Newsletter. July-Aug. 1975.
3. Brody, J. Inducing labor in childbirth: "Pernicious Practice" or safe and convenient benefit..." New York Times. March 10, 1976.
4. Caldeyro-Barcia, R. Some consequences of obstetrical interference. Birth and the Family Journal. Vol. 2, No. 2, Spring 1975.
5. Cetrulo, C., and Freeman, R. Problems and risks of fetal monitoring. In: Risks in the Practice of Modern Obstetrics (ed. S. Aladjem). St. Louis: C.V. Mosby, 1975.
6. Committee on Maternal Nutrition, Food and Nutrition Board, National Research Council. Maternal Nutrition and the Course of Pregnancy. Washington: Natl. Acad. of Sci., 1970.
7. Dunn, P. Obstetric delivery today: For better or for worse? Lancet. Apr. 10, 1976.
8. Epstein, J., et. al. A safe homebirth program that works. In: Safe Alternatives in Childbirth. Proc. of Natl. Assoc. of Parents and Professionals for Safe Alternatives in Childbirth Conference, May 15, 1976, p. 101.
9. Ferris, C. The alternative birth center at Mt. Zion Hospital. Birth and the Family Journal. Vol. 3, No. 3, Fall, 1976.
10. Finger Lakes HSA (exec. comm.). Standards for obstetrical care in Monroe County. Adopted June 22, 1976.
11. Goodman, M. Progress in low-risk normal childbirth care. Birth and the Family Journal. Vol. 3, No. 1, Spring 1976.
12. Haverkamp, A., et. al. The evaluation of continuous fetal heart rate monitoring in high risk pregnancy. Amer. J. Obstet. Gynec., Vol. 125:310-21, June 1, 1976.
13. Hobel, C. et. al. Prenatal and intrapartum high-risk screening. Am. J. Ob. Gyn. Sept. 1, 1973.
14. International Childbirth Education Association News. Maternity care alternatives. Vol. 14, No. 4, Winter 1975-76.
15. Kirsch, L. Letter to Elaine Ullian, Prog. Dir., Office of Health Facilities Level., Mass. Dept. of Public Health. May 12, 1976.

16. Klaus, M., and Kennell, J. Maternal-Infant Bonding. St. Louis: C.V. Mosby, 1976.
17. Knill-Jones, R.I., et. al. Anaesthetic practice and pregnancy. Lancet. Vol. 2, October 25, 1975.
18. Lancet editorial statement. Nov. 1974.
19. Laxova, R., et.al. A clinical service for prenatal diagnosis. Lancet. Vol. 2, Nov. 15, 1975.
20. Lechtig, A., et. al., Effect of moderate malnutrition on the placenta. Am. J. Ob. Gyn. Vol. 123, Sept. 15, 1975.
21. Lesinski, J. Editorial: High-risk pregnancy: Unresolved problems of screening, management, and prognosis. J. Ob. Gyn. Vol. 46, Nov. 1975.
22. Massachusetts Department of Public Health Regionalization of Maternity and Newborn Care Project. Perinatal regulations (draft).
23. Mehl, L. Home delivery research today: a review. Women and Health. Vol. 2, No. 1, 1977.
24. Mehl, L., et. al. Outcomes of early discharge after normal birth. Birth and the Family Journal, Vol. 3, No. 3, Fall 1976.
25. National Association for Mental Health. Primary prevention of mental disorders with emphasis in prenatal and perinatal periods: Action guidelines. Arlington, Va.: NAMH, 1800 N. Kent S.T.
26. Pennsylvania Department of Public Health. Preliminary study on the quantity and quality of maternal care in Pennsylvania with emphasis on the perspective of the consumer. Sept. 1976.
27. Pettigrew, A. Letter from the Massachusetts Maternity and Newborn Project.
28. Pfeufer, R. Communities, community hospitals, and regionalization of maternity care. Unpublished ms., 1975.
29. Pollner, F. "Homelike Delivery" center opens amid controversy. Ob. Gyn. News. Nov. 1, 1975.
30. Rush, D., et. al., Dietary services during pregnancy and birthweight: a retrospective matched pair analysis. Pediatric Research. Vol. 10, No. 4, April 1976.
31. Ryan, G. Improving pregnancy outcome via regionalization of prenatal care. JOGN Nursing. Vol. 3, No. 4, July-Aug. 1974.
32. Safe Alternatives in Childbirth. Proc. of Natl. Assoc. of Parent and Professionals for Safe Alternatives in Childbirth Conference, May 15, 1976. Arlington, Va.
33. Shaw, N. Forced Labor: Maternity Care in the U.S. New York: Pergamon Press, 1975.
34. Shearer, M. Fetal monitoring: Do the benefits outweigh the drawbacks? Birth and the Family Journal. Vol. 1, No. 1.
35. Shearer, M., Some deterrents to objective evaluation of fetal monitors. Birth and the Family Journal. Vol. 2, No. 2, Spring 1975.
36. Shearer, M., et. al., A survey of California OB-GYN malpractice verdicts in 1975 with recommendations for expediting informed consent. Birth and the Family Journal. Vol. 3, No. 2, Summer 1976.
37. Slome, C., et. al. Effectiveness of certified nurse-midwives — prospective evaluation study. Am. J. Ob. Gyn. Vol. 2. Jan. 15, 1976.
38. Special Delivery. News from Maternity Center Association. Vol. VI, No. 2, Autumn 1975.
39. Sugarman, M. Comments on the draft of "Perinatal Regulations." Sent to Massachusetts Department of Public Health Regionalization of Maternity and Newborn Care Project. Dec. 1976.

40. Sumner, P. Six years experience of prepared childbirth in a home-like labor-delivery room. Birth and the Family Journal. Vol. 3, No. 2, Summer 1976.
41. Walker, J. Prognostic value of antenatal screening. Am. J. Ob. Gyn. Vol. 1, Jan. 1, 1976.
42. Wennberg, J. Obstetric practices in Vermont. Unpublished ms.
43. Yanover, M.J., et. al. Perinatal care of low-risk mothers and infants: Early discharge with home care. NEJM. Vol. 294, 1976.
44. ACOG Task Force on Regional Planning and Health Systems Agencies. Statement on maternal health policy sent to Health Systems Agencies in the U.S. 1978.
45. Aleksandrowicz, M.K., "The Effects of Pain Relieving Drugs Administered During Labor and Delivery on the Behavior of the Newborn: A Review," Merrill-Palmer Quarterly, 20, 121-141, 1975.
46. Banta, H.D., "How Do we Deal with Technologies?" Public Health Notes, published by Public Health Association of New York City, Vol. 11, No. 29, Nov. 1976, p. 6.
47. Bonnar, J., "Selective Induction of Labor," British Med. Journal, 1, 651-52, 1976.
48. Boston Women's Health Book Collective. Appendix on regionalization to Chapter 18, "Women and Health Care," Our Bodies, Ourselves, Simon & Schuster, 368-70, 1976.
49. Browne, H.E., and Isaacs, G., "The Frontier Nursing Service: The primary care nurse in the community hospital," Am. J. Obstet. Gynecol., Jan. 1, 1976, Vol. 124, No. 1, p. 16.
50. Chalmers, I., "British Debate on Obstetric Practice," Pediatrics, Vol. 58:3, Sept., 1976, p. 308-11.
51. Chalmers, I., et al., "Obstetric Practice and Outcome of Pregnancy in Cardiff Residents 1965-73," British Med. J., pp. 735-738, 1976.
52. Chard, T., and Richards, R., eds., Benefits and Hazards of the New Obstetrics, Lippincott Co., 1977.
53. Cole, R.A., et al., "Elective Induction of Labor. A Randomized Prospective Trial," Lancet, 1:767-770.
54. Fleck, Andrew C., Jr., N.Y. State Dept. of Health, "Hospital Size and Outcomes of Pregnancy," unpublished paper, Feb. 1977.
55. Gabel, Harold D., "Alternative Birth Centers: Fact or Fantasy?" Virginia Medical, Nov. 1977.
56. Hack, M., et al., "Neonatal Respiratory Distress Following Elective Delivery. A Preventable Disease?" Amer. J. Ob. Gyn., 126, 43-47, 1976.
57. Haverkamp, A.D., "The Evaluation of Continuous Fetal Heart Rate Monitoring in High-Risk Pregnancy," Amer. J. Ob. Gyn., 125, 310-317, 1976.
58. "Increased Monitoring Conflicts with pressure for Homelike Atmosphere in Labor Suite," Ob. Gyn. News, Vol. 12, No. 4, Feb. 15, 1977, p. 31.
59. Kessner, David M., et al., Infant Death: An Analysis by Maternal Risk and Health Care. Washington, D.C.: National Academy of Sciences, 1973. (Two volumes.)
60. Kitzinger, S., and Davis, J.A., eds., The Place of Birth, Oxford University Press, 1978.
61. Kroener, W.F., "Changing Trends in Caesarian Section," Amer. J. Ob. Gyn., 125, 803-804, 1976.
62. Liston, W.A., and Campbell, A.J., "Dangers of oxytocin-induced Labour to Fetuses," British Medical Journal, 3: 606-607, 1974.
63. Lubic, Ruth W., "Comprehensive Maternity Care as an Ambulatory Service — Maternity Center Association's Birth Alternative," The J. of the N.Y. State Nurses Assoc., V. 8, No. 4, Dec. 1977.

64. Maternity Center Assoc., "Commentary on National Guidelines for Health Planning," Dec. 1977.
65. Neilson, Irene, "Nurse-midwifery in an alternative birth center," Birth Fam. J., 4:1:24, Spring 1977.
66. Rindfuss, Ronald R., and Ladinsky, Judith L., "Patterns of Birth: Implications for the Incidence of Elective Inductions," Medical Care, 14(8): 685-693, Aug. 1976.
67. Pfeufer, R., "For the Common Good of the Commonwealth? Regional Development of Maternity and Newborn Care Services," unpublished paper, Boston, April, 1977.
68. Slome, C., et al., "Effectiveness of Certified Nurse-Midwives," Amer. J. Ob. Gyn., 124, 177-182, 1976.
69. Sugarman, M., "Regionalization of Maternity and Newborn Care: How Can We Make a Good Thing Better?" unpublished manuscript, Boston, Sept. 1977.
70. Supplemental Hearing before the Subcommittee on Health and the Environment of the Committee on Interstate and Foreign Commerce, House of Representatives, Ninety-Fourth Congress, Second Session, on H.R. 12937, 14309, 114822 and 14497, Maternal and Child Health Care Act — 1976, September 13, 1976.
71. Tipton, R.H., and Lewis, B.V., "Induction of Labour and Perinatal Mortality," British Med. J., 1, 391, 1975.
72. Wennberg, J., National Health Forum, unpublished remarks presented in New York City, March 23, 1977 at the National Health Council.
73. Lubic, Ruth. Letter to Norma Swenson from Maternity Center Assoc., NYC, regarding screening criteria for childbearing center.
74. National Committee on Perinatal Health. Toward Improving the Outcome of Pregnancy, first drafted in 1970, later published by National Foundation for March of Dimes, 1976.
75. Pfeufer, R., and Land, D., Scientific, Philosophic, and Humanistic Approaches. Boston Assoc. for Childbirth Education Newsletter, July-August 1975.
76. Neutra, R. et al. The Effect of Fetal Monitoring on Neonatal Death Rates, presented at Am. Public Health Assoc., Washington, DC, Nov. 1977.

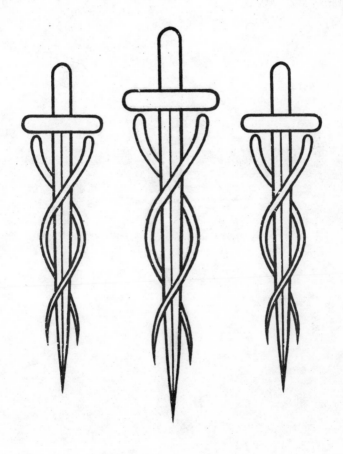

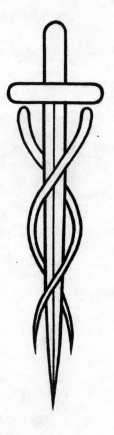

# Obstetric Intervention

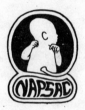

# CHAPTER ELEVEN

## FETAL MONITORING: FOR BETTER OR WORSE?

### By Madeleine H. Shearer, R.P.T.

For those of you who wonder what's next in obstetrical technology, there is a room-sized machine which was patented in the United States in 1963 by a man named Blonsky. For lack of a better name, I call this the obstetrical cyclotron. The woman is strapped in, and across her face is a gas mask. She gets rotated faster and faster until the centripetal force causes the baby to move down the birth canal and fall into a net basket between her legs.

Unlike this machine, which was never heard of again after 1963, electronic fetal monitors are still with us. By electronically picking up the fetal heart rate and pattern, and graphing it on a moving paper tracing, obstetricians hope to identify various components of the pattern which signify fetal distress, and intervene early enough to prevent fetal damage or death.

There is a photograph in the July, 1972, issue of Hospital Practice from Edward Quilligan's department at USC where the first "fetal intensive care" unit was established (1). It is a very typical scene of fetal monitoring: Mother on her back, nurse looking at tracing of the fetal heart. The lower belt has a buckle-like object on it. This is the ultrasound transducer which picks up the fetal heart beats. The upper belt has a strain gauge on it, which records abdominal tightening with each contraction. The paper strip chart has two tracings: the contraction and the fetal heart rate pattern.

### How Fetal Monitors Work

There are actually four ways to pick up the fetal heart rate (FHR) and two ways to record uterine contractions. You see that there are three types of external FHR pick-ups. Phonocardiography simply involves amplifying the sound of the FHR. It is used very little in labor now, because it picked up room noises and so forth and was unsatisfactory. The abdominal fetal electrocardiograph is used mainly in late pregnancy testing. Ultrasound is a third type of transducer. The fourth pick-up is an internal system, in which the electrode is attached directly to the fetus through the dilating cervix. The usual shape of the electrode is a spiral needle screwed into the baby's scalp (see figure 1). With this internal electrode the contractions can be recorded externally or with an internal catheter which is inserted past the fetus into the uterus.

It's almost like watching television to stand in a labor room and watch this monitor. The paper comes out and lies in folds in a drawer of the cabinet upon which the machine is set. A lighted green window up on the left of the monitor has an oscilloscope display of the fetal heart pattern. Then right next to that is the digital display in red, the numbers constantly flickering with each beat of the heart. I stand and watch and think to myself, "How can I possibly question this advanced technological breakthrough in obstetrics?" Just the added in-

Madeleine H. Shearer, R.P.T., is editor of the Birth and Family Journal, an author of many articles in the area of maternal-child health and a recognized authority on fetal monitors.

formation alone must be worth the effort. Each issue of the two major obstetric journals has two or three new research papers on interpretation of the fetal heart tracings.

Monitoring has become almost routine in obstetrics, in only eight years. Yet, during this same period an increasing exodus of parents from hospital obstetrical care has also taken place. Are these events connected? In one study of 111 home birth mothers, the most frequently cited reason for avoiding hospitals was that the baby was taken away after birth. The second most frequently cited negative factor was routine fetal monitoring. Monitor researchers are very angry with such women. In a recent article on monitoring in Patient Care (2), Dr. J.C. Hobbins said he thought women were being selfish and hedonistic to avoid monitoring for a few hours which might affect their child for 70 or 80 years. This is a view that was arrived at without asking women why they avoid monitoring. They are not convinced that monitoring is accurate or safe, and they feel sure that the same quality of care, or better, is available from frequent auscultation of the fetal heart. Growing numbers of doctors agree. Many obstetricians have voiced objections to routine fetal monitoring (36,37). They have been slow to adopt monitoring because they have found that they can detect serious fetal distress by using the traditional stethescope.

At our hospital in Berkeley, until very recently, monitors were seldom used, and the statistics for perinatal mortality were some of the best in the country. This reflected the fact that the hospital serves a population which is 85 percent middle class, professional and academic parents, as well as the fact that the city has attracted excellent obstetricians. Now, however, the hospital administration has announced plans to build a high-risk obstetrical unit and hire a perinatologist and a clinical nurse specialist in monitoring. When I asked some of the obstetricians how the hospital was going to pay for this unit and staff, with so few high-risk women to use it on, I was told that, with 70 percent of obstetrical care being paid for by government and insurance, and national health insurance promising to pay for all of it soon, the hospital can recover the cost of a $6000 monitor with the first 60 - 100 women monitored, simply by billing Medicaid and insurance $60 - $100 for that service separately. Then, revenue from subsequent monitorings and other intensive care tests and procedures (such as routine amniocenteses, serial ultrasound scans, prenatal stress and non-stress tests, and many others) will pay for perinatology staff, clinical nurse specialists, repair and maintenance staff, training and research programs, parent education to accept high-risk care — and the researchers have miles and miles of tracings to do research on.

Hospital obstetrical departments were money-losing places in the mid- to late 1960s. But with routine high-risk care that the government will pay for, large obstetric units have become lucrative. This explains in part some of the uncritical acceptance of monitors in academic obstetrics, and some of the bad temper of obstetrical professors toward criticism of fetal monitors. They remember back to 1968 when OB departments couldn't even replace worn out equipment, and obstetric residencies were going unfilled due to lack of interest — especially by the higher-graded medical graduates (3).

But, until that perinatologist arrives to convert the doctors of Berkeley to routine fetal monitoring, they will continue to believe that they can detect serious fetal distress by using a stethescope. Are they right? Here's the evidence for and against.

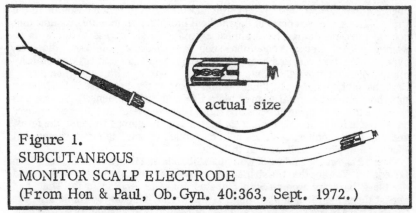

Figure 1.
SUBCUTANEOUS
MONITOR SCALP ELECTRODE
(From Hon & Paul, Ob. Gyn. 40:363, Sept. 1972.)

Editors' Note: The sharp steel helix on the tip of the probe (shown above) is thrust into the vagina, thru the cervix, screwed into the baby's head, and left there throughout labor. The helix is one of several metal devices for breaking the scalp of the newborn. All cause pain, as can be readily attested by any doctor or nurse who has had the misfortune of accidentally pricking themselves while handling one.

### Monitors vs. the Human Ear

Edward Hon, who started Corometrics Fetal Monitors in the late 60s, has published an experiment. It was intended to show that 15 experienced obstetricians listening to a recorded fetal heart rate over a microphone could not give an accurate count (4). Although Hon concluded from this data that obstetricians could not reliably determine fetal heart rates by stethoscope, this interpretation of the data may not be warranted. If you look closely at the range of counts for each of these eight heart rates, you see that these obstetricians were all within 10 - 15 beats of the precise rate, except for the extreme low and high rates. We know that in actual practice, when a doctor or nurse hears a very low or high fetal heart rate, he or she will check it again, and will base a sound clinical judgment on this and the total clinical picture presented by the mother and labor.

Benson (5) in 1968 compared auscultation chart notes with Apgar scores of the babies and found that auscultation failed to predict the infant outcomes except in extreme degrees. However, Haverkamp (6) found that when the fetal heart was auscultated very frequently — every 15 minutes — then the outcomes of 240 auscultated high-risk newborns were the same as those of 240 monitored ones. Haverkamp has since repeated his study with larger monitored and unmonitored groups, and found the same outcomes (7).

Now the question is: so what's the difference? If you can get equal results using two different methods, what's wrong with using the technological one? Hospitals do it all the time — you might even say that they are in the business of providing the most complicated technology possible.

What's wrong is that the cesarean rate has doubled since fetal monitoring has begun, and is now around 20 - 25 percent of all births in urban hospitals in the United States. Many reports in the medical literature on monitoring show that normal laboring women have almost as many fetal distress patterns as do women with high-risk conditions such as premature fetuses, diabetes, hypertension, toxemia, and heart disease (8 9). You and I and Dr. Jarzembsky might conclude from this that something is wrong with fetal monitoring. Perhaps monitors merely label normal heart rates "distress." Perhaps it somehow renders normal women more like high-risk women. There is much evidence that both these guesses are right. However, fetal monitor researchers have concluded from this finding that labor is a dangerous time for the fetus, and that fetal monitoring should not be confined to only high-risk women, but should be applied to all women in labor.

Figure 2 shows the finding of Edington, Sibanda and Beard from St. Mary's in London (8). You see that the striped bars represent normal women in labor, and the black bars are women with diabetes, toxemia, and so forth. They had almost the same rates of alarming FHR patterns, including variable and late decelerations of the heart rate, and loss of beat-to-beat variability — that nice bouncy line between beats on the tracing. Barry Schifrin (10) found that 80 percent of abnormal fetal heart rates using internal monitoring were in fetuses who were not in distress. At first, it was thought that if one checks all abnormal tracings with fetal blood acid-base tests, one could eliminate doubt and keep the cesarean rate down to the truly distressed infants. Beard in this study did manage that, but the only randomized, controlled study in which fetal blood sampling on distress patterns was routine — that of Renou (11) — found that the cesarean rate was still higher due to fetal distress with monitoring. Haverkamp (6, 7) found that there were two and a half times the cesareans in the monitored women as in the non-monitored women, and no differences in outcomes of the fetuses. Keith Russell (12), past president of District 8 of the ACOG, has written in July 1977:

> "Never before in the history of our specialty have so many cesarean sections been performed . . . on the (monitor) indications of 'fetal distress' with the subsequent delivery of essentially normal infants based on Apgar scoring. The universal increase in what may be termed 'unnecessary' cesarean sections has been a concern of even the most vocal proponents of universal intrapartum fetal heart electronic monitoring. Their current posture is that there has been widespread misreading and misinterpretation of fetal heart rate patterns (even while there has been extensive exposition of the various forms of tracings indicating 'fetal distress.')"

Dr. Russell also described several case histories of women dying from sepsis (infection) and fetuses dying from distress after doctors persistently relied on normal monitor tracings rather than on obvious clinical signs of trouble. He cited several lawsuits against hospitals, doctors and monitor companies based on the many fetal distress patterns on tracings which were really not distress at all (13).

Their evaluations of fetal monitoring point up the two big problems with it: inaccuracy and infections to mother and baby. The internal monitor is inaccurate by calling fetal distress not only to real fetal distress patterns, but to normal heart rates as well. In other words, it gives "false positives." This is not a new problem with electronic monitoring.

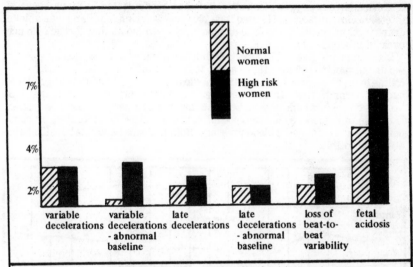

Figure 2.    COMPARISON OF SO CALLED "ABNORMAL" MONITOR TRACINGS BETWEEN NORMAL & HIGH RISK MOTHERS (Adapted from Edington, Sibanda & Beard, Brit. Med. Jour.,Vol. 3, p. 341, 1975)

### Brain Waves from Green Jello

It is possible to get brain waves by inserting electrodes into lime green jello (14). It was shown that electrodes pick up ambient vibrations and electrical potentials to the extent that it is hard to get a brain wave flat enough to declare a person dead, in some cases.

Ultrasound has the opposite problem from internal monitoring; it can make a dying fetus look normal on a monitor tracing. Doppler ultrasound has a unique property of vibrating in just the right frequency at times to make the ominous low fetal heart rates double and to cut in half the very high heart rates so they look normal (15). Most monitor researchers try not to use ultrasound fetal monitoring because of these inaccuracies, but most of all because it can make the tracing bouncy — as if the fetal heart has healthy beat-to-beat variability — when it does not, and when the fetus is actually in grave danger of death. This has been the basis of 4 lawsuits against monitor companies, hospitals and doctors which I have personally heard about.

### Complications of Immobility

Many parents who insist on not being monitored suspect that something about monitoring itself contributes to fetal distress patterns. There is much evidence that they are right. Probably the most well-known cause of fetal distress during labor is the mother's lying supine. Albert Huch of West Germany has developed a transcutaneous oxygen electrode which has been adopted in many neonatal intensive care nurseries. He used it on 200 fetuses during labor and was able to graph what happened to the fetal oxygen level when the mother turned onto her back in labor (16,17).

His results are given in Figure 3. Within two minutes fetal oxygen dropped to the danger point — 12 mm Hg — and it took 10-12 minutes of active therapy — rolling over, blood pressure elevating medication — to get the fetal oxygen level back to normal. This problem becomes extremely serious if the mother has been given epidural anesthesia, because then her sympathetic nervous system is unable to respond to lower blood pressure by vasoconstricting — by compensating and raising the blood pressure. Both maternal and fetal deaths have been due to this.

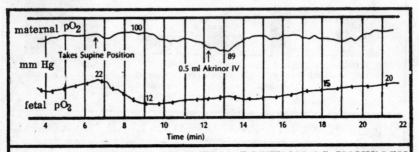

Figure 3.  EFFECT OF SUPINE POSITION AS SHOWN BY MONITOR TRACING. (Reproduced from  Hospital Pract. 11:6, June 1976)

Nurses especially are very aware of this problem, and try to get women to feel free to roll over when they have a monitor on. They offer to reposition the belts and so forth. But every treatise on monitoring admits that especially external monitoring causes the mother to be supine in order to get a good tracing. Even Corometric's patient handout says this. Often I hear that the problem is alleviated by elevating the bed 20 degrees. Many women still suffer pressure on the inferior vena cava to the heart at this angle. Also, this does nothing to help a second cause of lower uterine circulation: direct pressure of the heavy uterus on the lower aorta which serves the uterine artery. Ueland (18) and Caldeyro-Barcia (19) have shown by x-ray studies and volumetric studies that this mechanism does reduce fetal blood supply.

How important is immobility in causing fetal distress? Here is a quote from an article by Lee and Baggish (20):

"The cause of the only case of intrapartum death among the monitored group was a cord accident. On reviewing that case retrospectively the patient's monitor tracing revealed a long strip of unsatisfactory tracing during external monitoring, presumably due to the movements of both the mother and the baby."

Nearly every study of fetal monitoring reports a similar incident during monitoring. These deaths illustrate two points. First, they underscore Saling's finding that external monitoring failed to produce accurate tracings 44-63 percent of the time (21). Second is that intrapartum fetal death is not prevented by monitors; it is prevented by an alert nurse or doctor at the bedside of the laboring woman. Goodlin, who pioneered in monitor research 10 years ago, has said in 1977 that he had given up trying to get the monitor companies to produce an accurate machine. He concluded: (quote)

"One interpretation of our data and those reported elsewhere is that the healthy, term fetus tolerates labor, and although subject to certain accidents such as prolapsed umbilical cord, is not living through a particularly dangerous time period with regard to either death or permanent injury. When fetal accidents such as prolapsed cord or abruptio placentae have occurred on our service, they were diagnosed not by continuous FHR monitoring but by the standard technique of intrapartum surveillance and good nursing care." (22)

A third point is illustrated by that intrapartum fetal death reported by Lee and Baggish: that fetal monitoring has unique factors which can dispose fetuses to cord accidents. These are breaking the bag of waters to attach the scalp electrode to the fetus, and immobility. Gabbe (23) and Caldeyro-Barcia (24) found cord compression patterns with rupture of the membranes, in separate studies. Then some fascinating studies of internal monitoring in which women were able to walk around "radio-ing" the FHR to the monitor showed a virtual absence of cord compression patterns. Flynn and Kelly (25) reported the latest of these telemetry studies. When you realize that fetuses unexpectedly die of cord compression in labor, then when you read a study of cesareans and monitoring by Michael Hughey (26) of Evanston, and see that 43 percent of fetal distress patterns which prompted cesareans were cord compression patterns, then you realize how important mobility is in labor. In at least this way, the ancients knew much more than we: they did not immobilize their laboring women in labor.

## Monitors Increase Infections

I mentioned that infection was a problem with internal monitoring. With the internal system, the intrauterine catheter and fetal scalp electrode are connected by wires to a leg plate on the mother, from which the wires go to the monitor. In all but two studies of intrauterine and wound infection with monitoring, the rates of infection doubled over non-monitored women, ranging from about 3 percent in one study to 65 percent when monitored women had cesareans (27,28).

Figure 1 showed a fetal scalp electrode. It is rotated clockwise into the skin of the fetus through the dilating cervix in labor. Scalp abcesses occurred in 1 in 20-25 monitored newborns in a study by Winkel (29), and again in a study by Okada and Chow (30) last year. These abcesses develop after discharge of an apparently well baby, usually, and they often heal by themselves. However, sometimes they cause permanent bald spots, osteomyelitis, or generalized infection with death. There are also many accidents and injuries. Table 1 shows some of the injuries, accidents and infections from scalp electrodes.

Many expectant parents refuse to be monitored because they are not convinced of the safety of diagnostic ultrasound, which is used in the external monitor. Table 2 lists some of the possible effects. All 5 manufacturers of ultrasound monitors use 10 milliwats per centimeter squared at a frequency of 2 to 2.3 MH (megahertz). In this energy and frequency range we can find a number of animal studies in which alarming tissue changes occurred to adult and fetal animals. Note expecially the last in the list, the study reported last year of Barrett and Anderson (31) of the University of Missouri that 3 and 5 minute exposures to 8.5 mW:cm (2) reduced IgM antibodies in mice. Exposure times in the human in labor are not minutes but hours. The FDA is investigating diagnostic ultrasound at this time.

---

### Neonatal Scalp Complications with Internal Fetal Monitoring

● A scalp rash from the electrode — 85-90% of newborns

● Scalp abcess in 1 out of 20-25 monitorings (Okada & Chow)
- 34.2% contain aerobic bacteria
- 7.9  contain anaerobic strains
- 55.3  both
- 2.6  sterile

● neonatal deaths from infection in scalp wounds
- osteomyelitis
- gonococcal sepsis
- subgaleal abcess
- E. Coli sepsis

● Broken points needing surgical removal
- Placing electrode on fetal eye, genitalia, or in fontanelle
- Piercing meninges of the fetal brain with a stretched electrode
- Traumatic dislodgement of electrode, with neonatal hemorrhage
- Fetal death due to hemorrhage from blood sampling site

Table 1.  INJURIES, ACCIDENTS & INFECTIONS FROM FETAL SCALP ELECTRODES.

---

**What about all those "studies" that show benefits from monitors?**

I will close now with a brief discussion of the many studies published in the obstetric literature which attempt to evaluate the effect of fetal monitoring on perinatal mortality. All but 4 of these studies are from hospitals in which a period from the late 1960s before monitoring was compared to a period in the mid 1970s when monitoring was routine. With two exceptions — Stenchever's

(9) first and Shenker's (32) first studies — these show a reduction of perinatal mortality between these two periods, and the authors, who are obstetric department heads, claim that fetal monitoring reduced perinatal mortality. The fact is that perinatal mortality has dropped in these periods quite independent of any obstetric factors.

Two very nice studies illustrate this point. Jack Wennberg (33) studied perinatal mortality in Vermont among hospitals which use monitoring and those which do not. The mortality rate as a whole had dropped each year to a total of about 30 percent from 1968 to 1974, and the drop was identical among the institutions, regardless of monitoring. Iain Chalmers (34) studied perinatal mortality in Cardiff, Wales over a ten-year period ending in 1974, and found that it had fallen in this period. However, when hospitals which used liberal induction, advanced tests and sonograms and monitoring were compared with hospitals which used traditional methods, no difference was found in either the causes or rates of perinatal mortality.

### 1967-76 Experimental Effects of Ultrasound in Diagnostic Ranges (<10 mW/cm$^2$)

| Author | effect | Ultrasound intensity | exposure time |
|---|---|---|---|
| Macintosh et al | chromosome damage (in vitro) | 10 mW/cm$^2$ | 2 hours |
| Galperin-Lemaitre | breakdown of DNA (in vitro) | 200 | 2 & 5 min |
| Dyson et al | circulatory stasis (primates) | 20 | |
| Kremkau & Witcofsky | liver cell changes (mice) | 10 | |
| Tsutsumi et al | brain enzyme changes (dogs) | 1.5 | 3 min |
| Hu & Ulrich | EEG changes (primates) | 1.5 | 3 min |
| Murai et al | delayed reflexes and emotional reactivity (rats) | 2 | 5 hours |
| Sikov et al | delayed neuromuscular development (rats) | 10 | |
| Barrett & Anderson | reduction of IgM antibodies (rats) | 8.6 | 3 & 5 min |

Table 2. POSSIBLE DELETERIOUS EFFECTS OF DIAGNOSTIC ULTRASOUND.

There have been 4 studies which were better designed to evaluate fetal monitoring. One is that of Richard Paul (35) at USC, in which he found that small premature babies did statistically better with fetal monitoring. It is interesting to speculate whether the tiny babies are less affected by monitoring positional problems and the membrane rupture effects in causing fetal distress patterns. Paul did say that the normal fetuses in his study had a higher perinatal mortality than the high-risk monitored fetuses, but this difference was not statistically significant. The question which is always raised by Paul's finding is whether the high-risk women were given closer surveillance in labor. Was the improvement due to monitoring, per se, or by more attentive nursing? This is especially likely since monitoring was a novel technique during the period of the study, and USC had given over itself to demonstrating fetal intensive care units.

The only way to really find out if a new technique is beneficial or not is to randomly assign alternate women to a group which has the new procedure, and to another group which does not — in this case, to a non-monitored group. There have been three studies of monitoring based on this randomized, controlled design — two by Haverkamp (6,7) and one by Renou (11) of Australia. The big problems with this kind of study are three: making sure that, although selection for people in each group is random, the final two populations are indeed similar in every way except that particular event being studied, and making sure that there are enough people in each group so that the effects of chance are minimized. Finally, it is extremely important that those who tabulate the results do not know who was in the study group and who was in the control group — in other words, the evaluators must be "blind".

Renou's study of two groups of 175 high risk fetuses each is a favorite of the pro-monitoring doctors because it concluded that "The trial clearly showed that (fetal) intensive care is associated with improved neurologic and biochemical status of the neonate; however it is possible that this improvement results from the use of fetal diagnostic tests or some other factors associated with intensive care." In contrast, Haverkamp's first study of two groups each with 240 high risk women and his more recent study of two groups of 345 women each showed that the monitored fetuses had no difference in outcome from the non-monitored, but infections and cesareans were markedly increased in the monitored group. How do we explain this difference? All groups were internally monitored. All groups had only high-risk fetuses.

The most obvious question about Renou's study is that we do not know how the non-monitored group were cared for in labor. Haverkamp's were auscultated every 15 minutes. As with Paul's group at USC, Renou's group in Melbourne is involved in demonstrating fetal intensive care. The people tabulating the results are the same people who are developing the intensive care unit. There were two perinatal mortalities, one in each group, but this is not emphasized. The sample is very small compared to Haverkamp's, and one of the eight obstetricians withdrew his high-risk patients from the control group part of the way through the study, because he thought it was unethical to have high-risk patients in a non-monitored group. The study is interesting, but not conclusive. The only criticism of Haverkamp's first study has revolved around the issue of whether his two groups are similar, because there were so many more infections in the monitored group — even though a monitor had been installed in both groups, but was covered up in the "non-monitored" who were instead auscultated. A study by Weichetek (35) on infections showed that there were three times more vaginal examinations during labor in the monitored women than in non-monitored. This could explain the excess infections. Haverkamp also demonstrated clearly that the two groups were not statistically different.

## Conclusion

I believe that fetal monitoring has yet to show itself beneficial and without harm, and I join those expectant parents who are insisting on development of alternative birth settings where fetal monitoring will be replaced by skilled, close surveillance in labor.

## References

1. Quilligan, E.J.: The obstetric intensive care unit. Hosp Pract 7:161, 1972.
2. Chez, R.A., Fox, H.E., Hobbins, J.C. et al: Monitor every patient in labor? Patient Care 12:136, Feb. 1978.
3. Hodgkinson, C.P.: Challenge and response. (Presidential Address to the American College of Obstetricians and Gynecologists) Am J Obstet Gynecol 1 May, 1968.
4. Hon, E.H. and Paul, R.H.: Clinical fetal monitoring. I. Am J Obstet Gynecol 118:529, Feb. 15, 1974.
5. Benson, R.C. et al: Fetal heart rate as a predictor of fetal distress. Obstet Gynecol 32:259, 1968.
6. Haverkamp, A.D. et al: The evaluation of continuous fetal heart rate monitoring in high risk pregnancy. Am J. Obstet Gynecol 125:310, 1 Jun 1976.
7. Haverkamp, A.D. et al: Electronic fetal monitoring held no better than auscultation. Ob Gyn News 1 Jan 1978.
8. Edington, P.T., Sibanda, J. and Beard, R.W.: Influence on clinical practice of routine intrapartum fetal monitoring. Brit Med J 3:341, 9 Aug 1975.
9. Gabert, H.A. and Stenchever, M.A.: Continuous electronic monitoring of the fetal heart rate during labor. Am J Obstet Gynecol 115:919, 1973.
10. Schifrin, B.S. and Dame, L.: Fetal heart rate patterns: Prediction of Apgar score. JAMA 219: 1322, 6 Mar 1972.
11. Renou, P. et al: Controlled trial of fetal intensive care. Am J Obstet Gynecol 126:470, 15 Oct. 1976.
12. Russell, K.P.: Cries and whispers. (Presidential Address to the American College of Obstetricians and Gynecologists) Am J Obstet Gynecol 128:3, 1 May 1977.
13. Russell, K.P.: Comment after Goodlin R.C. and Haesslein, H.C.: When is it fetal distress? Am J Obstet Gynecol 128:440, 15 Jun 1977.
14. Page, H.: Jello shows 'life' when subjected to EEGs in an unusual teaching experiment. Medical Tribune Mar. 3, 1976, Page 9
15. Cetrulo, C.L. and Freeman, R.K.: Problems and risks of fetal monitoring. (In Risks in the Practice of Modern Obstetrics, 2nd edition, pp 86) ed. Silvio Aladjem. Mosby, 1975.
16. Huch, A. and Huch, R.: Transcutaneous, noninvasive monitoring of p O 2. Hosp Pract 11:6, June 1976.
17. Huch, A. et al: Continuous transcutaneous monitoring of fetal oxygen tension during labour. Brit J Obstet Gynaecol 84: Supplement I, 1977.
18. Ueland, K. and Hansen, J.M.: Maternal cardiovascular dynamics II. Posture and uterine contractions. Am J Obstet Gynecol 103.1, 1 Jan 1969.
19. Caldeyro-Barcia, R. et al: Compression of the aorta by the uterus in late human pregnancy. Am J Obstet Gynecol 95:795, 15 Jul, 1966.
20. Lee, W.K. and Baggish, M.S.: The effect of unselected intrapartum fetal monitoring. Obstet Gynecol 47:516, May 1976.

21. Saling, E.Z. and Dudenhausen, J.W.: The present situation of clinical monitoring of the fetus during labor. J Perinat Med 1:75, 1973

22. Goodlin, R.C. and Haesslein, H.C.: When is it fetal distress? Am J Obstet Gynecol 128:440, 15 Jun 1977.

23. Gabbe, S.G. et al: Umbilical cord compression associated with amniotomy: Laboratory observations. Am J Obstet Gynecol 126:353, 1 Oct. 1976.

24. Caldeyro-Barcia, R. et al: Adverse perinatal effects of early amniotomy during labor. (in Modern Perinatal Medicine, pp. 431, ed. Gluck, L. Yearbook Medical Publishers, 1974).

25. Flynn, A. and Kelly, J.: Continuous fetal monitoring in the ambulant patient in labour. Brit Med J 2:842, 1976.

26. Hughey, M.: The effect of fetal monitoring on the incidence of cesarean section. Obstet Gynecol 49:513, May 1977.

27. Gassner, C.B. and Ledger, W.J.: The relationship of hospital-acquired maternal infection to invasive intrapartum monitoring techniques. Am J Obstet Gynecol 126:33, 1976.

28. Hagen, D.: Maternal febrile morbidity associated with fetal monitoring and cesarean section. Obstet Gynecol 46:260, Sep 1975.

29. Winkel, C.A. et al: Scalp abcess: a complication of the spiral electrode. Am J Obstet Gynecol 126:720, 1976.

30. Okada, D.M., and Chow, A.W.: Neonatal scalp abcess following intrapartum fetal monitoring: Prospective comparison of two spiral electrodes. Am J Obstet Gynecol 127:875, 1977.

31. Barrett, J.T. and Anderson, D.W.: Suppression of the IgM response by ultrasound. (in press, available from the authors at the University of Missouri School of Medicine, Dept. of Microbiology, Columbia, MO.)

32. Shenker, L. et al: Clinical experience with fetal heart rate monitoring of 1000 patients in labor. Am J Obstet Gynecol 115:1111, 1973.

33. Wennberg, J.: Presentation at the 25th Annual National Health Forum. New York, March 23, 1977. ( in press, available from the author at Dartmouth Medical School, Hanover, NH).

34. Chalmers, I. et al: Obstetric practice and outcome of pregnancy in Cardiff residents, 1965-1973. Brit Med J 1:735, 27 Mar 1976.

35. Paul, R.H. and Hon, E.: Clinical fetal monitoring. V. Effect on perinatal outcome. Am J Obstet Gynecol 15 Feb. 1974.

36. Baker, A.: Technologic intervention in obstetrics: Has the pendulum swung too far? Obstet Gynecol 51:241, Feb 1978.

37. Hohe, P.: Routine fetal monitoring in normal labor and delivery. Am J Obstet Gynecol 125:573, 15 Jun 1976.

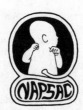

## U.S. GOVERNMENT REPORTS OPPOSING FETAL MONITORS

Two government studies of electronic fetal monitoring (EFM) have concluded that EFM has not been demonstrated to be of any benefit to the mother or her fetus. Both studies are free upon request. They are as follows:

FINAL REPORT OF THE MARCH 1979 ANTENATAL DIAGNOSIS CONSENSUS DEVELOPMENT CONFER- ENCE.

Request from Ms. Anne Ballard, Office of Research Reporting, Nat'l Institute of Child Health & Human Development, Bldg. 31, Room 2A34, Bethesda, MD 20014. Or call (301) 496-5133.

THE PREMATURE DELIVERY OF MEDICAL TECHNOLOGY: A CASE REPORT
by David Banta, MD, Group Manager, Health Program, Office of Technology Assessment.

Request the Banta Report from the Publications & Information Branch, Nat'l Center for Health Services Research, 3700 East West Highway, Hyattsville, MD 20783. Or call (301) 436-8970.

Note also that the Banta Study and Data are also published in the following form:

Banta, D., & S.B. Thacker. Assessing the Costs & Benefits of Electronic Fetal Monitoring, Ob. Gyn. Survey, 34:8, pp. 627-642, August 1979.

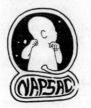

# CHAPTER TWELVE

## DOES ANYONE NEED FETAL MONITORS?

### By Albert D. Haverkamp, M.D.

Editor's note: The following is a transcript of the comments by Dr. Albert D. Haverkamp, an obstetrician and researcher at the Denver Medical Center, Colorado, made April 17, 1978 before the U.S. Senate Sub-Committee on Health. Dr. Haverkamp is well known for his important research comparing good nursing care with simple stethoscopes to electronic fetal monitoring. In a recent public statement by Dr. Helen Marieskind, currently engaged in research for the Department of HEW, she stated that she had reviewed over 400 technical articles on fetal monitors and only four (4) articles were based on valid scientific modalities. Two (2) of those four articles were the works of Dr. Haverkamp.

I am an obstetrician-gynecologist in a city-county hospital in charge of high risk obstetrics. I have been doing research on electronic fetal monitoring for the past four years. I would like to share with you my experiences and the results of my studies in this limited obstetrical area. The technique of electronic fetal monitoring involves the use of a mechanical system which records both the fetal heart rate and the mother's uterine contractions on a continuous graph paper, facilitating an analysis of the health status of the fetus during a delivery.

The obstetrician is increasingly using fetal monitoring for a number of reasons: 1. the sincere desire to improve infant outcomes; 2. the desire to base his or her actions on what appear to be objective clinical data, a graph rather than a nurse's report; 3. the seeming scientific value of more information; 4. the medical legal concern with not using a technique that a number of obstetricians state is necessary.

The obstetrical literature is replete with studies of intrapartum electronic fetal monitoring which suggest that this diagnostic technique improves perinatal outcome, reducing both mortality and morbidity of the infants (1, 2, 3, 4, 5, 6, 7, 8, 9).

Indeed, rather dramatic assumptions have been made about the potential reduction in the incidence of mental retardation if electronic monitoring were to be universally implemented. Quilligan, in an editorial in Obstetrics & Gynecology in 1975, stated "it seems reasonable to accept the premise that one-half of the intrapartum fetal deaths can be avoided. Likewise, assuming that brain damage is merely an intermediate point on the pathway to death, early recognition and elimination of fetal distress should reduce by one-half the incidence of handicapping disorders or mental retardation" (9). They further suggested that this was a cost-effective technique and that there would be significant economic advantage in electronically monitoring all labors which occur in hospitals (2, 10, 11, 12).

Such enthusiastic cost-benefit analysis, unfortunately, rests on some assumptions that are not justified either in the obstetrical literature or in the literature on mental retardation. These conclusions are based on data from obstetrical studies which were either retrospective or, when prospective, did not include truly comparable study groups nor the random assignment of subjects to various monitoring techniques.

Despite repeated suggestions that the differences in outcome of the infants might be somewhat subtle (5, 9) no long-term follow-up of electronically monitored versus unmonitored populations has been accomplished. Thoughtful researchers in the field have repeatedly noted the need for a carefully controlled prospective study. As Paul and Hon have stated: "To evaluate fetal monitoring fully, a well-designed obstetrical study, combined with comprehensive infant growth and development studies is necessary." (5).

Our studies, done in Denver, were the same studies Hon and Paul proposed at the University of Southern California in 1971, but which were not carried out. We wanted a study design in which all of the care given the pregnant patient was the same except for the technique of following fetal heart rate activity. Thus the patients would be treated at the same time, in the same institution by the same personnel. We began the study expecting improved outcome with the electronic monitoring and anticipating an ability to say just what the cost of fetal monitoring would be as well as being able to state what the perinatal gain could be with monitoring.

Maternal Child and Crippled Children's Services of HEW funded two studies, one from 1973-1975 and a second from 1975 which is still ongoing. In our first study we looked at the differential effects of electronic fetal heart rate monitoring and the more routine auscultation of fetal heart tones on perinatal or infant outcomes and maternal outcomes.

Our first study population consisted of 483 high-risk pregnant patients who were admitted during labor or who were to have labor induced. They were randomly assigned to one of the two groups, one in which the labor was followed by a nurse auscultating the fetal heart rate (i.e. listening with a stethoscope), and a second group in which electronic fetal monitoring was employed.

The study was explained to each patient and her consent was obtained before she was included in the study. The patient could withdraw from the study at any time. It was one-to-one care, nurse-to-patient, or nurse-machine-to-patient. The outcomes in which we were interested were particularly the Apgar scores and the biochemical status of the fetus. The Apgar rating is carried out at one and five minutes after delivery and evaluates the infant's condition by considering its color, heart rate, respiration, etc. A good score is 10; a baby without a heart beat has a score of zero. The condition of the infant can also be measured by the pH content of the blood from the umbilical cord. We expected that the electronically monitored infants would be in better condition than those who were merely auscultated since signs of distress could be acted upon more speedily. The results of that first study revealed no improvement in Apgar Scores in the electronically monitored group. Indeed, when we looked at the total number of low scores the auscultated group seemed somewhat better off. Nor did we find differences when we compared the two study groups as to their cord pH and blood gas results.

An interesting difference was noted in the methods of delivery used in the two groups. We found 16.5 percent of the electronically monitored patients apparently required Caesarean sections while only 6.6 percent of the auscultated patients were delivered in this way. This difference seemed to be the result of knowing about and taking quick action in response to a greater number of signs of fetal distress in the electronically monitored group. These results were contrary to our initial expectations. We therefore decided to pursue the matter further and commenced a second study with a tighter research design in July, 1975.

This research, "Fetal Heart Rate Monitoring and Scalp Sampling in High Risk Pregnancies" is a prospective study of a carefully controlled population of 690 high-risk obstetrical patients randomly assigned to one of three types of fetal monitoring groups. Patients experienced auscultation, electronic monitoring alone, or electronic monitoring with an option to obtain fetal scalp pH. The results of this study show no statistically significant differences among the infants from the three groups with regard to immediate perinatal outcome.

All groups had excellent infant outcomes. But, again, we found that the C-section rate for the auscultated patients was 5.6 percent, while for the electronically monitored alone 17.6 percent. This is a dramatic difference of almost 3 times the rate in one group. We concluded from these studies that:

1. There were no differences in neonatal outcome with respect to perinatal mortality, Apgar Scores, biochemical status, nursery course, or neurological status. Among our high risk patients, and under the circumstances of the study, electronic fetal monitoring, per se, was not associated with an improved outcome.

2. The Caesarean sectioned rate was markedly increased in electronically monitored patients (17 percent) in contrast with the auscultated group (6 percent). This was due to an increased diagnosis of both fetal distress and cephlo pelvic disproportion in the electronically monitored patients. The increase in C-sections was not associated with an improvement in perinatal outcome.

At a time when most thoughtful obstetrical authorities are urging universal electronic fetal monitoring, the study results appear unbelievable. However, if careful attention is paid to some other studies our findings do not seem so unrealistic.

Paul (13) found in analyzing some 50,000 deliveries at USC from 1970-1974 that there was no statistical difference in the perinatal mortality rate between monitored and unmonitored term size infants. Neutra (14) in a retrospective study of 20,000 patients at Beth Israel Hospital in Boston found no differences in term neonatal death rates between monitored and unmonitored patients, both being less than 1-1000.

I really believe we are over-selling our technology. Lilien (15) reported in 1970 from the Collaborative Perinatal study that term intrapartum (during labor) fetal deaths among low-risk mothers was exceedingly rare--less than 1-25,000 in that study. Yet, many hospitals won't allow a patient to labor without a monitor and many doctors won't accept a patient who will not have a monitor because of their medical legal fears. That is an awful lot of monitoring in normal term pregnancies to gain an unclear benefit.

From our study results and in looking at the obstetrical literature, in my opinion, there is no question that fetal monitoring increases the rate of C-sections. Paul found a primary C-section rate of 16 percent for monitored and 7 percent for unmonitored at USC from 1970-1974 (13). Of course, the groups are not truly comparable as the monitored patients were the high risk patients.

I have described this study in order to illustrate some of the problems we face in deciding which costs, benefits and risks to patients are warranted.

1. If we could extrapolate from the data of our study, we would suggest 6 in 100 women were undergoing unnecessary Caesarean sections.

2. The cost of delivery rises from $700 to $3,000, while women experience the morbidity (50 percent have some form of post-operative complication) and potential mortality of major surgery.

3. Further, they are required to undergo Caesarean sections with the next pregnancies and are separated from their new infants for a significant period of time. Recent writings by pediatricians have suggested that the early contact period between mother and infant is a crucial one in that "bonding" occurs. Studies have suggested a three-fold higher rate of child abuse and child deprivation in mothers undergoing Caesarean sections.

Monitoring, for the mother, increases not only the cost of her delivery, but decreases the naturalness of that delivery; decreases her mobility while in labor; requires that she receive care in a rather large hospital complex thereby limiting her choice of a place in which to have her baby; and significantly increases the probability that she will have major surgery (Caesarian section) during delivery.

I feel that fetal monitoring gives the doctor and nurse information. More information doesn't necessarily give a better outcome. It seems that in the OB patient, the more information you receive the more anxious you become about its significance and the more aggressive to ameliorate the problem so every piece of information that looks irregular problematically is like a red flag to a conscientious physician to get in there and do something. C-sections are done by conscientious people who are nervous, not knife-happy.

Our studies certainly do not answer all the questions about monitoring. What about the very small premature infant, especially those under 3 pounds who appear to benefit from monitoring? We excluded infants under 34 weeks from the study.

In our study, each mother was attended by a registered nurse who appeared to monitor her patients at least as well as the monitor. What if the nurse was not one-to-one, but could only intermittently check fetal rate tones of a laboring patient as so often happens on a busy labor floor? What if the same busy nurse intermittently watched a fetal monitor? If she cannot be with the patient all the time, she cannot watch the monitor continuously either. What if the nurse was not adept at auscultation of fetal heart tones? Many nurses and doctors so rely on the electronic monitors that they feel lost without them.

I believe that the technology and scientific development have enhanced our understanding of fetal stress during labor. Doctors Caldeyro-Barcia and Hon are distinguished men of science who deserve our admiration for their work. I would hope, however, that we also heed the comments of Dr. T. Almy who recently wrote an editorial in the New England Journal of Medicine (16) regarding the need for scientific trials in medicine. The reliance on clinical impression and comparison with past experience is an insufficient ethical basis for promulgating new therapies. It is because of my agreement with Dr. Almy that I wholeheartedly support Senate Bill 2466 for a National Institute of Health Care Research (Congressional Record S889), in which there is an expressed concern with the evaluation of technology, including "the study of the usefulness, cost, economic and social impact of medical practices and procedures."

I do have concern as to who will decide which studies are appropriate and relevant. As my own studies were turned down in 1972 by the March of Dimes and found disfavor with the people in Maternal and Infant Section of N.I.H. because fetal monitoring was already known to be necessary and totally effective, I feel that more controlled prospective studies are needed on fetal monitoring and I feel the need for continued support for our present studies so that the necessary follow-up as to possible later effects on the children will be done.

Finally, I fear that obstetricians may create a credibility gap and a crises of confidence by overselling the public on high technology and aggressive obstetrics, especially when a number of people are dropping out of the system altogether and having what appear to be reasonably healthy outcomes. This would be a grave disservice to the public and medicine.

## BIBLIOGRAPHY

1. Anonymous. "Is fetal monitoring worthwhile." Brit Med J 1: 515, 1971
2. Beard RW, Filshie GM, Knight CA, Roberts GM. "Intensive care of high risk fetus in labour." J Obstet Gynaecol Brit Commonw 78:865, 1971
3. Gabert HA, Stenchever MA "Continuous electronic monitoring of fetal heart rate during labor." Am J Obstet Gynecol 115: 919, 1973
4. Kelly VC, Kulkarni D: "Experiences with fetal monitoring in a community hospital." Obstet Gynecol 4: 818, 1973
5. Paul RH, Hone EH. "A Clinical fetal monitoring." Am J Obstet Gynecol 113: 529, 1974
6. Paul RH    Experience on a large clinical service. Am J Obstet Gynecol 113: 573, 1972
7. Amato, JC, "Fetal Monitoring in a Community Hospital." Obstet & Gynecol 50: 269, 1977
8. Renou P, Chang A, Anderson I, Wood C, "Controlled trial of fetal intensive care." Am J Obstet Gynecol 126: 470, 1976
9. Quilligan E, Paul R, "Fetal Monitoring: Is It Worth It?" Obstet & Gynecol 44: 96, 1975.
10. Bowe ET, in Fetal Growth and Development, Harry A Waisman and George Kerr, editors, New York City, McGraw-Hill Book Co., 1970
11. Saling, EZ, Dudenhausen JW. "The present situation of clinical monitoring of the fetus during labor." J of Perinatal Medicine 73: 144, 1973
12. Shenker L: "Clinical experience with fetal heart rate monitoring on one thousand patients in labor." Am J Obstet Gynecol 115: 1111, 1973
13. Paul RH, Huey JR, Yaeger CF, "Clinical fetal monitoring." Postgraduate Medicine 61: 160, 1977
14. Neutra R, Fienberg SE, Friedman E, "The Impact of Fetal Monitoring on Neonatal Death." APHA Meeting, Washington, D.C. Oct. 1977
15. Lilien AA, "Team Intrapartum Fetal Death." Am J Obstet Gynecol 107: 595, 1970
16. Almy, T. Editorial "Therepeutic Trials, Town and Gown, and The Public Interest," New England Journal of Medicine 29C: 280, 1977

140

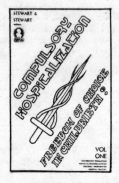

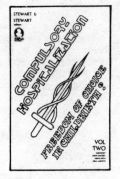

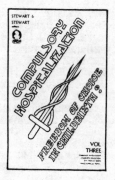

# A U.S. AGENCY TO REVIEW MEDICAL TECHNOLOGY

The FDA has long reviewed the marketing of drugs and food additives, considering their relative safety, efficacy, etc. Until recently, there was no similar review of technical devices used in health care. Thus, unproven devices such as electronic fetal monitors were freely promoted and sold to a gullible medical community which, in turn, sold the idea to their patients. Had the U.S. Government been authorized to regulate such devices and prohibit their promulgation unless proven safe and efficacious, EFM might not have swept the field of obstetrics as it did in response to unrestricted and aggressive marketing by their manufacturers.

The first step has been taken to create such a regulatory agency. It is called the National Council on Health Care Technology. It held its first meeting July 11-12, 1979. For more information concerning this Council, write to: National Institutes of Health, 5600 Fishers Lane, Rockville, MD    20857.

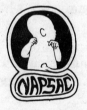

# CHAPTER THIRTEEN

## BENEFITS, LIMITATIONS, FALLACIES AND HAZARDS OF ELECTRONIC MONITORING OF THE HUMAN BODY

### by W.B. Jarzembski, P.E., Ph.D.

### Introduction

A paper on this topic should either be a single short paragraph or a lengthy tome. Anything in between must be an exercize in ego for the author. However, since so much of the treatment of this vast subject has been either superficial or of dubious scientific content, perhaps a discussion of a few salient topics will be of benefit to the reader. Due to the diversity of the readers, an attempt will be made to present the material in such a manner that most adult readers will be able to follow the concepts presented. Rather than follow the zig-zag path described by the title, this discourse will follow a more conventional didactic pathway by starting at the beginning.

"monitor — one who advises or cautions", Funk & Wagnalls, 1976. As used in clinical medicine, the word 'monitor' is normally taken to mean a device or function of relatively continuous service and includes functions of machines rather than of humans.

### Clinical Monitoring

Patient monitoring as a clinical entity had its beginnings with the introduction of bedside electrocardiographic (EKG) machines by Dr. B. Lown, a cardiac specialist in Boston. The EKG remains as the most widely used piece of patient monitoring equipment although many other devices have been added to increase the amount of information that is available to the patient monitoring team. At the time clinical monitoring was thus introduced (mid 1950s), few physicians had more than a cursory knowledge of the functioning of electronic devices and still fewer engineers had more than a passing interest in the physiological functions of the human body. Therefore for many years, and even today, a communications gap existed between these two important professions that prevented efficient utilization of the vast storehouse of technical knowledge that was available to the engineering profession.

Fortunately a few physicians and engineers recognized this hazardous bottleneck with the result that a new engineering specialty, Biomedical Engineering, was born. As with most new technology, this new engineering specialty needed both research and development as various educational techniques and strategies were developed and today, Biomedical Engineering is recognized as a separate engineering discipline with over fifty training programs in this country ranging from the baccalaureate to the doctoral level. Unfortunately there are almost fifty concepts of what constitutes the practice of

W.B. Jarzembski, P.E., Ph.D. is Associate Professor of Biomedical Engineering and Computer Medicine at Texas Technical University; former Chief Engineer for Advanced Research, Sunbeam Corporation; and has been an expert witness before congressional committee on medical devices.

biomedical engineering ranging from the repair of electronic devices to management of the technical functions within a hospital or medical center. It is the opinion of this writer that technology in health care delivery will come of age when all of the technological functions within the hospital are placed under the direction of an integrated engineering department staffed by professionals qualified to provide the numerous technologies involved ranging from technicians to Doctors of Engineering.

---

### PROBLEM SOLVING METHODOLOGY

When you need a Legal Problem solved,
                    Turn to.... A Lawyer
When you need a Baby Delivered,
                    Turn to.... A Nurse-Midwife
When you have a Tax Problem,
                    Turn to.... An Accountant
When you want Investment Advice,
                    Turn to.... A Stock Broker
When you have a problem in Mathematics
                    Turn to.... A Mathematician
When you have an Engineering Problem,
                    Choose One. A Lawyer
                                A Physician
                                A Mathematician
                                A Stock Broker
                                A Politician

---

It is interesting to note that few people turn to an engineer for the solution of an engineering problem.  Many of the errors in Fetal Monitoring application are due to ignorance of basic engineering principles on the part of those who apply them.  While engineers are the ones who design & develope such devices, engineers are seldom, if ever, consulted by physicians or nurses in their training for or clinical use of fetal monitors.

---

Figure 1.  SELECTION OF EXPERTS TO SOLVE SPECIFIC PROBLEMS.

To many in the health care delivery field any electronic black box that is sold as a "widget type A" is the same as any other "type A widget" sold by any other company. Even if true this would not be a good situation for it would essentially remove the good type of competition where companies compete on the quality of their goods and services as opposed to competing purely on the initial cost of the items. The State of Texas has a purchasing system that essentially eliminates quality as a consideration in competitive bidding to supply products purchased by the state. This results in a continual reduction in quality as well as an erosion of specifications with regard to function as purchasing specialists impose their will on the desires of the practicing professionals. This combination of lack of understanding on the part of the health care professional with an overzealous urge to save money on the part of purchasing professionals can indeed lead to a decrease in the efficiency of utilization of health care technology.

Perhaps it is time to look to the credentials of those who design and maintain these complex electronic and mechanical devices that hold so many lives in the balance. When congress passed the Medical Device Amendments to the Food and Drug Act in 1976, the physician was recognized as an essential ingredient of medical device development. In spite of testimony favoring some recognition of the qualifications of professionals involved in the actual development and design of these life critical devices, Congress chose to make no mention in this important area other than to require the Food and Drug Administration to solicit the advice of professionals in addition to physicians. There was no mention of any need to follow such advice and the current Director of the Medical Devices Bureau has made it quite clear that the Bureau considers such advice as just that, advice. Since the law does not address the question of qualifications of personnel involved in the development and design of medical devices the FDA had also stayed clear of such involvement.

Since the Federal Government has not seen fit to question the qualifications of persons doing development and design of medical devices, why is this topic germane to a paper such as this? It is the feeling of many as expressed by one high level Federal official that "since the physicians are the users of medical devices, they are the most qualified to determine the quality of such devices." Since the medical community has itself reached the conclusion that the scope of health care delivery is beyond the comprehension of one man and encouraged the individual physician to seek expertise in a specialty, and since the practice of engineering is so complex that the individual states typically require eight full years of training and education before an individual is considered qualified to practice engineering, it is not unreasonable to doubt that the physician has the expertise to make sound engineering judgments on the wide variety of devices that are currently available. If indeed the physician were so expert, would he be able to devote the time required to make a sound evaluation of these complex devices especially in view of the fact that few health care centers are equipped to make such an evaluation?

As a Professional Engineer I can easily design several versions of a device to perform a given function, all of which will meet any criteria that may be evaluated by testing or controlled through good manufacturing practices. These various designs could easily represent several levels of manufacturing costs, ease of use and long term reliability Based on many years of product design, field engineering and reliability experience I can unequivocally state that the professional with maturity in the field will design a more satisfactory device that the novice who is learning the basics while trying to produce mature designs. This is equivalent to saying that the experienced driver is more able to avoid an accident than the novice who is devoting a great deal of his mental effort to the act of driving.

With respect to electronic fetal monitoring, one can therefore justifiably ask if most physicians in obstetrical practice are qualified to evaluate one make of monitor over another. To do so requires an understanding of both medicine and engineering. Do they understand that different makes have different levels of reliability? Are their choices based upon the device's engineering capabilities to do the job or are they based upon other influences such as cost or superficial design?

## Parameters to Measure

If various electronic instruments are to be used to monitor signs to increase the effectiveness of health care delivery, which parameters (life signs) shall the physician measure? Quite clearly he must restrict himself to those parameters for which appropriate electronic devices are available and with which he is familiar. One of the functions of the biomedical engineer is to work with the medical community to determine which parameters are capable of being measured and to work with the medical device industry to insure that the medical needs are properly communicated to the manufacturer. Not the least of the tasks facing the biomedical engineer is the coordination of testing to determine that the concept carries a reasonable and realistic benefit-risk ratio.

As with any other walk of life, there is a tendency for the medical community to order and use devices that have been used before. A physician once told me that the true value of the biomedical engineer lies in the ability to help the physician choose new parameters that will yield more useful information with less risk. The biomedical engineer has training in the life sciences to supplement a basic engineering foundation. The doctorate in biomedical engineering often includes the first two years of medical school or a substantial portion thereof and is ideally equipped to serve as an interface between the doctor and the pure engineer. The final decisions must of course be made by the individual physician but the research may well be carried out by the biomedical engineer so that the physician can be well informed before making his decision. Unfortunately at this time there are not more than a hundred or so well qualified biomedical engineers in the country.

Current medical technology is capable of measuring over a thousand parameters on or in the human body. In order to be useful to the medical community, normals must be established for each parameter with appropriate corrections for factors such as age, sex, familial history, personal history, size, etc. It is also necessary to know the effects of various diseases on each of the parameters.

Another factor to be considered in the selection of parameters to be monitored is the sensitivity of the particular parameter to the patient's condition. Quite obviously the more sensitivity the parameter exhibits, the more suitable it would seem to be. On the other hand the parameter chosen should not exhibit wide changes due to causes that are not necessarily good indicators of a physiological or disease state. When one considers that, of the thousand parameters that can be measured, over three hundred may be measured, and that there are several hundred diseases, the problem of classifying parameters with appropriate correction factors and in determing the parameters that most nearly approximate changes in physical state becomes prohibitively large. For example, the process of birth is very complex involving the synchronization of innumerable maternal and fetal physiological processes. Most of these processes are unmeasurable and little understood. Electronic fetal monitoring involves the measurement of fetal heart rate, uterine contractions and sometimes fetal blood gas. Since this is only two or three of the countless possible relevant parameters, one can justifiably ask: (1) if these are sufficient? (2) if these are necessary? and (3) if electronic devices are the best way to obtain such data?

Fortunately most diseases may be characterized by the use of a relatively small number of parameters and only a few of these are suitable for monitoring purposes. To be suitable for monitoring purposes, the parameter must be capable of being measured on a continuous basis with as little interference with the normal functioning of the patient as possible. The more nearly obtunded the patient, the more physically restrictive the monitoring device may be. The trend however is toward development of monitoring devices that provide more information with less obstruction.

Chart I shows most of the parameters that are currently available for monitoring. Those marked with an asterisk are in most common use although new development is slowly changing this list. The most common devices used for routine clinical monitoring are those that show cardiac and pulmonary function be it adult, fetal or pediatric patients.

### Physical Quantities Used for Measurement of Physiological Parameters

Although the list of disease related parameters that may be measured on the human body seems endless, only a few have been demonstrated to be of value and suitable for patient monitoring. To further ease the burden on those who must keep up to date on the theory and operation of these devices, it is possible to monitor several different parameters with a single basic type of physical measurement. Thus even fewer concepts of physical measurements must be understood to maintain a high level of competence in understanding many different monitoring devices. Although the number of new and-or improved techniques is continually increasing, the number of physical quantities is hardly changing as most of the new developments are due to improved methodology using the same basic concepts and improved use of the data through use of the massive computational power available with the newer computers.

For practical reasons it is fortunate that several physiological parameters may be measured directly as electrical quantities and several more may be elicited, or evoked, by applying external currents to the body. This is fortunate as it allows the massive body of information developed by the electronics and electrical engineering profession to be applied to improve signal processing resulting in such improvements as automatic detection of arrhythmias and analysis of EEG signals.

All chemical activity involves a shifting of electrical charges. In the case of an electrical cell(unit of a battery) the chemical activity is designed so as to provide a useful output of electrical energy. In the human body there is a fantastic interaction between the chemical activity and electrical activity. In all cases of chemical activity, there is an associated shifting of electrical charges, or electrical activity, and good use may frequently be made of this electrical

## PATIENT MONITORING PARAMETERS

### NON-INVASIVE

| | | |
|---|---|---|
| *Temperature | - | Surface, Cavity |
| *Heart | - | Electrical Activity, EKG |
| *Pulmonary | - | Rate, Volumes, Gases, Edema |
| Vascular | - | Pulsatile Pressures, Traditional Pressures |
| Chemistry | - | Blood Oxygen, $CO_2$ |
| Brain | - | EEG, Specific Pathways (evoked), Edema |
| Nerve | - | Total Function, Conduction Rate, Nerve/Muscle Junctions |
| Respiratory | - | Apnea (newborn) |
| Physical | - | Anatomy |

### INVASIVE

| | | |
|---|---|---|
| *Heart | - | Pressure, Chemistry, Fetal EKG (fetal monitors) |
| *Uterus | - | Uterine Pressure (a standard measurement with fetal monitors) |
| Blood | - | Fetal Blood Gases, $PO_2$ |
| Brain | - | Pressure/Edema |
| G/I System | - | Chemistry |

Chart 1.  MOST COMMONLY USED PATIENT MONITORING PARAMETERS.

activity to monitor the state of the body. Examples of such measurements are the monitoring of hydrogen ion concentrations (pH) and the concentration of certain vital chemicals such as potassium and chlorine.

There are also many activities in the human body where there is a beneficial interaction between chemical and electrical activity. The entire nervous system depends on this interaction for the transmission of nervous impulses from the brain to any part of the human body in a few milliseconds (1:1000 sec.). It is important that there is a basic difference between chemical activity

| | |
|---|---|
| Electrical Potentials | - EEG, EKG, ERG, EMG, pH |
| Electrical Currents | - Blood Gases ($PO_2$, $PCO_2$) |
| Electrical Resistance | - Uterine Contractions, Galvanic Skin Resistance, Peripheral & Central Blood Flow, Blood Clots, Lung & Brain Edema, Brain Function, Lung Function |
| Photic | - Blood Gases |
| Weight | - Rapid Fluxations (lung fct.) |
| Pressure | - Cardiac Pressures |
| Ultrasound | - Edema of Brain & Uterine Cavity, Abnormal Tissue Growth, Getal Growth Rate, Fetal Heart Rate, Heart Valve Functioning, General Fetal & Adult Imaging |
| E.M. Radiation | - Transmission for General Imaging, Autoradiograph for Tissue Selectivity |

Chart 2.  PATIENT MONITORING METHODS--
PHYSICAL QUANTITIES MEASURED.

and electrical activity that is all too often neglected in the comparison of the two systems. Many chemicals that are found in the human body are capable of passing through cell membranes and so able to pass throughout the human body via the vast network of the vascular system. Depending on the molecular size there will be a selective process at the various cell membranes but eventually some fraction of almost all chemicals will arrive at every cell in the body. The transmission time varies from a few seconds to many hours. The endocrine system, as an outstanding example, furnishes the body with some very sophisticated control functions with timing that ranges from a few seconds in the 'fight or flight' case to many years in the case of menopause. Due to the fact that the chemicals involved (hormones) pass throughout the entire body, it is frequently possible to monitor the current state of a particular hormone by chemical analysis of the urine or blood.

Electrical activity, on the other hand, is a completely different story. It is not realistic to compare the two by discussing complexity for both chemical and electrical activity are confoundingly complex. Whereas the medical community has for hundreds of years recognized the complexity of the chemical side of life, there is still a naive belief that the electrical side of life is relatively simple with currents passing from point to point as if there were a few simple wires inside of the body.

Unfortunately this is not the case. With the notable exception of electrical batteries, most of the experience with electrical activity consists of experience with relatively simple electrical circuits where electrons flow within discrete conductors that are for all practical purposes completely insulated one from the other. Also acting in our favor is the fact that, for analysis, these circuits may be partitioned so that relatively small modules of the apparatus may be examined physically and analyzed for function. Another important aspect of electric circuits is that they are usually accessible for examination and electrical instruments may be connected to various parts of the circuit for measurements.

The human body, on the other hand, is what is known as a volume conductor. Although electrons are involved, the actual establishment of electrical fields and electrical currents depends on ions (molecules that carry an electric charge) which move quite slowly as compared to electrons. Every charge establishes an electric field that extends throughout space. The electric field at any particular point is the algebraic sum of the effects of all charges in the universe. Fortunately many of the contributing fields are of reverse sign and the effects cancel while the vast majority are too far distant to have a measurable effect, or more important to affect the measurement of the effect of specific charges. At this point, please allow me to take poetic license and digress. The understanding of electric fields is so complex that it is considered by many electrical engineers to be their most difficult subject and only a small handful of electrical engineers become expert in this field. Let it suffice to say that every electric charge has an infinite field that decreases in intensity with distance and that every electric field exerts a force on each charged particle. Some charged particles are free to move under the influence of this force and other particles are not. In a volume conductor such as the body, charges will move under the influence of electric fields but will remain within the body unless physical contact is made with other masses. Charges that are stationary create static electric fields known as D.C. (direct current) fields whereas moving charges create changing fields, both of which are of interest to the electrophysiologist.

At the cellular level, the ability of certain ions to pass through the cell membrane more easily than others causes a concentration of negative ions within the cell that is greater than the concentration of negative ions outside of the cell establishing a potential difference across the cell membrane. Many of the world's top scientists have spent decades studying these membrane potentials looking for information that will unlock some of the secrets of cell function so that we may better understand the basic functioning of the body systems.

The cummulative effect of this transmembrane potential throughout the body allows the practicing physician to make relative simple electronic measurements that give him insights to the condition of the physiological systems contained therein. The relationship between physiological event is not always clear but in many instances the inference of physiological function is great enough to be of use in diagnosis and care. For example the EEG (encephalogram) is a body surface measure of the gross activity of the brain. Since the surface electrical potentials represent a summing of all of the brain's electrical activity and since there are more electrical connections within the human brain than in all of the telephone systems in the world, it is clear that measurements made at the surface of the head can yield only very gross information relative to the condition of the brain. There are however several disease conditions that yield very distinct changes in the EEG, such as epilepsy.

On the other hand, the electrical activity of the heart is comprised of a coordinated system of relatively few components which acting in unison produce a surprisingly clear picture of the internal electrical events when measured at the chest surface. These electrical events have been shown to exhibit a remarkable correspondence to disease states which accounts for the fact that Dr. Lown's first choice of a physiological parameter for monitoring obtunded patients was the EKG. Although the basic EKG remains one of the most valuable tools for electrodiagnosis, several developments in the measurement of cardiac activity in the past decade have made this an even more valuable area for the physician's use. The most useful of these has been the so-called 'vector cardiography' in which additional electrodes placed at different locations around the chest have allowed the physician to study different aspects of the cardiac electrical activity.

Another area where electrical activity may be monitored at the surface of the body is the EMG (electromyography) which is the measure of the electrical activity of certain muscle groups. Although potentially of great value as a means of chronic monitoring (continuous) currently little use is made of this mode except for on the spot measurements of muscle activity or in biofeedback programs designed to teach control of certain muscle groups. There is no reason, however, not to consider the information that may be available for monitoring on a continuous basis.

Up to this point we have considered the measurement of electrical activity that occurs spontaneously within the body. During the previous decade, research has been directed toward evoking certain responses which then modify the electrical activity producing more useful information for the researcher and clinician. The major purpose behind the evoked response studies is that electrical computer techniques are available to greatly reduce the effect of other electrical activities on the desired electrical signals. With this technique, heretofore unavailable information has become easily measured. It is now possible to assess the ability of peripheral nerves to communicate with the brain and produce a physical response such as moving a certain muscle. It is also possible to assess the integrity of the links between the brain and the peripheral nervous system. This technique has been shown experimentally to be an early indicator of the effects of certain drugs on the brain, and as such, holds promise of being a suitable candidate for future monitoring study.

A third use of electrical measurements for monitoring purposes is the electrical quantity known as 'impedance'. This is a complex measure of how well electrical currents may be carried by a volume conductor. It is analogous to the term 'electrical resistance' as used with wire conduction systems, but since the passage of current in a volume conductor such as the body is carried by charged ions which are many times larger than electrons, the impedance to flow is affected by such things as ion size, electrical field strength, obstructions such as membranes, and availability of ions.

To measure electrical impedance on the human body, very tiny currents are injected into the body by means of electrodes similar to those used for EEG or EKG measurements. These electrical currents range in value from about a millionth of an ampere to a thousandth of an ampere. Most of the apparatus in use today uses alternating current with a frequency of about 100,000 hertz (cycles). Work by this writer and others indicates however that additional information may be available if frequencies as low as 100 hertz are used.

It would be desirable for the currents to pass through certain specified parts of the body, but due to the measurement of pulsatile current flow in an entire forearm. It is at this point that an accurate knowledge of the actual current pathways within the tissue would be very desirable, but today this knowledge is not available and little if any research is being done to relieve this critical lack of information. This writer has been searching for research funds to complete work started in this area. Among the reasons given for refusal to support research in this area was the statement that such research was too late, physicians are already using these methods.

There are three basic mechanisms whereby physiological functions cause changes in electrical impedance of the human body that are of interest to the physician and researcher. As the heart pumps blood through the vascular system, the pressure changes from a maximum during systole to a minimum during diastole. These pressure changes are evident in the change of diameter of various blood vessels. Since blood is a better conductor of electrical currents than tissue, these changes in diameter are accompanied by changes in electrical impedance. Thus a measure of electrical impedance will show a relationship between impedance change and pulsatile blood pressures and there is a known relationship between pulsatile blood pressures and the actual flow of blood under given conditions.

Pooling of blood (hematoma) or water (edema) in tissue will affect the ability of the tissue to conduct electrical currents. Since each of these conditions is relatively slow to develop and change, it will change the measured impedance slowly and will show up as a change in baseline impedance as opposed to pulsatile changes. This characteristic may be used in monitoring to detect changes in lung and brain edema or hemorrhage, and it is also used to detect the pooling of blood in limbs due to a clot. A similar technique has proven to be very effective in pulmonary monitoring. Although there is still controversy as to the relationship between lung volumes and measured impedance, there is little doubt as to the value of impedance monitoring to detect changes in pulmonary function.

The third area of interest in electrical impedance measurements of the human body lies in the fact that impedance measurements may very well reflect rather subtle changes in membrane properties. Edema may very well take place in two forms, one where the excess water is distributed primarily outside of the cells but within the interstitial spaces or it may be primarily within the cell itself. This distribution may well change in time and it may change even though the amounts of water present are quite normal. The writer has measured changes in impedance that were a result of such shifts that gave variations as great as ten to one. This area of impedance measurement has not yet moved out of the research laboratory primarily due to the small amount of funding that it has received in spite of the fact that the measure of electrical impedance accounts for a far larger number of monitoring parameters than any other modality.

This paper will not discuss the various types of monitoring that are possible using ionizing radiation such ax X-ray or gamma ray. Due to the teratogenic properties of these means, they have been found to be entirely unsuited for chronic monitoring, even short term.

This brings us to the clinical apparatus popularly known as 'ultrasonics' or ultrasound. This is a method that employs the mechanical properties of sound waves as opposed to the electrical properties of electromagnetic fields. Ultrasound has been useful in medical practice for several decades but it has just been in the past few years, thanks to the efforts of the National Science Foundation for an intensive research effort, that really effective apparatus has become available to the clinical physician and today it is possible to visualize internal structures without the harmful effects generally attributed to ionizing radiation.

Ultrasonic devices make use of the fact that certain materials exhibit a piezoelectric effect; that is, they change in size (one dimension) when placed in an electric field. When the electric field is alternating, the change in size follows the change in field and the surface becomes a source of sound waves at the particular frequency. If the surface of the piezoelectric device is placed against the surface of the body, the sound wave will be transmitted through the tissue. As in the case of volume conduction, this transmission of sound waves through tissue is a far more complex physical phenomenon than the mere transmission of sound through air. This is due to the fact that air is a relative homogeneous mass (uniform) whereas tissue is a very heterogeneous mass varying from point to point in its ability to propagate sound. In fact, the sound will be reflected from any surfaces within the tissue where there is a change in properties. It is in fact this reflective property that makes the medical use of ultrasound valuable.

The most simple type of ultrasound device is the 'A' Scan apparatus where a single transducer (piezoelectric unit) sends a series of short bursts of ultrasound energy into the body from a single location without movement of the transducer. The reflections (echoes) are detected by the same transducer in between bursts and displayed on a video monitor as vertical pips from a horizontal baseline. Each pip is indicative of an interface between two different types of tissue or a membrane. This system is of limited value although it has been used quite successfully to display the movement of inner surfaces such as the beating of a heart.

The next variation comprises a movement of the transducer to produce a series of echo producing traces. To maximize the effectiveness of viewing, the video display is arranged so that each transducer position produces a line of image but rather than have pips to represent echoes, the intensity of light produced depends on the strength of the echo. The screen then takes on a light and dark pattern that is representative of the tissue being viewed. The 'B' Scan as this device is called is actually capable of producing images that may be recognized as actual images of the anatomy within the field of view of the transducer.

A critical aspect of the ultrasound system is the coupling of ultrasonic energy from the transducer to the tissue. This becomes even more critical when the transducer is moved so a recent development is the use of multiple transducers with electronic switching from one element to the next. Systems employing over a hundred elements are currently available. With the advent of small, very low cost microcomputers, the multiplicity of information available from such an array of transducers may now be utilized for mathematical analysis which is capable of producing images far superior to anything yet seen. It is now possible to determine the sex of a fetus during the first trimester as the genitals become visable.

At the current state of the art, it is possible to make relatively accurate estimates of fetal maturity by measuring skull growth, to determine the sex of the fetus, to determine multiple gestation, and to determine certain disease conditions of the reproductive organs. False pregnancies may be determined with a high degree of certainty.

### Hazards of Clinical Monitoring

From fetal monitoring to geriatric monitoring, there is no area with more false information widely disseminated than in the area of patient safety! Scare tactics have frequently been used to gain personal gratification (perhaps through ignorance). In either event, it is the patient who loses. If an instrument or device is truly dangerous without compensatory benefit, the truth should be known to save the patient from harm.

Recently a newspaper syndicated article appeared on the subject of electroconvulsive therapy that was highly critical of the entire process. The article was based on an interview with a young physician and, assuming that the article was an accurate reflection of the views of this physician, very little was known of the process involved or the electronic equipment used to give the treatments. This highly critical treatment was given front page space. A carefully prepared rebuttal of this article was sent to the local newspaper but there was no response, not even an acknowledgement. It was ascertained that the editor did indeed receive the rebuttal but 'usually reliable sources' reported that the editor wouldn't touch the rebuttal with a ten foot pole because it was critical of a physician and written by a non physician.

The field of health care delivery is too important and too complex not to bring together teams of experts from the appropriate technical disciplines. We can no longer assume that the physicians have the requisite knowledge to make decisions in regard to matters that are complex far beyond their abilities in fields in which they have little if any training. If ever there were an area in which the expression "a little knowledge is dangerous" applies, it is in the area of health care safety. The physician with an undergraduate degree in engineering, the engineer with virtually no education in the life sciences and the lawyer with no training in either field can completely destroy the effectiveness of a health care safety team.

What are the actual hazards associated with clinical monitoring? It is the belief of this writer that the most significant hazard lies with the aforementioned penchant of the American public, if the news media does represent the public, to accept the cries of alarum raised by the self proclaimed protectors of the public, be they government or private, without examining the credentials of these experts.

Real hazards do exist with almost all of the various modes of monitoring. These will be covered in some detail below. However we must again look to other than material things if we are to find the real villains. The most important single factor when looking to safety in the hospital is the acceptance of safety as a way of life. Each and every individual in a medical setting must accept some responsibility for maintenance of a safe environment.

### Electrical Hazards

The safe use of electricity in any environment demands a knowledge of the various aspects of electrical engineering. It is often surprising that the most common cause of electrical hazard in the medical environment is the improper use of the grounding conductor that normally carries little or no current. It is well to understand that most electrical power circuits have two wires that are essentially without voltage with respect to the building ground. One of these wires is intended to carry the current from the actual use of power and is colored white. This wire is properly called the 'neutral'. The other wire, colored green, is called 'ground' and is primarily in the circuit to provide safety. In the event that the electrical power 'hot' wire (black, red or some other color) should actually become connected to the instrument case or internal circuit, the 'ground wire' provides a path to ground to either detect the current for a 'fault detection circuit' or provide a pathway to 'blow' the circuit fuse. In the rare event that the power 'hot' wire touches the case of the device and the green wire is actually not grounded, the case of the device may become hot. Any person touching the case and a ground simultaneously would then be subject to severe shock.

With the probability of both wires being faulty as low as it is, one would wonder why all the fuss. The answer is twofold. First, the probability is not all that low. Surveys a few years ago showed an alarming number of faulty cables as determined by x-rays of typical medical devices in service in hospitals as well as a large number of poorly wired receptacles in the hospitals. The second reason is that this is an easily understood problem for the pseudo experts to yell about for their own personal gratification. In this particular instance, there were sufficient grounds for concern.

Of still more concern however is the use of electrical stimulating currents for the relief of pain without an accurate understanding of the actual current pathways. For the male and nonpregnant female, the use of electrical currents to relieve pain has been one of the outstanding developments of recent biomedical engineering research. To date there has not been the least bit of evidence that these currents when properly used can cause any known deleterious effects. There is however some doubt as to the safety of these currents when used in the first trimester of pregnancy, but only when the currents are used abdominally. There is no direct evidence of hazard under these conditions but there is a certain feeling among some experts in the field that there may be danger.

Any discussion of electrical safety must take into consideration test methods that are used to determine the safety of a new device before it leaves the factory, and continued testing in the field as time erodes away the protecting insulation. To understand the appropriate test methods for a particular electrical device or system requires a broad understanding of the physical principles underlying the concept, design and fabrication of the device. All three areas are susceptible to premature failure if sufficient expertise is not utilized. In particular an analysis of failure modes by a knowledgeable professional can yield surprising results with respect to unsuspected long term failure modes. Virtually all insulation systems have a time-temperature lifetime expectancy, and an insulation system that stands up to all tests today may well be predicted to have too short a time-temperature life for a particular application.

## Mechanical Safety

All too often, in the eternal quest for unsafe electrical condition, the question of mechanical hazards is overlooked. When one considers however the sheer physical size of many of today's clinical devices, it becomes apparent that physical mountings must have long term reliability, and devices must be designed with centers of gravity that will prevent tipping under abnormal conditions. A certain emergency cart appears to be quite stable until one too many drawers is pulled open at which time the entire cart falls on its side. Suppose this happened at the time that defibrillator paddles were being applied during cardiac arrest.

The mechanical hazards that can exist in a medical center are too myriad for listing. They range from too little head room, horizontal control panels that will admit spilled coffee on to an electronic circuit, sharp corners that tear as persons rush past during an emergency, and even the monitor that is placed on a wall mounted bracket that may break from excessive vibration.

## Ultrasound Hazards

This paragraph could easily be labeled "Ultrasound Hazards — Are There Any?". It is self defeating to compare the possible dangers of ultrasound with the fact that for many years there was no danger associated with x-ray. All too many of those who wish to discuss ultrasound hazards bring out this fact and point to the almost certain knowledge that we now know x-radiation to be hazardous. It should be pointed out however that there is considerably more knowledge available today with respect to the mechanisms of damage due to ionizing radiation. There is also a considerable store of knowledge with respect to the mechanisms of action of ultrasound in the transmission and reflection of sound waves in tissue. In the early days it was assumed that x-radiation was safe whereas the medical use of ultrasound was considered as a potential hazard from its inception so that many tests have been conducted in many independent laboratories to detect any hazards.

Since ultrasound is a non-ionizing radiation, the mechanism of damage would either be due to local heating or to some unknown process. Damage due to heating of the tissue at the levels currently in use is highly unlikely based on the research to date which has not turned up definitive evidence of damage even at power levels considerably higher than diagnostic levels. Based on the evidence to date, it is quite reasonable to assume that ultrasound as currently used is clinically is safe.

Research continues, however, by highly competent scientists in several laboratories around the world. These men do communicate with each other to gain the synergistic effect that often results when great minds are rubbed together, but they do maintain a fierce independence. Paul Carson works in Colorado to determine the best way to actually measure ultrasonic power, Padmakar Lele investigates biological effects of ultrasound on tissue in Cambridge, Massachusetts, and the FDA maintains a citizen advisory panel of qualified scientists to maintain vigilance on these vital matters of safety in ultrasound.

To probe deeper into the safety aspects of ultrasound involves three distinct areas. First is the question of quantifying the amount of energy for each experiment and then correlating the results of several experiments. To describe an ultrasound waveshape requires a description of the length of each burst, the frequency of the pulses within each burst, the peak instantaneous power during the burst, the shape of the burst envelope and the number of bursts per second. To describe the effect of the ultrasound also requires a knowledge of the duration of application in any one setting and then the cummulative application time for the particular subject. To further complicate the problem, there is not a definitive relationship between the animal or tank model and the human maternal-fetal model. To thoroughly confuse the matter, consider the fact that many of the investigators consider the electronic black box that produces the ultrasonic energy as just that, a black box about which they know very little.

The next area to consider is the difficulty of ascertaining if there is any damage. Research to date has virtually eliminated the possibility that there are any gross abnormalities generated by the application of ultrasound, even during the first trimester. If anything, it has been demonstrated that the information generated has been life saving in some instances. This leaves the area of very subtle defects. It is possible to conjecture that the mechanical vibration at a molecular level could conceivably effect the process of mitosis resulting in a change in the manner in which the myriad brain cells find their individual pathways. But then if this did happen, is it bad or good? If we accept the premise that virtually all stimuli affect the way that neural connections are made, then we may presume that ultrasound will have some subtle effect, but this effect may well produce superior cerebration.

The last area of consideration is that of people who must furnish the information with respect to experimental results, whether research laboratory or clinical research. Science in a difficult area like the one at hand demands nothing but the best if the chaff is not to outweigh the wheat. The clinical investigator must have his mind on the need for collection of good data. Perhaps this is too much to ask of the clinical investigator who is primarily concerned with the safety and well being of the patient. If the only model available that can produce positive results is the actual mother and fetus, it may be necessary to have trained scientific investigators working along side of the medical clinician.

There have been recent findings that ultrasound may affect growth of human cells. Pinamonti has found that in vivo sonification (ultrasound irradiation) of erythrocytes (red blood cells) did change the permeability of the cell membrane to certain substances. This was attended by a shift of the oxygen dissociation curve to the right, indicating that the capacity of the cells to transfer oxygen was diminished. It is too early to assess the value of the work as the ultrasound used (8MHz, 8mw-cm2) did not have parameters that are common for diagnostic work. The sound power level (8mw-cm2) is considerably higher than normal and the burst characteristics are not described. The lack of information relative to the burst characteristics and the lack of complete information relative to the total time of irradiation in the report makes it difficult to integrate this particular experiment into the total pattern.

Other authors have suggested that ultrasound irradiation has decreased the growth rate of cells in vitro (outside the body) that were removed by amniocentesis for genetic study. Miskin, et al, present evidence that the use of ultrasound had its beneficial effects when used to guide the needle for amniocentesis in that the number of bloody taps and failed cultures was reduced.

## Computer Aided Monitoring

One of the greatest developments in medical history has been the development of the small computer element known as a microprocessor. This tiny, inexpensive electronic device has had a great impact on patient monitoring in that it allows much more complete information to be made available to the attending physician in a small fraction of a second. It is possible to save the complete monitoring history in full detail and present it in the form of graphs and charts with no effort on the part of the hospital staff other than the encoding of a short message to the computer via the computer terminal. The computer is also able to analyze the data as it is entered and inform the staff by means of lights and audible alarms if any unusual conditions occur.

## Summary

The subject of patient monitoring, even when limited to fetal and infant monitoring, is a vast, complicated subject encompassing many clinical and scientific disciplines. There is little doubt in the minds of professionals as to the need for clinical monitoring in many areas. Early ultrasonic monitoring of the fetus allows the physician to determine many fetal abnormalities so that early corrective action may be taken. Maternal and infant monitoring can also alert attendants to abnormal conditions.

The reverse of the coin is not the hazards of monitoring that seem to worry so many but rather the fact that excessive monitoring may take support from other important areas of health care delivery. Also medical support personnel may develop an over reliance on the monitoring devices with an attendant lack of personal attention to the patient. Personal attention may have more therapeutic value than the gathering of information by the monitor.

Having been asked many times to develop designs that are "idiot proof," this writer wonders if in so doing he is helping to raise a generation of idiots. Will medical support personnel become more proficient in the operation of machines to only become less proficient with their knowledge of the needs of the patient?

Another area of concern is the fact that while we look with great concern at the qualifications and credentials of our physicians, we pay little if any attention to the education and credentials of those who make important life or death decisions as to the design, testing and maintenance of the apparatus used by the physician. At present, neither government, physician nor industry seem to consider this an area for concern. In fact, although 56 states and territories require proof of professional competence in order to become licensed to practice engineering, most of these laws specifically exempt those who design medical apparatus under a blanket manufacturing exemption. The rationale is that our corporate managers do really have our best interests at heart and they will make sure that competent engineers really do the design work. If you agree with this philosophy, it is hereby suggested that you read Business Week, Forbes, The Wall Street Journal and Juris Doctor where the rule seems to make a fast buck without regard to normal ethics.

## REFERENCES

**1. Clinical Instrumentation**

1.1 Thomas, H.E., Handbook of Biomedical Instrumentation, Reston Press, 1974

1.2 Welkowitz, W and S. Deutsch, Biomedical Instruments: Theory & Design, Academic Press, 1976

1.3 Strong, Peter, Biophysical Measurements, Tektronix Corp., 1970

1.4 Cromwell, L. et al, Medical Instrumentation for Health Care, Prentice Hall, 1976

**2. Technology & Health Care**

2.1 Bronzino, J.D., Technology for Patient Care, Mosby Press, 1977

2.2 Rushmer, R.F., Medical Engineering, Academic Press, 1972

**3. Ultrasound**

3.1 Ultrasound in Medicine, Plenum Press, Vol's 1-3, 1975

3.2 Wells, P., Ultrasonics in Clinical Diagnosis, Churchill, Livingstone Press, 1977

**4. Scientific Papers**

4.1 Jarzembski, W.B., "Safety in the Hospital," Proc. 26th Ann. Conf. on Engineering in Medicine & Biol., Vol 26, No. 1, 1973

4.2 Jarzembski, W.B., "Pathological Implications of Changes in Transcranial Impedance" Proc. 2nd Int'l Conf. on Bioelectric Impedance, Lyon France, 1977

4.3 Jarzembski, W.B., et al, "Hospital Engineering Management - an Educational Program," J. of Clinical Eng., Vol 2, 67-72, 1977

4.4 Miskin, M., et al, "Ultrasound in Prenatal Genetic Diagnosis," Ultrasound In Medicine, Plenum Press, Vol 1:201-212, 1975

4.5 Lele, P., "Application of Ultrasound in Medicine," New England J. of Med. 286:1317, 1972

4.6 Lele, P., "Presentation to the FDA Panel on Review of Obstetrical-Gynecological Devices (acoustic), Washington, D.C., 29 Sept., 1975

4.7 Sunden, Bertil, "On the diagnostic value of ultrasound in obstetrics and Gynecology, Acta Obstretricia et Gyn Scand., Vol XLIII, 1964

4.8 Carson, Paul, "Exposure measurements on diagnostic ultrasound measurements" Presentation to the ultrasound committee of the OB-GYN Device Classification Panel of the FDA, 22 Jan. 1976.

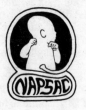

# CHAPTER FOURTEEN

## LASTING BEHAVIORAL EFFECTS OF
## OBSTETRIC MEDICATION ON CHILDREN
### Research Findings & Public Policy Implications

### By Yvonne Brackbill, Ph.D.

Editor's Note: This article is a copy of the testimony of Dr. Brackbill before the U.S. Senate Subcommittee on Health and Scientific Research presented on April 17, 1978, in Washington, DC. For a thorough and meticulous documentation of Dr. Brackbill's statements here, see her chapter in the book, "Handbook of Infant Development," J.D. Osofsky, Editor, New York: Wiley, 1978, which contains 168 references. A list of these references is also available from NAPSAC. Please send $2.00 for copying and postage.

Mr. Chairman and Members of the Subcommittee:

My name is Yvonne Brackbill. I am a Graduate Research Professor of Psychology and Obstetrics and Gynecology at the University of Florida.

I thank you for this opportunity to speak about the lasting behavioral effects of obstetric medication on infants and children--a research area in which I have been involved for the past decade.

Back in the 1960's, one of my graduate students told me that she wanted to do a thesis on the effects on infant behavior of obstetric medication, i.e., the anesthetics and analgesics given mothers during labor and delivery. (By behavior, I mean the ability to see and hear, the development of motor skills, language ability, intelligence, and so on.) She explained that she had been bothered by the prospect of brain damage from obstetric medication since her second child was born and that she was motivated by her lingering anger at having been given such medication against her will at the time. I told her I thought the question would already have been thoroughly researched by obstetricians since they had been using anesthesia for delivery for a century and since the question of possible damage was such an obvious one. The graduate student proved me wrong: there was no body of literature on the subject.

The study that she and I conducted was the beginning of systematic research on obstetric medication effects on infant behavior. At present there are some 35 studies on that topic. The investigators are a diverse lot, and the labs are scattered throughout the United States and Great Britain. Nevertheless, the major findings are clear, consistent, and unequivocal. I will summarize these for you. Full documentation is available in the supporting material which I request your permission to insert in the record as part of my statement.

Yvonne Brackbill, Ph.D. is a professor at the University of Florida engaged in the supervision of graduate research with the departments of Psychology and Obstetrics and Gynecology. She is co-author of the monograph, "Effects of Obstetric Medication on Fetus and Infant" in the book, "Handbook of Infant Development," and is author or co-author of many papers in this area of research.

The basis for the problem is this: The human baby's anatomical and physiological development is not complete at the time it is born. Apropos of obstetric medication, there are two very important ways in which the newborn is immature. One concerns the central nervous system. Important areas of brain are still undeveloped at birth. The production and development of neural elements probably continues ·in the cerebellum for 1.5 years and in the hippocampus for 4.5 years. During this period of rapid brain growth, the brain is especially vulnerable to damage. Also, it is especially easy for toxins to reach the brain in neonates because the so-called "barrier" between blood and brain is immature as well.

The second important way in which the newborn infant is immature, as far as obstetrical medication is concerned, is that the liver and kidney — the organs most needed for drug metabolism and excretion — are not fully functional at time of birth.

So, then, the situation is this. The newborn human being is an organism poorly positioned for dealing with drugs. They cross the placenta rapidly. They lodge in brain structures that are still developing and are therefore at high risk to damage. They are not readily transformed to nontoxic compounds since the necessary liver functions are immature. And they are not readily excreted because of inefficient kidney function.

From all these considerations, it would be small wonder if obstetrical medication agents did not inflict some mischief on the infant.

What are the behavioral effects of obstetric medication and how have they been studied? The 35 investigators I mentioned have studied healthy, full term babies who came from low-risk pregnancies and whose deliveries were normal and uneventful. (In this way one avoids confusing the effects of drugs with the effects of pre-existing disease or complications.) Most of the studies have been done on newborns, though a few have seen older babies. The most important study in NIH's Collaborative Perinatal Project, a longitudinal study of over 50,000 children which Congress authorized in the 1950's. Dr. Sally Broman and I have finished analyzing the results of this study for 3500 of its most healthy babies tested at 4 months, 8 months, and 12 months. We are now analyzing obstetric medication data for the same children tested at 4 years and 7 years.

Looking at the results of all 35 studies, almost all have found statistically significant behavioral effects of obstetric medication. Furthermore, the direction of these effects is uniformly, without exception, toward behavioral degradation and interference with normal function. NO study has ever demonstrated or even suggested that obstetric medication improves normal functioning.

A second general finding is that obstetric medication effects are more pronounced in some behavioral areas than others. During the first year of life, the strongest effects can be seen in the development of gross motor abilities — e.g., the ability to sit, to stand, and to locomote. They can also be seen in certain emerging cognitive functions, principally the development of inhibitory ability — e.g., the ability to stop responding to redundant signals, to stop crying when comforted, to stop responding to distracting stimuli. During later years, the strongest effects can be seen in the development of language and associated cognitive skills. At all ages, the effects are more clearly visible when tasks are difficult, i.e., when they require the child to exert itself, to make an effort, to cope with problems.

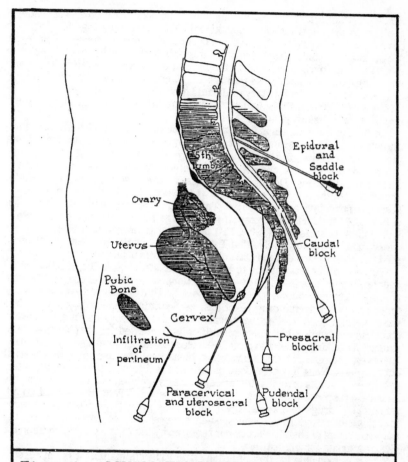

Figure 1.    SCHEMATIC DIAGRAM OF VARIOUS
GENERAL BODY LOCATIONS FOR DRUG INJECTION
FOR ATTEMPTS TO BLOCK OBSTETRICS PAIN.
(Adapted from Williams' Obstetrics, Hellman, et al.,
eds., 14th edition, Ch. 17, p. 438, 1971).

A third general finding is that the behavioral effects of obstetric medication
are dose-related and potency-related. That is, stronger drugs and larger doses
of a single drug produce stronger behavioral effects. For example, general
anesthetics have stronger effects than local anesthetics, and local anesthetics
have stronger effects than no anesthetic at all.

The most important general finding is that the behavioral effects of obstetric medication are not transient. They persist. Within the age range for which we have data — 1 day to 7 years — there is some evidence of decrease for a few drugs. But for other drugs, most notably inhalant anesthetics, the adverse effects are as strong at 4 years as they are at one year. It is difficult to avoid concluding that the damage is permanent. There are more details on adverse drug effects in the documentary material I have filed with you.

Now I will address three issues that help pull these empirical data into the perspective of health policy and planning.

The first of these issues is the increase over the years in obstetric drug administration. There seems to be a widespread misconception among the medical and nonmedical community alike that the number of drugs administered during labor and delivery is decreasing. This is not true. In point of fact, it is increasing. Documentary statistics are described in my appended material. On the whole, I estimate that 95 percent of births in United States hospitals nowadays are medicated. This means 3,500,000 medicated births out of 3,700,000 total births per year. If the average IQ loss per medicated birth is four points, this means 14,060,000 IQ points lost to new United States citizens every year. Cummulatively, that figure should put the problem of obstetric medication at the head of the class of national health priorities.

The second important issue to bring to your attention is the question of accountability in monitoring adverse reactions from these drugs and in controlling their distribution for clinical use. The United States does not monitor these or other adverse drug reactions, as Senator Kennedy pointed out last year. Neither does it effectively control the use of drugs commonly used in obstetric medication but never scientifically evaluated for that purpose. The drugs I'm talking about have all been cleared for clinical use by the FDA. However, the research that served as a basis for FDA clearance was carried out on adults. None has been done using infant subjects. Pharmacological test results from adults cannot automatically be extrapolated to infants because the neonate's response to drugs is often qualitatively different. If we insist on administering drugs to infants, the infant itself must be the object of pharmacological study. Nevertheless, such studies are not carried out by the manufacturers of obstetric drugs nor required by the FDA as a precondition for clearing drugs for clinical use.

Who is responsible for this situation? The FDA claims that it is not responsible for policing the uses to which a drug is put. The drug industry claims that it is not responsible for testing a new drug for all potential uses. From the perspective of child health and welfare, the issue of monitoring and controlling obstetric drugs exists in a vacuum of accountability.

The last policy issue to bring to your attention is a consumer issue: who decides what if any drugs a mother will take and how much? The medical community claims that mothers receive medication only when they request it for pain or when there are birth complications. Although there are no data allowing direct evaluation of this claim, there are indirect sources of evidence. (I have summarized these in my documentary material.) Collectively, they indicate that mothers do not receive adequate information on adverse drug reactions, on differences among drug risks, or on alternatives to drugs for relief from pain. They also indicate that women have little voice in deciding which if any drugs they will consume.

For many illnesses today, drug therapy is the only effective therapy. Under these circumstances, there's very little real decision making involved. But pregnancy is not an illness. Childbirth is not an illness. Administering drugs prenatally and perinatally is more often optional than essential, and there is plenty of room for decision making.

One additional point about the mother as decision maker. In a very real way, the physician protects himself-herself by allowing the mother to share in the decision making process: When the mother takes more responsibility for decision making, the physician takes less responsibility and to that extent makes himself-herself less vulnerable to charges of malpractice.

There are remedies for these problems. Among the potential solutions, I submit two basic recommendations for your consideration.

My first recommendation stems from the fact that the mother is a consumer. She must be treated as an intelligent human being, capable of understanding information on drugs when it is written in plain English, capable of evaluating drug risks and benefits, and capable of choosing alternatives to drugs. Furthermore, she has the right to this information — just as a smoker has the right to know that tobacco is injurious to her-his health. It is currently within the power of the federal government to achieve these goals. The DHEW has two offices to deal with consumer information and education. One is the Office of Health Information and Health Promotion; the other is the soon to be established Office of Health Technology. I recommend that DHEW prepare two versions of obstetric medication information: one appropriate for the consumer and one appropriate for the professional. I further recommend that the information be made available to all consumers through the Office of Health Information and Health Promotion and to all professionals through the Office of Health Technology.

My second recommendation is that you request the FDA to require long term, behavioral testing of new drugs on immature animals prior to drug clearance for clinical use. Let me emphasize each of the key elements in this recommendation. First, immature animals. As I've pointed out, the young organism's response to drugs is often qualitatively different from the adult's and cannot be predicted with certainty from the adult's response to drugs. The second key element is long term. Not all behavioral abnormalities are apparent immediately after birth. Many behaviors do not develop until later. As I mentioned, it now appears that obstetric medication has adverse effects on language ability; we did not know this previously because all studies had been done on young infants, prior to the age at which they begin to use language.

A third key term is behavioral testing of new drugs. Behavior is the most vital concern in human development and welfare. Our problems as a nation are underachievement in school, criminal acts, breaches of moral conduct, psychotic behavior, socially maladaptive acts. These are behaviors, and they are not equivalent to the physical and physiological measures traditionally used in drug evaluation. Blood gas parameters do not predict reading achievement. Apgar score does not predict language skills. Respiration rate does not predict motor ability. In order to predict such behaviors or to evaluate them, we must collect behavioral data. Behavioral teratologists have established that many substances toxic to the developing central nervous system cause measurable and permanent behavioral abnormalities in the absence of visible structural change or measurable physiological change.

Great Britain and Japan already have legislation requiring that the behavioral teratology of new drugs be studied before the drugs are marketed.

The United States leads the world in pharmaceutical research and development. We must regain our leadership in testing drugs for safety and effectiveness to ensure the mental health, physical health, and welfare of our children.

Thank you again, Mr. Chairman and members of the Subcommittee, for this opportunity to speak to you about the lasting behavioral effects of obstetric medication on infants and children.

---

Note: It is possible for the FDA to require long term, behavioral testing of new drugs on immature animals prior to drug clearance for clinical use without additional legislative authorization. The FDA already has available two routes. One route is via the Code of Federal Regulations, vol. 21, section 314.1 (section on reproduction and teratology studies). The second route is by way of the Federal FDA act, which empowers the Secretary of HEW to deny clearance for a new drug on the grounds that testing did not include all those tests which have reasonable applicability and for which methodology is available.

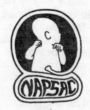

## U.S. GOVERNMENT REPORTS ON OB PRACTICES

Two important government reports were published September 24, 1979, concerning the questionable value of current obstetric practices.  They are:

EVALUATING BENEFITS & RISKS OF OBSTETRIC PRACTICES, HRD-79-85, A Report to Congress by the Comptroller General of the U.S. General Accounting Office.

A REVIEW OF THE RESEARCH LITERATURE & FEDERAL INVOLVEMENT IN OBSTETRIC PRACTICE HRD-79-85A, A Study by the Staff of the U.S. General Accounting Office.

Both are available from the U.S. General Accounting Office, Room 1-30, Park Building, 12420 Parklawn Dr., Rockville, MD 20857.   You may write directly for a copy or request a copy through your senator or congressman.

Also available is a bibliography of references that goes with the two above studies.  For some reason, it was published separately instead of being included as parts of the above.   It is entitled:

BIBLIOGRAPHY OF ARTICLES ON OBSTETRICS PRACTICES

This bibliography contains about 1,000 citations in the areas of induction of labor, pain relieving drugs in obstetrics, forceps, vacuum extraction, fetal monitoring, cesarean section, and other topics.  It may be obtained from the same address given above.

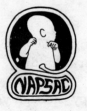

# CHAPTER FIFTEEN

## EPISIOTOMY: FACTS, FICTIONS, FIGURES, AND ALTERNATIVES

Carol Brendsel, R.N.
Gail Peterson, M.S.S.W.
Lewis E. Mehl, M.D.

### Acknowledgements
The help and encouragement of Doris Haire, D.M.S. is gratefully acknowledged, as is her pioneering inspiration to open to question practices assumed true. The help of Benjamin Graber, M.D. and Georgia Kline-Graber, R.N. in providing information regarding methods, questionnaires, and answering questions, is also gratefully acknowledged, along with the statistical assistance of Ammon Igra, Ph.D., and the help of our Administrative Assistants Gail Penso and Bridget Scadens, and the excellent typing services of Jana Reiser and Super Typing Service. We also wish to acknowledge the American Foundation for Maternal and Child Health who furnished part of the support for this research by a grant.

### Introduction
Episiotomy has been the norm in American obstetrics since about 1930. One of the rationales for this has been the widespread belief among physicians that doing an episiotomy protects against later pelvic relaxation and prevents the need for corrective surgery later in life. We could find no scientific justification for this in the literature although in 1920 it appeared in William's Obstetrics textbook stated as a belief and has been there ever since. By the 1975 edition of William's Obstetrics it is stated as fact. Other stated rationales for doing an episiotomy include the belief that the episiotomy protects the infant's head from unnecessary, and possibly damaging, head compression against the perineum and that the episiotomy prevents later sexual dysfunction. There is no evidence regarding either of these positions. The belief that the baby's brain will be damaged from being on the perineum is an interesting one and psychohistorically may relate to a fear of women and may relate to castration anxiety in a fear of being engulfed in the vagina. There does not seem to be any logical rationale for the image of the baby's head as a battering ram against the perineum, especially since, with a normal birth, the baby's head descends two steps forward and then ascends one step backward, each time stretching the perineum more and more in a gradual process, rather than against the perineum.

---

Carol Brendsel, R.N. is a researcher and practicing nurse at The Center for Research on Birth and Human Development (CRBHD); Gail Peterson, M.S.S.W., is a psychologist, Director of Family Research at the CRBHD and author of several papers on birth alternatives and the psychological aspects of birth; Lewis E. Mehl, M.D., is Director of Research at the CRBHD and author of over 40 articles, coauthor of several books on alternatives in childbirth, including "The Place of Birth," Oxford Univ. Press.

The need for doing an episiotomy has been used as a block against change in birth practices. Doctors state that they cannot do a delivery except on a delivery table because it will be hard for them to do an episiotomy on anything but a delivery table and it would be even more difficult to repair an episiotomy on anything but a delivery table. Likewise, this has also prevented consumers from assuming different positions for delivery besides the usual flat on the back dorsal, lithotomy position. It has also prevented avoiding stirrups for delivery and prevented the delivery from being a sterile surgical affair. Without routine episiotomy there becomes very little need for the surgical asepsis that is usually practiced. Even then, when an episiotomy is necessary because of fetal distress, a sterile field can be quickly created on a normal, comfortable double bed for the repair without increasing the incidence of infection.

A common argument used in favor of episiotomy has been that the incidence of pelvic relaxation and the need for vaginal reconstructive surgery has been on the decline in the last 40 years. This is similar to the argument used to advocate routine hospital delivery, stating that because there have been more hospital deliveries than at home in recent years and because perinatal mortality is improving, hospital delivery is the cause of improved perinatal mortality rates. This is the same specious argument which is applied to most procedures in modern day obstetrics which have no scientific justification. It is the argument of trends. The episiotomy rate in American obstetrics in recent years has been almost 100 percent. Interestingly, however, the incidence of pelvic relaxation has also dramatically declined in Holland where the prevalence of episiotomies has not changed in recent years. This suggests to us that other factors operate besides episiotomy in determining pelvic relaxation.

The purpose of the research that we will be presenting today is to explore the objective basis, if any, of the use of episiotomy to prevent pelvic relaxation.

### Methods

To find subjects we approached childbirth educators to obtain the names of students who had delivered with or without an episiotomy. The childbirth educators themselves were also asked to participate. Subjects were contacted by telephone and the details of the study were explained. If they were interested in participating we obtained information from them regarding their age, race, parity, length of time since delivery, pattern of previous episiotomies, if any, and socio-economic status based on their number of years of education. We did a prospective matching so that each woman that was selected for inclusion in the group with no episiotomies had a counterpart in the group with episiotomies who was of the same age, race, parity, length of time since delivery, pattern of previous episiotomies, socio-economic status, nursing status, and pregnancy status. Prospective matching means that before including a woman in this study she had to be matched with another woman in the other group so that they would be a pair and would be compared together. If a match was obtained between two women they were contacted regarding participation again and an interview and examination time was scheduled. Our acceptance rate for subjects was 80 percent. It is interesting that those who declined to participate seemed to be those who were afraid of the sexual implications of being examined and also seemed to be somewhat closed. All of our examinations were done in the subject's home and we obtained informed consent for proceeding. This informed consent took the form of explaining to subjects why we were doing the study, what we were interested in, and what would be done. All of the examinations were done by our nurse practitioner. The minimum time since delivery for being included in the study was one year. The range of time from delivery to the time of examination was 1-13 years for the women in the study group. We did the exams in the subject's home to minimize the anxiety effects and to make them the most comfortable. In addition, all of the exams were done by the same person, who was a woman, for the same reasons.

So that our results would be accurate, before beginning, we conducted an initial training session between us to be sure that the criteria we were using would be those that would be obtained by separate examiners. After we agreed exactly for 10 subjects the training period ended.

The method of examination used was to perform the exam in the subject's home, which lasted between 2 and 3 hours. The first phase of this contact consisted of an oral interview in which subjects were asked questions related to sexuality, sexual attitudes and functioning, their previous deliveries, their couple's relationship, and the like. This questioning period helped to develop rapport between our examiner and the subject. Next a thorough pelvic exam was performed, followed by time for the woman to become comfortable with the use of the perineometer. Three contractions of the vaginal muscles were then measured with the averaging of the initial reading and the maximal reading. In addition, women were asked to sustain as hard a contraction as possible for as long as possible. This resulted in the sustained perineometer reading and the second sustained measure. Following this, women who did not know how to do a proper Kegel exercise were instructed in how to do so. We then left a questionnaire for them to complete regarding their sexual attitudes, past history, level of sexual functioning and symptomatology. The oral interview also included a review of symptoms in terms of the pelvic organs.

We coded data onto Fortran coding sheets and entered them into the computer.

## Results

The mean number of pregnancies of women in our study was approximately 2.3 for both groups. Twenty-nine women in both groups had had one child, 19 women had had two children, and 2 women had had three children. Eighteen percent of the women in both groups were currently pregnant and 26 percent of the women in both groups were currently nursing. All of the women were of a middle socio-economic background. Obviously our study contains no information regarding the effects of multiple births on pelvic relaxation.

In terms of the results of clinical examination, we found no statistical significant differences between the two groups in the incidence of rectocele (weakening of the muscles of the posterior vaginal wall with protrusion of the rectum into the vagina), poor vaginal muscle tone (pubococcygeus), poor Kegel contraction, undissolved sutures, turned labia, clitoral adhesions, or significant sensory discomfort around the vagina. There were more cystoceles in the non-episiotomy group, but regression analysis (a statistical technique which allows one to see to what extent a group of variables contributed to one particular outcome measure such as cystocele) showed that this was not related to having no episiotomy. There were 31 labial scars in the non-episiotomy group compared to 8 in the episiotomy group, and these did not cause any symptoms. There were 48 perineal scars detected in the episiotomy group compared to 8 in the non-episiotomy group and there was significantly more vaginal numbness in the episiotomy group with 10 cases compared to 1 case in the non-episiotomy group. Eleven women in the episiotomy group complained of vaginal discomfort compared to 5 in the non-episiotomy group.

The importance of doing more sophisticated statistical investigation is emphasized by these tables. Without the regression analysis one might have concluded that episiotomies did, in fact, decrease the incidence of cystocele (prolapse of the bladder into the vagina from weakening of the muscles in the anterior vaginal wall). Obviously, frequency tables must be interpreted with caution without further statistical techniques such as regression analysis, since, in any new area of study, important influences may not be recognized and not controlled for in a matching study. Frequency tables set the stage for multivariant techniques such as regression analysis which provide more reliable indications of the relationships between variables being measured and of the extent to which unmeasured variables may be influencing one's results.

There were no statistically significant differences in the results of the perineometer readings between the two groups. The perineometer consists of an apparatus inserted into the vagina which the woman squeezes by tensing her Kegel muscle. The device is attached to a pressure meter from which the pressure of the muscle tightening can be read. The perineometer has been shown in other research to be a good indicator of vaginal muscle tone and strength of the pubococcygeus muscle. There were no statistically significant differences in the initial reading on the perineometer, the maximum reading, the reading which could be sustained, and the duration of time which this reading could be sustained between the two groups. This indicated no statistical significance on the basis of physiological measurements.

We also found no statistically significant differences in pertinent history factors between the two groups. The average number of Kegel exercises done before birth, in the first three months postpartum, and at the time of the exam was not statistically significantly different between the two groups. The same number of women in both groups had light hair and fair skin, and the mean time since the first delivery for the non-episiotomy group was 3.2 years and for the episiotomy group was 3.6 years. The number of lacerations was the same between the two groups, but the episiotomy group had one third degree laceration and four fourth degree lacerations, while the non-episiotomy group had none.   Research published in the proceedings of the 2nd NAPSAC Conference, "21st Century Obstetrics Now." showed  a 10 percent incidence of combined 3rd and 4th degree lacerations in 1000 patients receiving episiotomies compared to none in 1,000 patients who have not received an episiotomy.

Cononical correlation analysis (another multivariant technique) showed that there was a relationship between the combination of having a low sustained perineometer reading, having a rectocyle, and having sensory discomfort with the combination of increased parity (number of births), doing Kegel exercises in the fourth trimester, having a significant laceration, not doing Kegels at the time of examination, increasing gravidy (number of pregnancies), and having had an episiotomy. There was also a correlation between the combination of having vaginal numbness, labial scars, and poor vaginal muscular tone with increasing parity and with lacerations of increasing severity.

Regression analysis showed the following results. For cystoceles, the significant predictor variable was having had an episiotomy with the first delivery ($p \leq 0.005$). This variable predicted 9 percent variance of cystocele for a significance of .01. This means that 91 percent of the reasons for having a cystocele are due to factors others than the ones we measured, which means that they are due to non-birth related factors, since we also included length of labor, birth weight, and the like as potential variables which could show up. For the prediction of whether or not a woman would have a rectocele, the important variables were: the severity of any laceration she may have had with the first delivery ($p \leq 0.0009$), doing Kegels postpartum in the fourth trimester ($p \leq 0.005$). This combination of variables predicted 27.7 percent of the variance of rectoceles, leaving 72.3 percent of the reasons for having a rectocele to be accounted for by non-birth related factors. The significance of this prediction was less than 0.0009

For vaginal discomfort we found that doing Kegels before the birth decreased the incidence and having red hair and a fair complexion increased the incidence. This combination of variables predicted 15.3 percent of the variance of vaginal discomfort for a significance of 0.001. For the initial perineometer reading we found that the more pregnancies a woman had the lower the reading would be, and the more severe the laceration might have been with the first birth, the lower the reading. This combination of variables predicted 14.1 percent of the variance of the initial perineometer reading for a significance of 0.01. Red hair and fair complexion predicted 4.3 percent of the variance of the maximal perineometer reading for a significance of 0.039. With increasing time since the first delivery, the maximum time that the highest reading could be sustained seemed to increase, and this variable predicted 6.9 percent of that reading. For sensory discomfort this was predicted by the severity of the laceration at the first birth and was decreased by increasing time since the first birth. These two variables predicted 18.3 percent of the variance of sensory discomfort for a significance of less than 0.0009.

### Conclusions

Our initial hypothesis was that obstetrical factors per se would be significant contributors to postpartum pelvic symptoms. That this was not the case is apparent from our data. This forced us to reconsider our prior hypotheses and to generate some new ideas from the data. Most importantly, pelvic symptomatology, including sensory discomfort, cyctocele, rectocele and the like, is multifactorily determined. Many factors seem to interact together to produce these clinical conditions. While some obstetrical factors are significantly important, they only account for a small portion of the factors contributing to pelvic symptoms.

Our sample seemed reflective of middle class women having three children or less and probably reflects the population most private physicians encounter. It was interesting that both groups had the same total number of lacerations when episiotomy extensions are considered. From these results we can conclude that the patient's interest seems to be served by avoiding episiotomies and lacerations, especially for those of increasing severity. Clinically, sometimes an episiotomy may be useful to avoid more severe tearing. In our practice we avoid lacerations and episiotomies by teaching clients perineal massage prenatally as physical therapy for the tissues. Women and their partners are instructed in massaging the perineum, vaginal area and labia for ten to fifteen minutes daily for the last three months of pregnancy (in the hope they will use this at least 3 or 4 times weekly). Our clinical impression, and that of others using this, is that it is effective in preventing tears. In addition, a slow, controlled delivery of the head (assuming a stable fetal heart rate) is an essential part of avoiding lacerations. The active help of the woman through her own sensations by decreasing or stopping pushing when she feels burning during the time of crowning is an integral part of preventing tearing.

Kegel exercises during the pregnancy and after the fourth trimester seem to be beneficial. Many of the women we studied were not doing Kegel exercises with maximal effectiveness, so their benefits may be underestimated. Kegel exercises in the fourth trimester seem to have a mild deleterious effect. Further research needs to be done to substantiate this or to determine if it is artifactual or because of another complicating variable.

Having red hair and fair skin seemed to increase the possibility of having vaginal discomfort. Increasing time since the first birth decreased the severity of sensory discomfort and increased one of the perineometer readings. This would indicate improvement with time. The cononical correlation findings show that the number of pregnancies as well as the number of deliveries had an effect. Perhaps this is hormonally mediated.

In summary, further research to delineate the predictors of pelvic relaxation need to be more broad and to consider social factors in more detail than obstetrical factors. From our research we can conclude that episiotomy is definitely not prophylactic against pelvic relaxation and is merely another factor in a large multifactorial process.

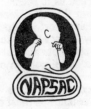

### References

1. Logan, T.G. The vaginal clasp: A method of comparing contractions across subjects. University of Nevada, Las Vegas, unpublished manuscript, 1976.
2. Kegel, A.H. Physiologic therapy of urinary stress incontinence. In Carter, B.N. (ed) Monographs on Surgery 1952. Williams and Wilkens, Co., Baltimore, Md. 1952.
3. Kegel, A.H. Stress incontinence and genital relaxation. CIBA Clinical Symposia 4 (2), February - March, 1952.
4. Kegel, A.H. Early genital relaxation. New techniques of diagnosis and nonsurgical treatment. Obstetrics and Gynecology 8 (5): 545-550, 1956.
5. Kegel, A.H. The physiologic treatment of poor tone and function of the genital muscles and of urinary stress incontinence. Western Journal of Surgery, Obstetrics and Gynecology 57: 527-535, 1949.
6. Wharton, L.R. The nonoperative treatment of stress incontinence in women. Journal of Urology 69 (4): 511-519, 1953.
7. Kegel, A.H. Physiologic therapy for urinary stress incontinence, Journal of the American Medical Association 146 (10), 915-917, 1951.
8. Kegel, A.H. The nonsurgical treatment of genital relaxation. Use of the perineometer as an aid in restoring anatomic and functional structure. Annals of Western Medicine and Surgery 2 (5): 213-218, 1948.
9. Graber, B. and Kline-Graber, G. Diagnosis and treatment procedures of pubococcygeal deficiencies in women. In Lo Piccolo, J and Lo Piccolo, L. In press, 1977
10. Graber, B. and Kline-Graber, G. Differential diagnosis in screening patients with sexual complaints. University of Wisconsin, Madison, unpublished manuscript, 1977.
11. Graber, B. and Kline-Graber, G. (University of Wisconsin, Madison) Epidemiological report on clitoral foreskin adhesions. Paper presented at the Second Annual Conference of Sex Educators, and Counselors, University of Texas Medical School, Galveston, Texas, March, 1975.
12. Kline-Graber, G. and Graber, B. (University of Wisconsin, Madison) The pubococcygeus muscle and sexual functioning: and update on Kegel's work. Paper presented at the Second Annual Conference of Sex Educators and Counselors, University of Texas Medical School, Galveston, Texas, March, 1975.
13. Mehl, L.E. Research on home confinement from the United States. In Kitzinger, S. and Davis, J. (eds.) The Place of Birth. Oxford University Press. New York, 1978.

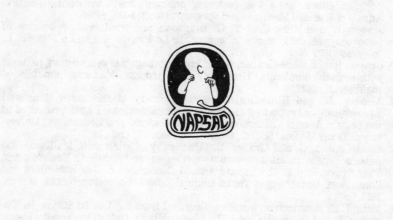

# CHAPTER SIXTEEN

## UNNECESSARY CESAREANS:
## DOCTOR'S CHOICE, PARENT'S DILEMMA

Susan G. Doering, Ph. D.

The Collaborative Perinatal Study, reviewing more than 50,000 births which occurred between 1958 and 1965, cites an overall cesarean section rate of 5 per cent (1). Obstetric and nursing textbooks have, for generations, called a 4 - 5 per cent rate normal. As Kroener said, in 1976,

> One of the long held principles of obstetrics has been that the cesarean section rate was inversely proportional to the quality of obstetrics practiced. Any physician with a high section rate was evaluated for the quality of his obstetrical care and accused of trying to pad his financial remuneration (2).

In other words, one could judge a physician by his section rate: the lower it was, the better obstetrician he must be.

But things have changed. A study of 204 selected hospitals, conducted by the Commission on Professional and Hospital Activities, reports on two million deliveries for the period 1967 to 1974 (3). In 1967, the section rate was 5.1 percent, ranging from 4 percent in small hospitals to 5.4 percent in large hospitals. In 1974, the overall rate was 9.8 percent - more than double - having increased to 6.7 percent in small hospitals and to 10.4 percent in large hospitals.

Evrard and Gold, reporting on Rhode Island hospitals, noted a 6.4 percent cesarean rate in 1965, which rose to 14 percent in 1975 (4). Gibbons, studying Baltimore hospitals, found that 5.4 percent of the live births in 1968 were delivered by cesarean section, while the rate had gone up to 10.2 percent in 1973 (5).

In other words, by the early 1970s, the overall rates of cesarean section had at least doubled in the United States, and the trend had not yet leveled off. One physician, writing in the American Journal of Obstetrics and Gynecology, says,

> I well remember the stress and concern of the surgeons and internists at Good Samaritan Hospital in Los Angeles when, in 1956, we were placed on probationary status by the Joint Commission on Accreditation because the hospital section rate was almost 10 percent. The entire obstetrical staff was almost drummed out of the Corps (2).

Things have changed a lot since 1956. Now it often appears that hospitals and obstetricians hold the opposite value: the higher their cesarean section rate, the better their obstetrical care. Gluck, writing in 1977, called the rise in rates astonomical, and said that in some hospitals the rate was even in excess of 20 percent (6).

Susan G. Doering, Ph.D. is a Research Scientist at Environmental Programs, Inc. and Project Director of the First Pregnancy Study, Johns Hopkins University, Baltimore.

## Why Is the Cesarean Section Rate Rising?

What has caused the rapid and sudden rise in cesarean section rates in recent years? There is no one simple explanation; the cause appears to be a complicated interaction of several recent changes in obstetrical procedures and practices. These include the following: widespread fetal monitoring, liberalization of indications for surgical delivery, (including repeat sections), increased intervention in the natural physiology of labor and greater fear of malpractice suits.

### Widespread Fetal Monitoring

There are many studies which show a direct correlation between the rise in the use of fetal heart rate monitors and the rise in incidence of cesarean section (7-14). The link between the two could be seen as a positive change, if one believes that the monitor reveals fetal distress which would have gone unnoticed by the nurse with her fetoscope, thus enabling us to save babies who otherwise would have been born dead or damaged. Unfortunately, this is not the case, as Haverkamp and his colleagues have shown in their carefully controlled 1976 study (7). Haverkamp randomly assigned high risk mothers in labor either to be in an electronically monitored group or to a group auscultated periodically by nurses using the standard fetoscopes. Infant outcomes were equally good for both groups; the only significant difference was that the electronically monitored group was sectioned at a rate of 16.5 percent, while the nurse-monitored group's rate was a very low 6.6 percent, (considering that the mothers were all high risk.)

Edward Hon, the inventor of the fetal monitor, has pointed out that proper use of the machine should lead to lower cesarean section rates, because more accurate diagnoses of fetal distress could be made. He feels that the recent rise in the rates is due to the fact that so many physicians and nurses are "inexperienced" at interpreting fetal monitor tracings (15). Furthermore, as Shenker et al. point out, the fetal monitor produces as many as 40 percent false positives, i.e. signals fetal distress when, in fact, the baby is fine (16). So even when medical attendants are competent to read the monitor tracings, it appears that there still may be many errors.

Add to this the fact that unfortunately, machine malfunctions are a fairly common experience. Many a laboring woman has been completely panicked when her monitor "sounded funny" or stopped, thinking that her baby was in trouble or actually dead (17). Even if she can eventually be reassured that her baby is fine, it is often difficult for her to regain her control and relaxation.

### Liberalization of Indications for Cesarean Delivery

Because cesarean surgery is safer for the mother now than it used to be, physicians are far more likely to resort to it when in doubt, particularly if the alternative might be a difficult vaginal delivery (10). Thus, if a baby is presenting breech or with some rarer malpresentation (5, 8, 11, 12), if the mother shows signs of toxemia or eclampsia (8), if she's an "elderly" primipara (18, 19), or if there is prolonged rupture of the membranes (20), doctors will decide sooner on a surgical delivery, sometimes without even allowing a trial labor. Cesareans are done more quickly for suspicion of fetal distress (8, 10-12, 20) and also for what is variously called uterine dysfunction or dystocia or "failure to progress" (8, 10-12, 20). This last category often includes laboring women who "fail" to progress fast enough for their attendants, as some physicians misinterpret the Friedman normal labor curve (21, 22), treating it not as the average that it is, but as if it were an outer limit on labor time (23). In addition, of course, cesarean sections are still used for the old indications: cephalopelvic disproportion, placenta previa and abruptions of the placenta, but these emergencies account for only a small proportion of current cesareans (5, 10, 11).

### Repeat Cesarean Sections

If the rate of primary cesarean sections is rising, and if most American doctors persist in the old 1914 dictum: "once a cesarean, always a cesarean" (11, 24, 25), it stands to reason that repeat sections will contribute increasingly to the rising cesarean section rate.

Outside of the United States, women who have had one cesarean delivery are not routinely sectioned with succeeding births. Trial labors are common and success rates vary from 37 percent to 69 percent of previously sectioned women managing a safe vaginal delivery, depending on which research you read (26-29). Success depends on the indications for the first cesarean surgery and on the type of uterine incision used, as well as on the philosophy of the medical attendants.

The main fear voiced by the American medical community is that the old uterine scar will rupture, but this turns out to be a very rare occurrence (0-0.5 percent), and furthermore, approximately half of the ruptures that do occur, happen during the pregnancy, and thus could not have been avoided by elective repeat cesarean section in any case (26, 27, 30, 31). The slightly more likely outcome is a partial separation of the old scar, which appears to occur in approximately 1 percent of all cases and is reported to have no dangerous consequences to either mother or infant (26-28). A British physician states:

> Many repeat cesarean sections have been done for inadequate reasons, in particular, for fear of scar rupture. Rupture of the lower segment scar is too uncommon to justify repetition of section for that reason alone (27).

When vaginal delivery is attempted after cesarean section, success rates differ greatly depending on why the original section was done. For instance, if the previous section was done for cephalopelvic disproportion, 58 percent of McGarry's mothers and 59 percent of Morewood's were able to deliver vaginally. If a cesarean had been done for prolonged dysfunctional labor, 67 percent and 74 percent managed vaginal deliveries. When failed induction was the cause of the first, only 44 percent and 35 percent were able to avoid a second cesarean. But when non-repeating indications such as fetal distress or malpresentation caused the first section, about 80 percent of both groups achieved vaginal deliveries.

The type of uterine incision will make a big difference in the feasibility of attempting vaginal delivery also. The old classical (top to bottom) incision is far more likely to rupture in succeeding pregnancies than is the new low cervical incision. In both McGarry's and Morewood's sample, mothers with classical scars were not even allowed to attempt a vaginal delivery; they were all sectioned electively. Since the vast majority of cesarean sections are currently being done with the low cervical incision, many more women are good candidates for trial labor and possible vaginal delivery after cesareans. It is up to American physicians to pay more attention to the foreign research literature (or to generate some of their own) and to stop insisting that a previous cesarean dictates surgical deliveries for all future pregnancies.

### Increased Intervention in the Natural Physiology of Birth

Interfering with the natural physiology of labor and delivery is becoming more and more common in the United States (32, 33). We have already discussed widespread fetal monitoring, and of course, delivery of a baby by abdominal surgery is the ultimate in intervention with nature's plans. But let us turn now to two common interventions which can cause situations like fetal distress or dysfunctional labor, which are then "cured" by resorting to cesarean section.

One such common intervention is the use of oxytocin for induction or stimulation of labor. The longer, harder, stronger contractions caused by oxytoxic drugs such as Pitocin are known to often cause fetal distress, by interfering with the uterine blood flow (20, 34-36). The studies of fetal monitoring in high risk groups automatically place women receiving oxytocin into their "high risk" category, even though nothing else is wrong with them (7, 16, 23, 24).

Use of oxytocin can and occasionally does cause the rupture of a perfectly healthy unscarred uterus (23, 27) resulting in an emergency cesarean section to try to save both mother and baby. Failed inductions are also a common cause of cesarean delivery (23, 27, 28).

Induced or stimulated labor is not only harder on the baby, it is much harder on the mother. Women report greatly increased pain from contractions stimulated by oxytocin, making it more likely that they will require analgesia (33, 38, 39). Since many of the drugs commonly given laboring women can cause fetal distress and-or uterine dysfunction, more cesareans are the result.

Epidurals are one of the most common ways of dealing with the pain of late first stage labor nowadays, so it is important for women to be aware of how the epidural will affect her labor (and indirectly, her baby). Epidurals slow and weaken contractions considerably for at least a half hour after each dose (40, 41). Since fresh doses are commonly given about once every 60 minutes, the result is often a drug-caused dysfunctional labor. This result is so widely recognized that many physicians routinely combine epidurals with oxytocin stimulation, hoping to counteract the effects of one drug with the other (39-40). When they do not succeed, instead of letting the epidural wear off, the patient is often sectioned for "dystocia" or "failure to dilate."

Epidurals often interfere with the flexion and descent of the baby's head during labor, probably through the mechanism of weakened or ineffectual contractions )37, 42-44). And again, instead of letting the epidural wear off and even getting the patient up and walking about, the answer is often a cesarean section for "arrested descent" or "failure to dilate."

### Greater Fear of Malpractice Suits

Jones, when asked to write on the use of cesarean section in present-day obstetrics for the American Journal of Obstetrics and Gynecology, sent questionnaires to representative medical school department chairmen, professors and practicing obstetricians in order to include their opinions (10). He says that almost 100 percent of the fifty replies he received mentioned fear of malpractice suits as one of the main reasons for the recent increase in cesarean section rates. And, indeed, physicians have good reasons for these fears. In a recent case in Virginia, $1.5 million was awarded to a four year old boy, whose parents argued that his cerebral palsy was caused by being delivered vaginally when a cesarean section was called for. (The settlement was later overturned by a higher court.)

Given that so many of the indicators for cesarean section are a matter of interpretation rather than clear cut categories, one can see why many physicians, when in doubt, might choose surgery rather than less drastic alternative measures first.

### A Curious Diurnal Variation

Because the cesarean operation is seen as safer and easier now than it was in the past, and because indications such as "failure to dilate" and "fetal distress" are often a matter of interpretation rather than simple black-or-white decisions, there is a growing concern that unnecessary surgery may be occurring among obstetrical patients as well as among other types of patients in the United States (39, 45-47). Although direct evidence of unnecessary surgery is very difficult to gather, some interesting indirect evidence is available. In some of my own research on 123 primiparous women, I found an inexplicable diurnal variation in cesarean section rates. Twenty non-elective (emergency) sections occurred in the sample, and one would expect to observe that approximately half should occur during the day and half during the night. Instead, four emergency sections were done between 8 p.m. and 7:59 a.m. while sixteen were performed during the day (8 a.m. to 7:59 p.m.). This is a large and significant difference, even in a sample as small as twenty cases. If we were observing elective (planned) cesarean sections, naturally we would expect to find most of them occurring during the working day, when there is improved anesthetic and pediatric coverage, but it is hard to understand why 80 percent of the obstetrical emergencies requiring surgery would happen during the day, while only 20 percent happened at night.

A diurnal variation was also observed in Gibbons' data on 3,489 first births in two Baltimore hospitals in the years 1968 and 1973 (5). 390 women in the above sample were delivered by cesarean section. In 1968, when the section rates were 5.4 percent in Baltimore, no diurnal variation was observed; about 50 percent of the cesareans occurred in each 12-hour period. But in 1973, when the rates had gone up to 10.2 percent, Gibbons observed that private patients showed a significant variation. 58 percent of these women were sectioned between 7 a.m. and 6:59 p.m., while only 42 percent were sectioned between 7 p.m. and 6:59 a.m. Interestingly enough, the clinic patients in her sample still showed about 50 percent cesareans during the day and 50 percent at night. Clearly, further research is needed in this critical area.

### The Effects of Surgical Birth

What difference does it make in the long run if more babies are now arriving through an abdominal incision rather than through the birth canal? Physicians, selling modern advances, tell us that cesarean surgery has never been safer for the mother and that they are saving our babies, delivering "better products", as they put it, by doing so many cesareans (23, 39, 48). Is this true? Let us look at the effects of cesarean section on mothers and babies and decide for ourselves.

### Effects of Cesarean Section on the Mother

First of all, the statement that cesareans have never been safer for the mother, simply means that the surgery is safer now than it was 20 or 50 years ago. That is certainly true. For instance, we now have antibiotics to control (but not prevent) the many infections which commonly occur after cesarean delivery. But no one has ever claimed that surgical delivery is safer for the mother than vaginal delivery. Women do still die in childbirth, although it is rare. Evrard and Gold found that the mortality rate for women delivered by cesarean section (in the 1970s) is 26 times greater than the mortality rate for women delivered vaginally (4). The morbidity is far higher also, approaching 50 percent in several reports (10, 11). That means that half of all new mothers delivered surgically have some serious illnesses such as infections or hemorrhage, etc. (49)

Douglas, reviewing data on 3,295 women with previous cesarean sections, concluded that those who had repeat sections had higher morbidity and mortality rates, and thus it was safer for a mother to have a vaginal delivery after cesarean section than to risk a repeat section (24).

Not only are 50 percent of surgically delivered women actually sick post-partum, but virtually 100 percent experience a great deal more pain, weakness, problems moving around, and difficulties in holding or caring for their newborns. In my own research, I observed that women who had been delivered by cesarean were significantly more negative about their birth experience, were much more miserable physically, required far more drugs postpartum, experienced more serious and longer lasting depression, and did not "feel like a mother", (a measure of attachment and bonding) till much later than the vaginally delivered women (50). Many other researchers have reported on the shock, deep disappointment, feelings of failure and other negative emotions experienced by cesarean mothers postpartum (48, 51, 52). Surgery is never a pleasant experience, but becoming a mother through major abdominal surgery is particularly difficult. Helpless dependent newborns cannot wait until their mothers "recover"–they need mothering at once.

### Effects of Cesarean Section on the Baby

This brings us to the baby's side of the story. Is a surgical delivery safer and easier for the fetus as some physicians claim? Or is it at least equal to a vaginal delivery? It is a difficult question to test, because when cesareans are done for complications, when you compare outcomes. it is hard to say which ones were caused by the original complications and which can be blamed on the surgical delivery itself. It has been shown that term babies delivered by cesarean section are more likely to require stimulation to begin breating, and that they have more fluid in their lungs than vaginally born babies (53).

R.D.S. (respiratory distress syndrome) is reported by many as the biggest problem of infants delivered by elective cesarean section (6, 23, 54, 55). The cause of this problem is that estimates of fetal maturity were incorrect, (i.e. the baby was premature). The problem occurs even after careful use of ultrasound and testing of the L-S ratio, the most sophisticated techniques currently available. In other words, the beginning of labor is still a more accurate indicator of when the baby is ready to be born and survive on its own, which is why European doctors, even when planning a repeat cesarean section, wait until the woman goes into labor.

In order to study the fetal outcome of being subjected to cesarean delivery,

Benson and his colleagues did their research on a group of mothers who all had repeat sections with no labor first, thus ruling out results caused by medical complications (54). Because miscalculation of fetal maturity is so common in repeat sections, Benson dropped all premature babies from his sample. Thus any differences in mortality or morbidity that he found are even more striking, because he has removed the highest risk infants from consideration. Nonetheless, he did still find significant differences. Neonatal mortality (death) was twice as high in the surgically delivered infants when compared to a vaginally delivered control group. Four times as many cesarean babies had dangerously low 5 minute Apgars (0-3 range). And at both the four-month and the one-year pediatric-neurologic exams, significant differences between the groups were found. The author states:

Reasons for favoring vaginal delivery were evident at four months and this was substantiated at the one year pediatric-neurologic examinations (54).

Cesarean delivery also requires that the mother receive fairly large amounts of drugs, which promptly affect the immature fetus, of course. Whereas, with preparation for childbirth classes and a vaginal delivery, a woman stands a very good chance of needing no drugs or only a local and thus delivering an undrugged, responsive baby. The deleterious effects of all obstetrical drugs on babies has been thoroughly documented elsewhere and does not need to be reviewed here (56-61).

### Conclusion

While cesarean sections are clearly more hazardous to the life and health of the mother, it appears that, other things being equal, delivery by cesarean is not safer for the infant either. It is time to call a halt.

### References

1. Niswander, K.R. and M. Gordon, The Women and Their Pregnancies, Philadelphia: W.B. Saunders, 1972.
2. Kroener, W.F., discussion following Hibbard, L.T., "Changing Trends in Cesarean Section," Am J Ob Gyn 125: 804, 1976.
3. Klassen, D.F., "Cesarean Section Rates: Time, Trends and Comparisons Among Hospitals Sizes, Census Regions, and Teaching and Non-teaching Hospitals," PAS Reporter 13: 1, 1975.
4. Evrard, J.R. and E.M. Gold, "Cesarean Section and Maternal Mortality in Rhode Island," Ob Gyn 50: 594, 1977.
5. Gibbons, L.K., Analysis of the Rise in C-section in Baltimore, unpublished doctoral dissertation, School of Hygiene and Public Health, the Johns Hopkins University, 1976.
6. Gluck, L., "Iatrogenic RDS and Amniocentesis," Hosp Practice (March 1977), pp. 11 - 17.
7. Haverkamp, A.D. et al., "The Evaluation of Continuous Fetal Heart Rate Monitoring in High-Risk Pregnancy," Am J Ob Gyn 125: 310, 1976.
8. Lee. W.K. and M.S. Baggish, "The Effect of Unselected Intrapartum Fetal Monitoring," Ob Gyn 47: 516, 1976.
9. Tutera, G. and R.L. Newman, "Fetal Monitoring: Its Effect on the Perinatal Mortality and Cesarean Section Rates and Its Complications," Am J Ob Gyn 122: 750, 1975.

10. Jones, O.H., "Cesarean Section in Present-Day Obstetrics," Am J Ob Gyn 126: 521, 1976.
11. Hibbard, L.T., "Changing Trends in Cesarean Section," Am J Ob Gyn 125: 798, 1976.
12. Hughey, M.J. et al., "The Effect of Fetal Monitoring on the Incidence of Cesarean Section." Ob Gyn 49: 513, 1977.
13. Koh, K.S. et al., "Experience with Fetal Monitoring in a University Teaching Hospital," Ob Gyn Survey (Sept. 1972), p. 594.
14. Paul, R.H. et al., "Clinical Fetal Monitoring: Its Effect on Cesarean Section Rate and Perinatal Mortality: Five Year Trends," Postgrad Med 61: 160, 1977.
15. Wunderlich, C., "Cesarean Deliveries Increasing," ICEA News 15: 1, 1976.
16. Shenker, L. et al., "Routine Electronic Monitoring of Fetal Heart Rate and Uterine Activity During Labor," Ob Gyn 46: 185, 1975.
17. Starkman, M. "Psychological Responses to the Use of the Fetal Monitor During Labor," Psycho Med 38: 269, 1976.
18. Kane, S. "Advancing Age and the Primigravida," Ob Gyn 29: 409, 1967
19. Shapiro, S. et al. Infant, Perinatal, Maternal and Childhood Mortality in the United States, Cambridge: Harvard University Press, 1968.
20. Hausknecht, R. and J.R. Heilman, Having a Cesarean Baby, New York: Dutton, 1978.
21. Friedman, E.A. "Primigravid Labor: a Graphicostatistical Analysis," Ob Gyn 6: 567, 1955.
22. Friedman, E.A. "Patterns of Labor as Indicators of Risk," Clin Ob Gyn 16: 172, 1973.
23. Sutherst, J.R. and B.D. Case, "Cesarean Section and Its Place in the Active Approach to Delivery," Clinics in Ob Gyn 2: 241, 1975.
24. Douglas, R.G. "Pregnancy and Labor Following Cesarean Section" in Reid and Barton (eds), Controversy in Obstetrics and Gynecology, Philadelphia: W.B. Saunders, 1969.
25. Donavan, B. The Cesarean Birth Experience, Boston: Beacon Press, 1977.
26. Kuah, K.B. "Labour and Delivery after Caesarean Section," Aust N Z Ob Gyn 10: 145, 1970.
27. McGarry, J.A. "The Management of Patients Previously Delivered by Cesarean Section," Ob Gyn Brit Comm 76: 137, 1969.
28. Morewood, G.A. et al., "Vaginal Delivery after Cesarean Section," Ob Gyn 42: 589, 1973.
29. Ranade, V.R. et al., "Analysis of Labor Following Previous Cesarean Section," J Postgrad Med 18: 79, 1972.
30. McGaughey, H.S. et al., "Pregnancy and Labor Following Cesarean Section," in Reid and Barton (eds.), Controversy in Obstetrics and Gynecology. Philadelphia: W.B. Saunders, 1969.
31. Pauerstein, C.J., "Once a Section, Always a Trial of Labor?" Ob Gyn 28: 273, 1966.
32. Turnbull, A.C. "Introduction" to Card and Richards (eds.) Benefits and Hazards of the New Obstetrics. Philadelphia: Lippincott, 1977.
33. Dunn, P.M. "Obstetric Delivery Today: for Better or for Worse?" Lancet (April 10, 1976), p. 790.
34. Alvarez, H. et al., "Induction of Labor - Part II," J Reprod Med 6: 17, 1971.
35. Fields, H. "Complications of Elective Induction," Ob Gyn 16: 476, 1960.
36. Editorial: "A Time to be Born," Lancet (November 16, 1974) p. 1183.
37. Beacham, W.D. et al., "Rupture of the Uterus at New Orleans Charity Hospital," Am J Ob Gyn 106: 1083, 1970.
38. Kitzinger, S. "Effects of Induction on the Mother-Baby Relationship," practitioner 217: 263, 1976.

39. Randal, J. "Too Many Cesareans?" Parents (November 1978) p. 72.
40. Henry, J.S. et al., "The Effect of Epidural Anesthesia on Oxytocin-Induced Labor," Am J Ob Gyn 97: 350, 1967.
41. Lowensohn, R.I. et al. "Intrapartum Epidural Anesthesia: an Evaluation of the Effects on Uterine Activity," Ob Gyn 47: 129, 1976.
42. Friedman, E.A. and M.R. Sachtleben, "Station of the Fetal Presenting Part: Arrest of Descent in Nulliparas," Ob Gyn 47: 129, 1976.
43. Holt, J. et al., "Lumbar Epidural Analgesia in Labour: Relation to Fetal Malposition and Instrumental Delivery," Brit Med J 1: 14, 1977.
44. Ralston, D.S. and S.M. Shnider, "The Fetal and Neonatal Effects of Regional Anesthesia in Obstetrics," Anesthesiology 48: 34, 1978.
45. Clark, M. et al., "Too Much Surgery?" Newsweek (April 10, 1978) p. 65.
46. Bombardier, C. et al., "Socioeconomic Factors Affecting the Utilization of Surgical Operations," N E J Med 297: 699, 1977.
47. De Jong, R.H. "Too Many Surgeons?" J A M A 237: 267, 1977.
48. Brody, J.E. "Personal Health" N Y Times (March 8, 1978) p. 22.
49. Editorial: "Complications of Cesarean to Mother" B F J 4: 103, 1977.
50. Doering, S.G. and D.R. Entwisle, The First Birth. Final Report to NIMH, August 1977.
51. Affonso, D.D. and J.F. Stichler, "Exploratory Study of Women's Reactions to Having a Cesarean Birth," B F J 5: 88, 1978.
52. Cohen, N.W. "Minimizing Emotional Sequellae of Cesarean Childbirth," B F J 4: 114, 1977.
53. Saunders. R.A. and A.D. Milner, "Pulmonary Pressure-Volume Relationships During the Last Phase of Delivery and the First Postnatal Breaths in Human Subjects," J Ped 93: 667, 1978.
54. Benson, R.C. et al., "Fetal Compromise During Elective Cesarean Section," Am J Ob Gyn 91: 645, 1965.
55. Hack, M. et al., "Neonatal Respiratory Distress Following Elective Delivery. A Preventable Disease?" Am J Ob Gyn 126: 43, 1976.
56. Abrahamson, K. and I. Joelsson, "The Effect of Pharmacological Agents Upon the Fetus and Newborn," Am J Ob Gyn 96: 437, 1966.
57. Aleksandrowicz, M.K., "The Effect of Pain Relieving Drugs Administered During Labor and Delivery on the Behavior of the Newborn," Merr-Palm Q 20: 121, 1974.
58. American Academy of Pediatrics: "Effect of Medication During Labor and Delivery on Infant Outcome," Peds 62: 402, 1978.
59. Ralston, D.H. and S.M. Shnider, "The Fetal and Neonatal Effects of Regional Anesthesia in Obstetrics," Anesthesiology 48: 34, 1978.
60. Scanlon, J.W. "Effects of Local Anesthetics Administered to Parturient Women on the Neurological and Behavioral Performance of Newborn Children," Bull N Y Acad Med 2: 231, 1976.
61. Standley, K. et al., "Local-Regional Anesthesia During Childbirth: Effect on Newborn Behaviors," Science 186: 634, 1974.

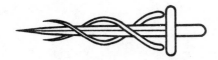

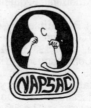

# CHAPTER SEVENTEEN

## WHAT EVERY PREGNANT WOMAN SHOULD KNOW ABOUT CESAREANS

### Lynne R. Browne

### Preface

This article comes as an attempt to work out my feelings about what I now consider to be a cesarean that was perhaps caused by labor intervention and was certainly due to lack of support and sensitivity to the essence of the birth experience.

I began pregnancy enjoying my changing body (even when it meant nausea) because I sensed a deep inner connection between my baby and me, and me and the universe. As my "belly" grew, my sensitivity grew. I dreamed of a birth surrounded by love and togetherness, awe and celebration.

My labor began irregularly after a few "false labors", and in order to keep me calm about "When is this baby coming?" I entered the hospital. My membranes were artificially ruptured at about four centimeters. I was then attached to a fetal monitor and given oxygen. My labor was intense, and like every other labor, difficult at times. But I cannot remember a time that I reached such spiritual awareness and connection as I did while my body was within the force of giving birth.

Then came transition and pushing. I pushed for three and a half hours (although I later read in the operative report that I was only dilated to nine centimeters), flat on my back, with no one attempting to answer my questions or support me in any way. When I was told they would do a cesarean, I was grateful to know the baby would come out. Finally, someone was going to do something for me!

Only, days....months....years later I am left to struggle with the loneliness, the disconnection of my body from me, my baby from me, my husband from me, my very being from the universe. The price one pays for technology and for releasing one's own responsibility for one's own body to a stranger!

I write this article hoping that I can alleviate some of my own pain, to know that other women will not suffer from the same lack of education, and therefore lack of responsibility, for the birth of their own babies--that they themselves will give birth (not the doctor) joyously--connected to and loved by all who are present at the birth of new life.

### The Role of Childbirth Classes

In most "natural" childbirth classes rarely are the truly psychic changes that birthing women experience discussed fully and openly. Childbirth education needs to become more than breathing techniques and a discussion of labor and birth physiology. Labor is not simply dilatation and expulsion, as most medical texts would have us believe. It is, in fact, a total human experience--physical,

Lynn R. Browne is co-founder of the Central New Hampshire Cesarean Educational Alliance and a childbirth educator teaching classes to former cesarean couples who want to have a subsequent vaginal birth. Ms. Browne is mother of two--the first by cesarean and the second vaginally.

intellectual, emotional and spiritual. And in order to understand the process we must educate ourselves in all aspects.

At the same time we need to reexamine our jargon and philosophy. Quite often the expression, "stay in control" is used by educators and parents alike when describing the optimum labor experience. I suggest that no one is ever "in control"–that we were never meant to be–that the force of labor is the true controller. Like the tides of the sea, the waves come upon us–and we can choose to either scream for our lives or flow with them, "To stay in control" is only our human fallacious attempt of gaining power over the all-encompassing force of nature–of staying in control of our own mortality. May I suggest in place of control, we choose to "let go"–to let go of our fears, our egos, and our very desire to control. To let go of our self-consciousness that we may be lifted by the birthing experience to a level of consciousness we have never before attained. For there is, oh, so much more, than dilatation and expulsion!

With the intensity of the entire natural birthing experience in mind, let us now consider the ultimate unnatural birthing experience–cesarean section. In recent years, with the rise in cesarean rates all across the country, many "natural" childbirth educators are now including "cesarean education" in their class series. Cesarean education usually includes a discussion of indication, methods and procedures used during preparation, operation, and recovery. The idea here is that if a woman is "prepared" to have the natural birth experience taken away from her she won't experience the anger, guilt, or serious depression often resulting from unexpected cesareans. Though there is no doubt that it is always better to be prepared for any experience, I question the validity for what we prepare these women. For which is the better adjustment–to be "educated" to accept any cesarean regardless of its cause as simply an alternative method of childbirth, or to be educated to be a discerning client about necessary and unnecessary procedures, interferences, and operations–taking on the responsibility for one's own life, and in particular, one's own birthing experience?

It is my premise that the psychic phenomenon of birth, the medical interventions in the normal process, and the ultimate interference–cesarean section — are deeply interconnected. We can no longer afford to ignore that relationship. The purpose of this article, then, is to bring this subject to the forefront in the minds of all concerned with the experience of childbirth.

### The Cesarean Emergency Scene

Emergency! Fetal monitor registers less than 60 beats per minute! The doctors and nurses fly into action. General anesthesia, classical incision--a much-needed cesarean section–Birth! APGAR score - ONE! Still more rushing–to the neonatal center half-way across the state. Three weeks later–healthy baby home with Mom and Dad. Another miracle of modern medicine!

In recent years the cesarean birth rate has climbed from a mere 2-4 per cent to a national average that is presently above 12 per cent, and approaching 30 per cent in some big city hospitals. Why? Can it be true that suddenly in the past ten years so many of the women in this country are not capable of giving birth to their own babies?

If a choice could be made without endangering the life of herself or her baby, a mother would, almost without exception, choose to give birth herself. This instinct to give birth comes from a power deep within the psyche of the birthing woman. However, its balance is delicate and can be easily interfered with, often resulting in cesarean sections. Along with knowledge about the technical aspects of childbearing, doctors, nurses, midwives, childbirth educators, and especially the expectant couples themselves must take on the responsibility of knowing and teaching about this delicate balance, and the possible consequences of interfering with it. Only then will an expectant parent be truly "prepared" for the total experience of birth.

With this in mind, let's begin this cesarean birth story again--this time at the beginning.

Mother reports leaking membranes to the doctor, who tells her to go for a walk to bring on contractions. Forty-eight hours later, still no contractions....into the hospital to be induced (standard practice to avoid infection). Pitocin drip, fetal monitor. Head is high....Bandal's ring (oxygen to fetus through the placenta is cut off due to very strong contractions, particularly common with induced labor when head is not yet engaged). Fetus aspirates meconium, heart rate drops to 60.

Could this cesarean, and even more importantly, the actual indication for the cesarean, have been avoided? Indeed, what was the cause of the drop in the fetal heart rate? Bandal's ring. Labor was induced before the baby's head was engaged. The balance of the timing of the birth was interfered with. Induction was an unnecessary interference in the natural process of the birth. True, leaking membranes can increase the chance of infection. However, a woman can be instructed as to the necessary measures to avoid infection (such as no intercourse, no baths, no crowds, no internal exams, remaining in her "home" environment), and to conscientiously take her temperature every four hours so that if infection did occur, then the necessary measures of induction or cesarean could be taken immediately. I know of one woman whose water broke who received and followed the above instructions from her midwife, and gave birth over a month later to a healthy vibrant baby. It is possible that labor interferences such as induction, often-times done to avoid problems which in fact do not yet exist, may be primary causes of indications for cesarean delivery!

Now let's say you are in labor, and find yourself in the following situations:

### Induction of Labor

What will you do if your doctor wants to induce your labor? In most cases induction is an unnecessary interference--an interference which can be quite dangerous. Other than induction to avoid infection (discussed above), "reasons" for inducing labor are: convenience for the mother, convenience for the doctor, over-due (remembering that the due date is only a calculated guess, not an unequivocal fact), and slow progress or lack of progress (otherwise known as "uterine inertia").

There are generally two types of induction: artificial rupture of membranes, and pitocin (artificial hormone stimulation). Artificial rupture of membranes removes the natural cushion surrounding the fetus which protects him from the pressure of labor contractions. Therefore the fetus is more likely to develop signs of fetal distress following artificial rupture of membranes. Pitocin wafers or drip is usually used when rupture of membranes fails to stimulate contractions adequately. Because it is artificial and not produced by the mother's body, neither the mother nor the baby are prepared for the birth. Both react with distress. Instead of a mother feeling a greater sense of trust of her body, she trusts technology and IV's. This undermines the instinctual process of birth--instead of curing "uterine inertia" we cause "mind inertia". And finally, cesarean section for failure to progress or fetal distress result.

I cannot emphasize enough the fact that all of these "reasons" for induction are simply man's way of attempting to control the truly uncontrollable forces of labor. We want to predict and control when labor will happen and how fast it will happen. In general, Western man sees himself in a constant "battle" with nature, and he will win only when the whims of nature are conquered. Perhaps we might do better to review our position within nature: that we are dependent upon nature, and can only "win" by becoming more in touch with ourselves and the universe in which we live. Within the realm of birth, then, perhaps we might do better to accept that as long as the mother is healthy and the fetal heart tones are strong, that nature is a far better controller than man.

## Cervical Dilation and State of Mind

How will you assure that the psycho-spiritual climate created by your birth attendants remains positive towards you and the type of birth you wish to give?

As labor becomes more intense, the mother's focus becomes more and more within. As the cervix dilates (as she "opens up" physically), the mind dilates (she "opens up" psychologically). The protective walls which normally act as a filter of thoughts and vibrations (feelings), drop away--she is left totally open to all psychic vibrations. If those she is with truly love and support her, this openness is a great asset to the progress of her labor and her ability to give birth in a more open and relaxed environment. But if her birth attendants or nurses are ambivalent, or, even worse, negative towards the mother or her ideas of birth, the psycho-spiritual climate can be devastating. Husbands, especially be aware of the psychic energy present with your wife! During intense labor all her energy is focused on getting the baby out, and she can no longer think clearly about outside matters. (If someone told her they were going to throw her out the window to help the baby to be born, she would probably say, "That'll be fine.") Therefore, you, as her husband and most beloved birth attendant, must take on the responsibility of protection for both her and the child. All those present at a birth need to tune into the force of energy which brings life into this world.

## Fetal Monitors

What will you do if your labor is "normal", but the doctor wishes to attach the fetal heart monitor as a matter of routine? Let us first remember that such advances in technology were created for monitoring high risk labors, and proved to be a great asset. However, it does not necessarily follow that what is good for high risk birth will be even better for normal labors.

The most damaging effect of the monitor is that it diminishes the mother's trust of her own body, her own feelings, her own instincts, replacing that trust with a trust of machines. To be attached to a machine denies one's humanity, one's connection to the universe, and to the force which holds that universe together--the very force which is the true controller of the labors of all mothers bringing new life into this world. In other words, in being connected to a machine, the mother loses touch with the force of her labor, with herself--an interference of great significance.

In addition to the psychological effects of the monitor, it is physically uncomfortable (painful at times), confines you to bed at a time when it is important to move about, and can be easily misread.

We might also do well to consider the possible effects of the monitor on the birthing child. The most "fool-proof" monitor is the internal one. In order to be attached, the membranes must be ruptured. (We have already discussed the possible correlation of rupture of membranes and fetal distress). Do the electrodes implanted in the scalp of the baby cause unnecessary additional pain to the already difficult process of being born?

Finally, the supposed purpose to fetal monitors is to avoid severely distressed babies, thereby having "better babies" by performing emergency cesareans, whenever the heart rate drops below the "safe" level. However, although the cesarean rate in the United States has increased to such appalling percentages, the United States is still 15th in the modern world for maternal-infant mortality. If the fetal monitor and cesarean sections were really so effective, I would hope that the maternal-infant death rate would reflect that effectiveness.

### Prolonged Second Stage

What will you do if second stage is prolonged, and a cesarean is suggested? The controversial question involved here is, "What constitutes a prolonged and dangerous second stage?" The medical establishment usually defines prolonged as any labor in which there is "failure to progress" after "X" hours. This attitude places the mother under tremendous pressure; and birth was not meant to be a "pressure" event. In contrast, for most midwives, as long as the fetal tones remain strong, a mother is supported and encouraged with almost ritual instinctual vocalizing, gentle massaging, and helped to find positions which are comfortable and effective.

This attitude of support and encouragement in contrast to one of tremendous pressure to perform is probably the most significant factor in a mother's ability to give birth safely without interferences. Without this support women become more easily discouraged, tune into their exhaustion rather than their purpose, and tend to totally give up–to ask for the "help" of the hospital such as medication, anesthesia, forceps and even cesareans! Of course, they are seeking help, but perhaps the help they really seek is emotional attention and support.

In order to cope with this lack of support, expectant parents anticipating a hospital birth must know more, understand more, and trust themselves even more than perhaps a home birth couple. The greatest second stage preparation a couple can give themselves is understanding that hospitals often treat second stage as if it were totally disconnected from first stage. However, we must be aware that although the function and feeling of second stage contractions are totally different, the same principles of relaxation, trust in oneself, and instinct to give birth apply to second stage as well as first stage labor.

Let's now deal with some of the particulars of second stage. Most Lamaze courses teach that the cervix must be fully dilated in order to start pushing. Even that basic education teaches couples of the danger of pushing too soon. Yet in many hospitals today doctors are instructing a woman to begin pushing even though her cervix has not reached full dilation (as long as push contractions are present). This is an incredibly dangerous policy that can lead to cervical tears, cervical edema, and cesarean sections (indication–failure to progress, cephalo-pelvic disproportion). Obviously, there can be no progress–as the pressure on the cervix from bearing down will not allow the cervix to dilate that last centimeter, and the presenting part of the baby cannot pass through a nine-centimeter pelvimetry. Therefore, what may appear to be cephalo-pelvic disproportion (CPD) may in fact be "pushing too soon." The difficulty here in terms of coping with this situation is that very few couples have the experience to recognize full dilation. Therefore they must ask knowledgeable and direct questions about the progress of her labor and the amount of dilation, and make the final decision themselves regarding when she will begin pushing. In order to do this, the mother must listen closely to her body. Does it seem like it is time to start pushing, or do you feel you could wait a little longer? Many midwives ask the laboring mother to wait til she can wait no longer--thereby assuring full dilation.

The next area of understanding is how to push. In some classes we are taught to curl around the baby and push with all our might. However, it is possible to push incorrectly, or too hard. Once again, we must be guided primarily by our inner feelings. How does my body want to push? Shiela Kitzinger, midwife in England for many years, says that a mother should never push, only lean (implied in that statement is trusting one's own body, trusting the force of nature that will bring this baby into the world, and relaxation of the mother with this force.) Ina May, midwife on The Farm in Tennessee, says, "A lady should push with a soft mouth--a relaxed mouth means a relaxed puss." Birth attendants can aid a mother's relaxation with strong positive psychic vibrations, lots of close contact, massage of tensing pussies, and warm compresses and gentle massage of the perineum.

Position is also a factor in second stage effectiveness. NEVER lie flat on your back. The traditional Lamaze position (partial sitting) is good for many women. However, hands and knees position is great for posterior presentation because it takes the pressure off the spine. Posterior babies usually take longer as the presenting part is larger. Squatting is the most effective for very prolonged second stage labors--the position actually enlarges the pelvic opening by one to one and a half centimeters. Plus, you have the added advantage of gravity being with you.

Finally, don't be afraid to "make noise". It is false to believe that making noise indicates that you are "out of control". The grunts and groans, and primal sounds many women hear coming from their mouths may seem to be shocking and embarrassing. On the contrary--they are the beautiful sounds, the "right" sounds, the instinctual sounds that make our every sense aware that the birth of a new life is imminent.

### Breech

What will you do if the baby is in breech position? It is sometimes possible to externally turn a baby, but often it is not. You will then be faced with a big decision: schedule a cesarean? Wait for the onset of labor, then perform a cesarean? Or attempt a vaginal delivery? The advantage (and, believe it or not, you do have an advantage) to this situation is that the birthing couple is now able to make the choice while their minds are still relatively clear (before the onset of labor). It is most important to realize that you truly do have a choice, that although a breech delivery is in fact more difficult for mother, baby, and doctor, that many babies have successfully entered this world bottom first. The couple must weigh the importance of vaginal delivery against the difficulty of breech presentation. If you then choose a cesarean, you have a period of adjustment in which you can come to terms with and accept a cesarean in place of a vaginal delivery. (You can expect something close to what you will get). You are also in a position to "bargain" with the doctor and hospital about the atmosphere of the cesarean birth.

## Cephalo-Pelvic Disproportion (CPD)

What if during one of your pre-natal exams the doctor feels that the size of your baby and the measurement of your pelvis are disproportionate (CPD) and he wants to schedule a cesarean? First, realize that cephalo pelvis measurements are educated guesses. Although better than an uneducated guess, the true test of disproportion cannot be made until it is time to push that baby through the pelvis. (See discussion of prolonged second stage). Once again, it is a decision to be weighed; and the couple has the advantage of being informed of the possibilities prior to labor.

Other indications for cesarean section, such as placenta previa, prolapsed cord, and abruptio placenta are life endangering situations to mother and-or baby. At these times we can be very grateful for the skill of trained obstetricians and the modern technology of safe cesarean sections. However, as these situations are not usually known in advance, all expectant parents should not only prepare themselves, their doctor and their hospital for the kind of natural birth they want, but also should make arrangements in advance in case an emergency cesarean is truly necessary, to have the best possible cesarean experience — father with mother in OR, spinal or epidural anesthesia, mirrors in OR, baby held and touched by both parents in the OR, baby examined within the sight of the parents, baby with parents in recovery room, rooming in (with the aid of father, friend, or nurse). For try as we may, everything does not always go our way.

But I wish to emphasize that my point is that pregnant couples anticipating natural births must be informed about cesarean births (their indication, and the possible correlation of labor interferences with cesarean indications) — so that true choices can be made by each couple. For we can holler and stammer all we want about hospital policies and patients' rights, but only the informed client (not patient, for she is not sick — only having a baby), can be knowledgeable enough to make her own decisions about the birth of their child. The uninformed don't know enough to know what questions to ask. It is our responsibility therefore to ask the questions while there is still time to read and think, and make a true choice before labor begins.

## Conclusion

Labor is not time for gathering information and making decisions. It is time to swim with the current, ride with the waves — to let go of all thoughts, all words, all controls — to listen to the force from within. Giving birth is the time machine thrusting us back before words ever existed, to our instincts — our instincts would guide us through had we not been civilized. But now we have the subconscious to interfere with the instinct. The fears we hold hidden deep within us, are not cleared away by any man made technique no matter how complex. We must look beyond technique. We must look within ourselves, prepare our spirits for the coming birth of our child. For, like it or not, we will be returned to the primal sea — the birth of our very existence. The power of the universe is laid upon every woman as she bears her child. The awesomeness of that power can be frightening; or it can bring the birthing woman to a plane of existence she has never before touched.

For more information on cesareans, how to avoid them and how to cope with them should you have one, write: Cesarean Educational Alliance, Journey's End Rd., Francestown, NH 03043 (603) 547-2095

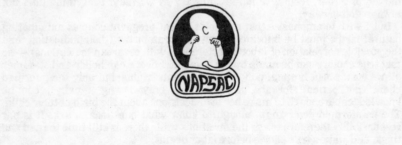

# CHAPTER EIGHTEEN

## VAGINAL BIRTH AFTER PREVIOUS CESAREAN SECTION
### BY J.R. McTammany, M.D.

Our interest in vaginal deliveries for previously sectioned mothers has been rewarding and productive. I first became seriously interested in 1977 when I heard an Audio-Digest tape upon which Dr. Berkeley S. Merrill from San Antonio, Texas, discussed their experience with their technique. Another report of the same material appeared in a 1978 issue of OB-GYN News by Dr. Charles E. Gibbe — a co-worker.

On this service, previously sectioned patients are allowed to labor and attempt vaginal delivery if their section was done with a transverse low cervical incision and if there was a normal post-operative course free of infection. The patient need not have had a previous vaginal delivery. About half of their patients achieved a successful vaginal delivery, the others being sectioned again for the usual indications. The uterine rupture rate was 0.5 percent, not the 3 percent we are taught. In those cases where the uterus did rupture, it was not a catastrophic event with pain, bleeding and shock, such as one might see in a primary uterine rupture. It was rather a relatively quiet disruption of the old scar. Diagnosis was at times uncertain, the only clue being a cessation of progress. Uterine rupture did not necessitate hysterectomy. Perinatal mortality was the same in both groups. After over 600 such cases, they are satisfied to continue their program, feeling that it represents a tremendous cost savings for consumers, that it obviates considerable morbidity which would be associated with so many repeat sections, and that it affords the successful couples great satisfaction.

In our hospital we have been doing the same thing for 18 months now and have had 24 previously sectioned couples attempt a vaginal delivery. We did not exclude patients with a previous diagnosis of CPD, feeling that many of these were more likely to have been dysfunctional labors, either intrinsically or due to medication or anxiety. In all patients we did insist that they be in the hospital. We used an IV to have a vein ready and we cross-matched blood in case it might be needed. Initially we monitored all patients, but we do it more selectively now. We have the operating room alerted for a "stat" section, but we try to "play down" their aspect of things in order to help the couple have a normal experience. We conduct the delivery in our birth rooms just the same as our regular patients, with bonding, quietness and dignity. Siblings are present, if the couple so desires.

In our small series, the results have been the same as that for the Texas group: Half have delivered vaginally and half have been sectioned for new primary indications. Those delivered vaginally were indistinguishable from the usual vaginally-delivered patients, except for our added measure of joy and release, as one might expect. These patients were mainly those previously

---

J.R. McTammany, M.D., is in private practice in obstetrics and gynecology and has incorporated midwifery and out-of-hospital alternatives into his services.

sectioned for fetal indications, malpresentation or prolonged rupture of the membranes.

The patients who were re-sectioned were largely patients who were first sectioned for dysfunctional labor or "CPD" — a diagnosis which we feel is actually more often a problem with dysfunctional myometrical activity. It seems that in this group of patients there is some intrinsic mal-function of the neuro-muscular activity of the myometrium. If such a hypothesis is true, it would not be surprising to see many of these patients experience the same outcome in a subsequent labor.

The re-sectioned couples, as a group, were not remorseful, but rather very grateful to have had the opportunity to "give it a try." Their post-operative adjustment to the circumstances was easy. We do employ a policy of having couples be together in the operating room for childbirth and letting them hold their babies for bonding. This accomplishes a great deal to preserve the fundamental significance of childbirth. At the end of this article is a reprint of a handout from our service going more into detail on the "Family-Centered Cesarean Birth."

We have had no problems at all with our program so far. There have been no ruptured uteri, or any other complications out of the ordinary.

We have offered vaginal delivery to a number of couples previously sectioned who decided to go ahead with a repeat section. They fear having a long hard labor, only to be sectioned again. They fear the need for an emergency section which would require general anesthesia, when they want to be awake. They are mindful of the fact that the medical profession generally does not approve of this practice. And finally, they are happy that their husbands may be present, take pictures and hold the baby in the operating room.

To quote Dr. Gibbe, we are not "evangelistic" about it. The procedure has settled down and become a comfortable part of our over-all practice. We employ it without anxiety when it is appropriate to do so, and this seems to us to be as it should be. We view it as another large step in the direction of making our methods of medical practice sensitive to the needs and feelings of our child-bearing couples. Their strong endorsement of the practice, and the lack of serious problems, has been rewarding to us and allows us to recommend it for practitioners elsewhere.

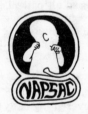

The following Appendix is taken from a leaflet given to couples planning a birth at Community General Hospital where Dr. McTammany is Chief of Ob.

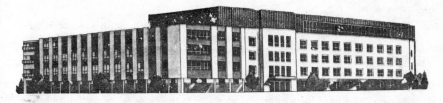

# COMMUNITY GENERAL HOSPITAL
145 North Sixth St., Reading, Pa. 19601 • Phone (215) 376-4881

Reading's Downtown Hospital  •  The Patient Is Our First Priority

## APPENDIX

### FAMILY-CENTERED CESAREAN BIRTH

Beginning in 1975, Community General Hospital in Reading, Pennsylvania developed a program of "Family-Centered Cesarean Birth." Briefly stated, this means allowing a parturient's husband or S.O.P. (significant other person) to be present in the operating room during her cesarean section so that the couple and their newborn child may share the birth experience.

Following is an outline of the procedure we have worked out over the years and presently employ. The couple is given as much explanation prior to the section as time permits. In "stat" sections where there is very little time, the father is still taken along if he wants to go, and explanations are given later. When the patient is taken to the O.R., her husband is taken to the doctor's dressing room where he changes clothes and waits until the induction of anesthesia (usually spinal) is completed. He is then brought into the O.R. and seated on a stool by his wife's left shoulder beside the anesthesiologist. The I.V. and B.P. cuff are both on the patient's right arm so her left arm and hand are free to use for maintaining contact with her husband, and later caressing her baby. The husband is invited to stand if he wishes, and watch or photograph all he chooses. Most of the time, however, they choose to remain seated except for the moment of birth.

When the baby is born, it is expeditiously suctioned and wrapped in a warm blanket. Care is taken to cover the child's head so heat loss from the wet scalp is reduced. Then the infant is placed in the arms of his father. The father then takes the child to his wife, and the three of them spend the next 20 or 30 minutes getting acquainted. Non-urgent chores such as wiping-off, footprinting, eye treatments and cord care are all delayed until after initial bonding is satisfactorily completed. Those procedures only upset the baby at a time when it needs the closeness and reassurance of his parents. When the baby feels safe and settled, these matters may be tended to, and the child is not usually as upset by them. Only significant medical problems alter this routine. Nevertheless, in almost every case, the couple may have just a few moments to hold and see the child — so very important! In some cases, their precious liberty taken was the only time a little premie was held warm and alive by its parents. It is unlikely that these few seconds would significantly jeopardize an infant's prognosis, and yet they mean so much to the couples.

Among their usual duties, the staff often help also with picture taking when couples plan pictures. When this initial phase of bonding is complete and the baby is ready, the nurse takes the child to the nursery. The father is given the choice of going along or staying in the O.R. until the operation is completed. Most elect to stay, even when their wife is asleep, but a few go to the nursery — especially if they are feeling a little "undone" by the whole affair.

Upon completion of the surgery, mothers go to the recovery room for an hour or so, and then back to their room where they have their baby and nurse if they desire. Some mothers who are feeling and doing well elect to skip the recovery room and go directly to their own room so they may have their baby sooner. Most do, however, require a period of time in the recovery room, and they are generally satisfied, having experienced good bonding in the O.R.

The post-operative routine is generally left to the guided discretion of the couple. Many recuperate with remarkable rapidity and go home in two or three days. Some choose rooming in and all basically care for their babies the same as mothers delivered vaginally.

We have felt that in cases where the patient is given a general anesthetic, it is even more important for her husband to be there because his eyes will serve as her eyes, as he later describes it all to her and fills in this blank area of her memory on this most significant event. Also, he bears the full responsibility for "Parent-Infant Bonding," which is so very important for all of them

We perform this type of childbirth once or twice a week, and have delivered hundreds of babies this way. Our experience has been overwhelmingly positive. We have seen no increase in infection, either infant, maternal, or among other O.R. patients. The only negative factor has been two or three fathers who experienced syncope. They sat down outside the O.R. briefly, and then returned to resume their duties. Curiously, most of these cases have been in husbands going in for their second section. With this exception, everyone including staff, doctors and couples have had a very positive and fulfilling experience. The babies also obviously have enjoyed it because they usually open their eyes, look around and are very contented, crying only when they are taken from their parents. From the standpoint of bonding and satisfaction on the part of the parents and baby, the results are the same as achieved in the delivery room — the surgery seemingly secondary and "behind the curtain." In fact, the intensity of the bonding and outpouring of mother's love often seems even greater, as all in the O.R. are trying to hold back tears.

The very active role taken by the parents in such a childbirth seems to be responsible for their accelerated post-operative course as they just continue the natural process of caring for their new baby. It has approximately halved the average length of stay for section patients and has prepared them much better for their new roles.

It should be pointed out that every one of these deliveries is different, as one would expect. Some work out beautifully and some are a bit of a struggle. The surgeon must add to the many things on his mind an additional concern — namely the husband and how he is doing. The others in the O.R., likewise, must be aware of and sensitive to additional factors. All of us here have had a good experience, however, and really enjoy sharing the joy of the couples. It makes us feel good to think that we have had a part in providing such a unique and fulfilling opportunity for the couples. We feel proud when they give us that certain look and a really sincere "thanks."

People drive from hundreds of miles away to have "Family-Centered Cesarean Birth" here. Many cards and letters are one measure of the success of the program. The Board and Medical Staff of the hospital have never regretted undertaking this bold program, and they recommend it for any group who want to provide and enjoy something very special in the field of obstetrics.

*J.R. Mc Tammany*

J.R. Mc Tammany M.D.
Chief, OB-GYN
Community General Hospital
Reading, Pennsylvania

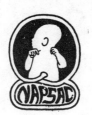

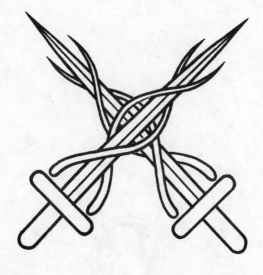

For parents concerned about how to avoid an unnecessary cesarean, see previous Chapters in this Volume by Doering & Browne. For information on emotional support for cesarean couples, see chapter in Volume Three by Drucker & Hoogerwerf, pp. 825-830.

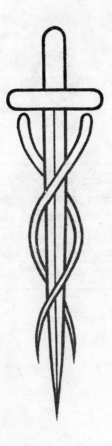

# Hospital Practice

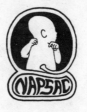

# CHAPTER NINETEEN

## HOW HOSPITALS DISRUPT THE PROCESS OF FAMILY BONDING

### Sheila Kitzinger

We may be in danger of approaching 'bonding' as if it were a kind of magic glue which makes a mother and baby stick together. It is being thought of by some as if the obstetrician can present a child to a mother and if he does it in the right way, gets a super-fixative, a special chemical adhesive which becomes active only under certain conditions. So much concern is now being shown about the way in which the mother bonds with the baby in the first hour after birth that we are even getting "the baby basher detectives" watching mothers carefully to see if they are doing the right things and responding in the "correct" way. I believe that this is yet another obstetric routine which stops women from being themselves, from feeling what comes naturally and doing what they want to do.

It very often happens that after a woman has delivered her baby she needs time to "become herself" again, to feel her separateness from the baby before she can reach out her arms to it. For many women that is a perfectly normal phase through which they pass in the moments after birth.

I believe profoundly that birth is a sexual experience, or that it can be, not only for the mother but also for the father. After any intense sexual experience there comes a time which we might call that of "recollection." Orgasm involves a psycho-physiological "ascent" to climax, attainment of the peak, release, and then a time following when the two bodies draw back and are separate from each other after the passion, before they reach out to touch each other in a new tenderness. Something very similar frequently happens after childbirth too. After the birth passion of the second stage a mother should be permitted to follow her own rhythms. She may not be ready immediately to reach out to touch her baby. (I say this even though I have myself helped to draw my own babies out of my body and have never needed that separateness to "be myself" again).

In hospitals today a woman is subjected to so many indignities, so many things are done to her, such a variety of machines fixed onto her, that she may have a great need to "find herself" again.

We sometimes get a very fragmented, mechanized view of the basic attachment processes between human beings when "bonding" is adopted as official hospital policy. It is infinitely more subtle than glue. It can and should exist not only between mother and baby but between father and baby, for as

---

Sheila Kitzinger is a childbirth educator, social anthropologist, international lecturer, former teacher, University of Edinburgh, author or coauthor of numerous works including the books, "The Experience of Childbirth," and "The Place of Birth." Her latest major work is a study of maternity hospitals and women's experiences in them to be published by Fontana, London, in 1979, under the title of "The Good Birth Guide." An authority on hospital practices, particularly in Great Britain, she has also given birth to her own children at home.

each child is born into the world there is born not only a new human being but a new family. It is not enough to get babies born safely. It is not enough even that a mother feels that the baby is hers. We must also provide an environment in which both parents feel safe to be themselves.

I have just completed a study of British maternity hospitals (1) in which I receive detailed reports of prenatal care, care in labour, postnatal care and help with feeding from 1500 mothers contacted through radio, television and the press who had their babies in hospitals all over Britain. This was followed by obtaining information from the hospitals concerned about their policies and the environment which they provided for labour and delivery. In many of the letters from the hospitals there were statements such as: "Bonding is encouraged;" "the staff understand bonding;" "time for bonding is allowed in the delivery room."

I would suggest that we need to look at the total environment which hospitals offer for birth if we are to make any assessment of opportunities for bonding, for what happens in the minutes following delivery depends on and is the outcome of everything that has occurred before.

In Britain today 30 to 40 percent are induced with oxytocin. This study revealed that most women who wrote (and these were not, for the most part, women in the childbirth movement, but ordinary members of the public) did not want to be induced unless it was absolutely necessary. A few liked the idea of induction for social convenience. But the vast majority of women, whether or not they wanted induction, said they had had little opportunity to discuss the matter with the obstetrician and when it was performed it was often done without explanation or consent. The result was that women often felt assaulted and the labour became a frightening experience. Some women were fortunate to receive explanations of what was being done because these were given over their supine bodies to students or nurses, and this sometimes led to a reduction in anxiety. But most of the women whose labours were induced found that the whole birth experience was tinged with a feeling of helplessness.

When official figures were requested from the hospitals it transpired that some of the hospitals did not know their statistics for induction and there was a delay of weeks or even months while these figures were processed by the records office. Comparison of the rates revealed that there was a very wide variation between hospitals and often between obstetricians in the same hospital. Some hospitals had as high an induction rate as 60 to 70 percent. Some were as low as 10 percent. The interesting thing was that there were similar obstetric populations in some of the highest induction rate and lowest induction rate hospitals.

The increased fetal distress in induced labours was demonstrated by Liston and Campbell (2), who also showed that babies were more likely to be admitted to special care units after induced labours and that this was directly related to the amount of oxytocin used. Whereas 4 percent of babies were admitted following spontaneous labour, 9 percent after labour started with artificial rupture of the membranes but no oxytocin, and 13 percent after labour was induced and maintained with a low dose of oxytocin, 24 percent were admitted after labour in which high doses of oxytocin had been used. The greater respiratory depression suffered by babies after induced labour was also revealed in the British Birth Survey of 1970 (3), a ratio of 9 where artificial rupture of the membranes plus oxytocin was used compared with one of four where labour was not induced. It must be remembered that the non-induced group includes prematures, who are the highest risk category of all. The 6 percent of babies born weighing 2500 g or less in the United Kingdom account for 60 percent of neonatal deaths (5).

The women in my study who wrote that their labours had been induced often said that they were left for long periods of time with their legs up in lithotomy stirrups. Some became very anxious; some got cold; it appears that postural hypotension and pressure on the vena cava may have occurred in some women, because a large number of them reported feeling faint.

A professor of Reproductive Physiology, Tim Chard, has commented about obstetrics in Britain that "spontaneous labour is now an abnormality" (4).

In 1976 the official average induction figure in British hospitals was 41 percent, but there are also a great many labours which are accelerated with an oxytocin drip. Statistics concerning these labours are not readily available so that the general public is unaware of the extent to which intervention takes place in labour or the outcome of these labours as compared with those in which no obstetric intervention takes place. Moreover, unless a specific research project has been carried out in a hospital, obstetricians and other doctors are usually not aware of the statistics or the comparative outcomes of such labours either. Some hospitals apparently have every woman linked to an intravenous drip.

One of the consequences of having an intravenous drip is that there is minimal or no mobility in labour. We know from the work of Caldeyro-Barcia (6) that this may be dangerous for the baby. Another result of augmented labour is that women experience rapidly recurring, powerful contractions which are difficult to handle. The letters from women whose labours had been accelerated revealed that the experience was particularly anxiety arousing and the contractions especially hard to cope with when they were not asked what they thought about having a drip set up.

The routine of doing artificial rupture of the membranes on admission seems to be increasingly common in British hospitals. Senior nursing officers often wrote saying that membranes were ruptured on admission or as soon as dilatation reached 3-4 cms if the head was engaged. There was no indication that they were aware that this might have deleterious consequences by removing the 'cushion' protecting the fetal head (7).

In the mothers' reports there was a good deal of description concerning the people who helped in labour. Many warm feelings were expressed about midwives, especially those who were able to give continuity of care, which is often very difficult in the hospital situation.

The elderly primigravida encountered special problems. She often went through the process of amniocentesis, of learning that her baby was "high risk" and came to think of herself as reproductively inadequate. It often seemed that a new diad came into existence, a new procreating couple, not the father and the mother but the obstetrician and the mother who collaborated with each other during the pregnancy and labour to get the baby born. Studies of the possible effects of this on the interaction between husband and wife need to be undertaken.

Nowadays it is a normal practice in Britain for husbands to be present during labour and delivery. On the other hand, many hospitals appeared not to know how to make husbands welcome and help them to feel comfortable. In some cases midwives tried to get women to collude with them, in effect to reject the man's help during labour, by saying things like "We women really understand each other; men can't know." There seemed to be a need for midwives and nurses to have more understanding of their own psychological needs in the work they are doing and occasionally their rejection of the men. They also need more education to understand the psychology of fatherhood. Throughout pregnancy and while his baby is being born a father is not merely an adjunct to a woman, not just a woman's "labour coach." He should not be there to be a worshiper at the shrine of the uterus. He is a man; he is a person too.

One British obstetrician has said that every woman should deliver in an intensive care situation(9)! Because of the amount of obstetric intervention which occurs today and the technological equipment involved in childbirth, machines often took the place of the fathers. The father was physically separated from the mother because the machine had to be pushed by the bed. Men were also turned out for many minor procedures; such as admission procedures, whenever the woman used a bedpan, every time a doctor came in to examine, when an I.V. was set up, etc. This meant that there was no continuity in the relationship between husband and wife (8). When she most needed her partner there he tended to be turned out.

There are increasing numbers of forceps deliveries. One study done in Oxford showed that when elective epidurals were used, forceps deliveries were 5 times more likely than when epidural anaesthesia was not given. It is usual in British hospitals to turn men out also for forceps deliveries. (We have not yet reached the point in Britain of thinking of a forceps delivery as a "natural" birth, as it is sometimes claimed to be in the United States)!

There is a marked contrast between the situation in which the man was a guest in the hospital and was allowed to be with his wife, and that at home in which the doctor and midwife are the guests.

Protective garments appeared frequently to fill a purpose of socially humiliating the man. A study by Roth (9) indicates that protective garments play a ritual role denoting status in the hospital hierarchy. The lower down in the hierarchy any individual is, the more protective clothing he must wear. Some hospitals insisted on gowns, masks, caps, and overshoes for husbands. Others omitted any of the last 3 of this list, though all insisted on gowns. A great amount of protective clothing sometimes seemed to produce a barrier between husband and wife. They could not kiss each other easily, for example. The mask used for longer than 15 minutes is no longer sterile. It, therefore, has limited protective function and we must see its use as having primarily a ritual function in denoting that the father has low status (9). When a study was done in one hospital comparing bacterial counts when overshoes were used and when they were not used, it was discovered that there was no statistically significant difference. That hospital has discarded their use. In British hospitals hair coverings rarely completely cover the hair. We might conclude, therefore, that they also have a ritual function.

In my study (1) it emerged that most women had choice as to whether or not to receive medication, although there was a substantial minority who felt they were under pressure to accept drugs in the middle of contractions, and sometimes staff used the peak of contractions, when the woman was under the greatest stress, to say "Don't you think you need an epidural?" Women were also told frequently that they had "a long way to go" in labour, or words to that effect, when in fact they were almost fully dilated; and there were some unfortunate occasions when a hypodermic syringe was pushed into a woman who was given a possibly high dosage of Demerol, and she said she was told, "Never you mind, we know what we're doing."

It was possible for many women to ask for mini-doses of medication, but it was clearly very difficult when a junior or student midwife felt she could not give a dosage lower than that which the obstetrician normally prescribed, and sometimes a woman had to choose between not having Demerol at all and having a dose of 150 mgs. This is enough to cause extreme drowsiness, nausea, vomiting, confusion, amnesia, visual disturbances and hallucinations in some women. It may make the baby slow to breathe immediately at delivery and may cause it to be sleepy during the days following birth and, therefore, to be slow at sucking, and interfere directly with the interaction between mother and baby and between father and baby in the all-important hours and days after birth.

In some hospitals women wrote that they felt that epidurals were "pushed" and they were frequently offered a "package deal" of induction and epidural anaesthesia. They said that they were told that even though they did not need pain relief when labour started they would be bound to need it later so they might as well have the epidural set up while the anaesthetist was available. Many women indicated that they were not informed of the side-effects of epidurals and were frequently surprised when their blood pressure suddenly dropped and they felt weak and faint, or when their bladders had to be emptied with a catheter. Some women also said that they did not realize that if they accepted an epidural there was an increased chance of a forceps delivery.

Another factor which emerged from this study was the difference between care in the daytime and at night in the hospital. Care at night appeared to be dramatically reduced to produce difficulties, especially for breastfeeding mothers who wanted to feed their babies when they woke. A completely different system regarding feeding was sometimes instituted when the night shift came on, which was frequently made up of agency nurses who were unaware of. or not interested in the ethos of the maternity hospital regarding care or the methods of the day sister on that particular ward. The result was conflict, mothers and babies at the receiving end. Even when there was no direct hostility, such an uncoordinated system always seemed to result in muddle and confusion. In some hospitals there was also very slack discipline at night, which meant that people were walking around and chatting and waking up mothers, and babies were left to cry. In these hospitals writers often reported that they left the hospital exhausted and longing for a rest and a good night's sleep.

In some hospitals women were not supposed to be in labour at night apparently, if they could help it, not, at any rate in advanced labour. Labour was supposed to occur in the right place, the labour ward, and at the right time, which seemed to correspond roughly with daytime office hours. In one hospital, for example, a woman on the prenatal ward with rapidly escalating contractions every four minutes said she was told to "go back to sleep and stop imagining things." The night sister recognized that she was in labour, however, because when she handed her over to the day staff she gave a message to the day sister who examined her immediately and moved her to the labour ward and then at top speed to the delivery room as, in fact, whe was in the second stage. In some hospitals, too, if a woman was admitted during the night she tended to be given sedation, her partner was told to go home, and she was put in a darkened room and told to sleep, unless it was recognized that she was in strong labour. For some women this meant that they were deprived of their partners' support and of help from the staff when they most needed it, and they either passed hours in anxiety and pain until the hospital started up again, or were subjected to a sudden dash to the delivery room in the early hours of the morning while being told to "stop pushing." Consequently also, their partners often missed the birth of the child.

It was interesting, too, that certain methods of managing labour, notably the acceleration of labour with oxytocin and the use of epidural anaesthesia, often seemed to depend on the time of the day in relation to the labour. A woman who was laboring during the night was unlikely to be accelerated or to have an epidural. On the other hand, if she started labour during the day, went through the night, and was still in the first stage when general activity started up in the morning and when the doctors' rounds were down, in many hospitals she was put on an oxytocin drip. That is, it seemed that the active management of labour related to the social divisions of time rather than to the overall progress of that particular labour. The impression was that a few women who could have done with some stimulus to their labours did not get it because it was nighttime, and that a much larger proportion of women who had had a weary night during which their morale had dropped, and who had been given inadequate emotional support, were then accelerated in the morning. This acceleration was given in place of other, more directly human support.

It was also at night that a woman was more likely to be told that she should not get out of bed, and was occasionally enjoined to "be quiet" and "not disturb other patients," when she longed to change position or move about. It is possible that her spontaneous urge to get on all fours, to rock her pelvis or to stand up would have produced more effective contractions and that, here again, oxytocin was introduced in place of rather than in addition to, or instead of, other simpler methods of stimulating labour.

In some hospitals night was also artificially foreshortened by rigid routines which meant that mothers were woken for feeding their babies but did not get the all-important English morning tea till half an hour after they had finished, and in one hospital they did not get breakfast till an hour after that. Or mothers were all woken at 5:30 or 6 a.m. regardless of the fact that some had been feeding their babies on demand during the night and had just dropped off to sleep again. It is probably staff recognition of the problem of getting adequate sleep in hospital that has led to the wholesale distribution of sleeping pills at night time, which one mother said were "dished out like candy."

Perhaps it is because nurses are so used to giving medication to sick people that they sometimes could not understand why a new mother should refuse sedatives at night, and failed to sympathize with women who were concerned that they would not hear their babies cry, that they would not be able to wake to feed them and also that drugs would contaminate their milk. This is one area where there needs to be much better communication between women in hospital, pediatricians and the staff on the wards.

Most writers who commented on their physical surroundings, even those who had had very positive birth experiences, said that they found the hospitals "forbidding", "clinical" or even "frightening" places. This was even more likely to be the case when the mother was in a large, modern unit than when she was in a small, old one. We do not seem to have solved the problem of how to design maternity hospitals which are attractive places to enter and be in. This is not merely a matter of putting up drapes, flowered wallpaper, or hanging plants. It is a question of the people in the hospital and the relations women have with them. That is far and away the most important thing.

On the other hand when sensitive, responsive people work in a hospital they soon realize that women usually do not like to give birth in boxes. I was appalled when I visited one large, modern hospital in the United States and was taken to see the labour and delivery rooms in the basement. There, amongst the plumbing, within tiled walls, tucked away below stairs in what would be the equivalent in British society of the Victorian servants' quarters, where the "domestics" lived underneath the ground without daylight, birth was taking place.

In this study many women appreciated being able to see growing, living things out of the window, gardens and trees for example. We have not given enough consideration to the surroundings for labour. Many hospitals have been built in which the labour and delivery rooms have no windows. This is unfortunately the case in some of the delivery rooms in the very splendid hospital in Oxford. There were some detailed descriptions of ceilings. When women are in bed the view may be more or less restricted to the ceiling. In some hospitals these were cracked, pitted, stained and otherwise marked. One woman said she encountered a blood stained ceiling above the delivery table, but luckily had been warned about it already by a friend who had a baby there two years previously! Some women also said that they were lying so that light was shining directly in their eyes.

It is very difficult to engage in a psychosexual activity with not only one's body but one's whole mind and to spontaneously give birth in such surroundings.

The second stage of labour, too, is far too often treated, even by childbirth educators, as an assault course on delivery. The tape-recorded sounds of what is happening in many delivery rooms make it appear that something analogous to a prize fight is in progress. We have lost respect for the spontaneous physiological rhythms which occur in the second stage, which are remarkably similar to the rhythms of lovemaking and orgasm.

In many hospitals it was possible for the woman, provided she made it clear that this mattered to her, to try and deliver without the need for episiotomy, but many women had episiotomies in the end because staff delivering them had no idea of how to help them deliver so that they did not need an episiotomy. There were many instances of women being urged to push harder and harder so that they lost touch with what was happening on the perineum and thus could not push out the baby's head with sensitivity and discretion.

Of almost every hospital mothers said that staff encouraged breastfeeding and often added that they were enthusiastic. Unfortunately advice and assistance given did not always match up to the enthusiasm and the biggest problem which women met in hospital after hospital was conflicting advice, which at times led to confusion and despair and resulted in the mother losing confidence and giving up breastfeeding.

The night after delivery was an ordeal for many women because they longed to have their babies with them and there were often hospital rules that the baby had to be in the nursery over the first night. Some women also missed their husbands during this night and felt they wanted to have them close to share the experience and to talk over the birth. I should like to see the day when all hospitals have very large double beds in which mother, father and baby can be together.

Bonding is not an emotional sticking plaster. It is the end result of a process which is best rooted in and nourished by an environment in which one can live through a very intense psychosexual experience.

Hospitals at present, and I suspect many of those which say they have "family-centered care" and "encourage bonding" are on the whole highly unsuitable places in which to have a baby. Birth needs to take place where not only a baby, but a family can be born.

Birth, like death, is a great, universal experience which we all share. It can either be a disruption in the flow of human existence, a fragment of time endured which has little or nothing to do with the passionate longing which created the baby, or it can be lived with beauty and dignity and labour itself be a celebration of joy. Birth is also part of a woman's very wide psychosexual experience and is intimately connected with her feelings, which can last a lifetime, about her own body, her relations with others, her role as a woman, her worth as a human being and her sense of personal identity. This is why the way in which we bear our babies is so important.

### References

1. Kitzinger, S., The Good Birth Guide, Fontana: London, 1979
2. Liston, W.A., and Cambell, A.J., Dangers of Oxytocin-induced labors to foetuses, British Med. J., iii, 606-7, 1974
3. Chamberlain, R., et al, British Births, 1970, Vol I, The First Weeks of Life, Heinmann, 1975
4. Chard, T., and Richards, M., Benefits and Hazards of the new obstetrics, Spastics, Internat'l Med. Pub., 1978
5. Alberman, E., Facts and Figures, in Chard, op. cit. (4), 1978
6. Caldeyro-Barcia, R., et al, Effects of Position Change on uterine contractions during labor, Am. J. Ob. Gyn. 80:284, 1960
7. Schwarez, R.L., et al, Fetal heart rate patterns with intact or ruptured membranes, J. Perinatal Med., 1:153, 1973
8. Kitzinger, S., Women as Mothers, Fontana: London, 1978
9. Roth, J.A., Ritual and Magic in the control of Contagia, Am. Soc. Rev., 22, 1957

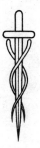

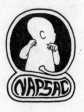

# CHAPTER TWENTY

## AN IN-HOSPITAL BIRTHING ROOM: ONE YEAR'S EXPERIENCE

### by Richard B. Stewart, M.D.; Asher Galloway, M.D., and Linda Goodman, C.N.M.

The Douglas Childbearing Center, also known as the Birthing Center or the Birthing Room, is part of a full-service obstetrical facility located in the Douglas General Hospital in Douglasville, Georgia, 20 miles west of downtown Atlanta. It was officially opened November 1, 1976.

The Center came into being as a result of a combination of factors. The first of these is my own commitment to the use of nurse-midwives in my practice. When I left Americus, Georgia, in 1975, Dr. Schley Gatewood Sr. and I had practiced with two nurse-midwives, using the team approach, for two years. I knew that I did not ever want to practice obstetrics again on any but a very limited scale without using this approach. I firmly believe that the best kind of delivery a woman can have is to be attended by a trained midwife, or a doctor who practices like a midwife. The trained midwife can recognize complications as well as an obstetrician, and she has the great advantage of remaining with the patient throughout labor.

So in Atlanta I made the rounds, looking for a hospital that would accept the idea of a nurse-midwife working with me as a team. I did not find one.

Finally I located the Douglas General Hospital, which was willing to consider the idea. I started going out there one day a week in April 1976. Meanwhile, the word had gotten out around Atlanta that there was a doctor who believed in midwives, and I began to get invited to meetings of home birth groups, NAP-SAC groups, and childbirth education groups, where I was delighted to find a great interest in alternatives to present obstetrical care, including delivery by midwives.

The alternatives being sought by these women are principally those having to do with family-centered maternity care, and include having the husband or other support person present throughout labor and delivery, not being separated from the baby and the husband after delivery, unlimited rooming in, and permitting children and other family members to visit the postpartum unit. Many prefer to be delivered by a nurse-midwife, and in December, 1976, I employed Linda Goodman, a graduate of the University of Mississippi School of Nurse-Midwifery.

---

Richard Stewart M.D., Asher Galloway, M.D. and Linda Goodman, C.N.M. all work as a team in the Atlanta area. They have an in-hospital birth center at Douglasville, Georgia, which is the topic of this paper. They also provide services in Decatur and Atlanta. In addition to births in the center, they offer prenatal care and back-up to couples desiring a home birth. This paper was first presented before the Georgia Ob-Gyn Society in Palm Beach, Florida, in December 1977, again at the NAPSAC Conference in Atlanta in May 1978, published in the Journal of the Medical Association of Georgia, pp. 631-633, and published here by permission of its authors. The Douglasville Childbearing Center started in November of 1976, and as of July 1, 1978, after its first 20 months, has had 502 births.

Other alternatives not necessarily related to family-centered care include:
1. No routine procedures such as prep, enema, or IV fluids unless indicated;
2. Labor and delivery in the same bed without transfer to a table where stirrups and straps and flat-on-the-back position are required;
3. No silver nitrate drops in the baby's eyes until there has been eye-to-eye contact for some time as advocated by Klaus and Kennell;
4. Early discharge.

Perhaps the most fortuitous circumstances of all then came into play as plans for a Birthing Room offering all the above alternatives proceeded rapidly between April and November. When the obstetrical unit at Douglas General was built, two large, well-equipped delivery rooms were installed, but only one small labor room. No one seems to know the reason for this, but it worked out just perfectly to take the delivery table out of one delivery room, install a regular bed, a few rugs, a bedside table and lamp, and a few wall hangings — in short, to create a bedroom-like atmosphere (except for the tile walls!). In addition, there is the installed oxygen, suction, mounted blood pressure apparatus, scrub sink and utility area. The small nursery is located across the hall.

Personnel was the other important factor, and for those who might be contemplating a set-up similar to this I would emphasize that it is probably the most important factor. We had a number of applications from excellent nurses who were looking for this type opportunity, so from the beginning we have had no disgruntled, unhappy nurses or aides walking around mumbling under their breath about "all these crazy, newfangled ideas." You can have the nicest facilities in the world available for family-centered care, only to have the whole atmosphere ruined by one person who walks into the area with an opposing spirit.

I cannot say enough in praise of our nurses, some of whom are childbirth educators, and all of whom know what is taught in CEA, Bradley and Lamaze classes well enough to act as support persons if the patient and-or her husband start to lose control of the situation.

In November we had five deliveries; in December, three; in January, seven. By the end of one full year we had had exactly two hundred.

One infant death took place at the Medical Center in Macon, Georgia, over a month following delivery. After it became apparent that this patient would need a cesarean section because of premature rupture of membranes and failure to progress in labor with IV pitocin, the Angel II team at Grady Memorial Hospital was alerted in accordance with previous arrangements we had made with them to transport any of our sick infants. During the cesarean section, the team had to answer another emergency call, and by the time they arrived the only bed available was in Macon, Georgia. The infant was operated on at a little over two weeks of age for patent ductus and died two weeks after surgery.

Because of this, we decided in the future to transfer all mothers before delivery if there seemed to be a good chance that the infant might be in trouble.

One such transfer was done when a mother presented in active labor, five centimeters dilated, with gestational age between 25 - 26 weeks. The infant was double footling breech. My partner, Asher Galloway, accompanied this patient to Grady Memorial Hospital where she elected to buck the odds and have a cesarean section.  The infant weighed 490 grams and is alive and apparently well at home today, thanks to super care given in the Grady Memorial Hospital

## DOUGLAS CHILDBEARING CENTER
### Nov. 1, 1976-Nov. 1, 1977

Total no. of deliveries ...................... 200
Total delivered in birthing room ............ 167
Age of mother
  19 and under .......................... 10 (5%)
  20-24 ................................. 90 (45%)
  25-29 ................................. 64 (32%)
  30-34 ................................. 24 (12%)
  over 35- .............................. 12 (6%)
Gravida
  1 ..................................... 61 (30.5%)
  2 ..................................... 84 (42%)
  3 ..................................... 29 (15.5%)
  4 or more ............................. 26 (13%)
Hours in labor
  0-4 ................................... 39 (19.5%)
  4-8 ................................... 91 (45.5%)
  8-12 .................................. 49 (24.5%)
  over 12 ............................... 21 (10.5%)
Hours postpartum to discharge
  0-6 ................................... 28 (14%)
  6-12 .................................. 114 (57%)
  over 12 ............................... 58 (29%)
Episiotomy ............................. 66 (33%)
Laceration ............................. 45 (22.5%)
Postpartum hemorrhage .................. 14 (7%)
  needing transfusion ................... 5 (2.5%)
Forceps deliveries ..................... 10 (5%)
Paracervical blocks .................... 13 (6.5%)
Saddle blocks .......................... 10 (5%)
Pts. on fetal monitor .................. 24 (12%)
Uncomplicated vertex deliveries ........ 174 (87%)
Breech ................................. 7 (3.5%)
Twins .................................. 4 (2%)
Cesarean sections ...................... 15 (7.5%)
  Repeat ................................ 4
  Primary ............................... 11 (5.5%)
    CPD ............................... 5
    Failure to progress ............... 2
    Breech ............................ 2
    PRM, failed induction ............. 1
    Transverse lie .................... 1
Patients transferred before delivery ......... 2 (2 live births)
Babies transferred after delivery ........... 5 (1 set twins)
Babies known to have been admitted elsewhere
  in first month of life .................... 6
Perinatal deaths ......................... 1 (5/1,000)
Previous C-sections delivered vaginally ...... 2

Neonatal Intensive Care Unit. We feel that it also helped that this mother came every day for months to the nursery to pump her breast and give the milk to the baby.

One other such case was that of a gravida three, Rh-sensitized mother who had amniocentesis twice in our facility. When her titers began to rise and her spectrophotometry showed her nearing the danger zone, she was transferred to Grady for possible intrauterine transfusion. She made it to 34 weeks without the intrauterine transfusion and was delivered of a live baby which did well after extrauterine exchange transfusion.

We feel that this has been a proper utilization of the concept of regionalization.

A word about follow-up of our infants. Since most mothers go home in less than 12 hours after delivery, we make every effort to know who their private pediatrician is and to see that they have the infant seen by him within 48 hours after discharge. We have identified the few groups of pediatricians in the Atlanta area who are comfortable with this arrangement and they have been very helpful to us also. Ninety-five percent of our mothers breastfeed, and the support of the pediatrician is indispensable. Of the six babies admitted elsewhere after discharge, five were for hyperbilirubinemia, one of whom was exchanged for ABO incompatibility. The other infant had slight pneumonitis which also gave an elevated bilirubin.

All mothers on discharge take with them a slip of paper with the results of the cord blood type, Rh, hematocrit, Coombs and bilirubin.

These are most of the elementary scientific facts. I would now like to make a few remarks about the non-scientific facts.

I stated as my primary conviction that attendance by a trained midwife is the optimum care that a woman can receive in labor. My second conviction is that the psychological and emotional factors in labor and delivery are at least as important, if not more so, than the medical factors. That is a conviction, not a proven scientific fact. It will probably never be proven as a scientific fact, since psychology and emotion are hard to put on graph paper.

But one thing is a fact. Women in fast increasing numbers are demanding to be heard, and respected, and treated individually. In the field of obstetrics, since it involves the most important event in a woman's life, giving birth, all the movements now gaining momentum — the feminist movement, consumerism, the revolt against the overuse of technology, dehumanization and impersonalization by hospitals, and the return to nature and natural processes — are coming to a head.

### The Home Birth Movement

Take the home birth movement. You may oppose it vehemently, but this movement, as one example of all the above, is here to stay. I get letters from doctors who send the records of patients transferring to me which state, "Since this lady has decided to have her baby at home, I have told her I do not offer this service and advised her to seek help elsewhere."

What service? Home delivery? I don't do home deliveries either, and neither does the nurse-midwife employed by me. The patient is asking for prenatal care. When she and her husband come to me for the initial consultation I talk a long time with them to explore their reasons for wanting home birth. I explain that we have an alternative that offers the warmth and comfort of home, with the added safety factor. In spite of this, some still decide to deliver at home. In my mind, that puts them at increased risk, and it behooves me to see them even more often for prenatal visits to pick up the least little thing that may go wrong.

If I do this — if I say, "I think you may be doing the wrong thing, but I respect your right to assume for yourself all this responsibility, and I will give you meticulous prenatal care" — then if anything does go wrong, when I suggest that they need an in-hospital delivery, they comply immediately.

If I send them away in a huff with some put down about their foolishness, I not only reinforce their negative attitude about cold, insensitive doctors, but I have given them an attitude that may make them stay at home in a critical situation way past the point at which they should call for help. No one likes to hear "I told you so," even when she is bleeding to death.

A number of hospitals in the Atlanta area are fast making arrangements for alternatives in labor and delivery and postpartum areas. This makes me very happy, because I feel deeply that what women are asking for today is not a whim or fad, but something they and the infant need.

The studies on maternal-infant bonding are proliferating, and I have to agree with one observer at a conference dealing with this subject who said, "Never have I seen such overwhelming and convincing scientific evidence for something so perfectly obvious."

I invite all of you to take a long and serious look at nurse-midwives, alternatives in labor and delivery, and the establishment of such facilities in your institution. Even if you are not philosophically committed to the ideas, but just trying to "keep up with the competition," I think in the end you will be happily pleased at what you discover.

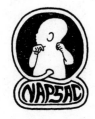

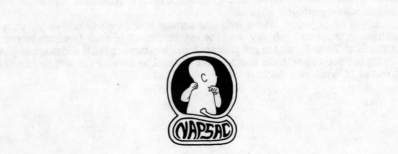

# CHAPTER TWENTY ONE

## MAKING HOSPITALS MORE LIKE HOME:
## OPPORTUNITIES FOR INNOVATIVE RESEARCH

### James R. Allen, M.D., M.P.H.

Many of the practices and routines instituted in hospital nurseries over the last century have been to try to prevent the spread of infections among infants in the nurseries. Compared with adults, older children or even babies a few months old, newborn infants are extraordinarily susceptible to a wide variety of infections. Medical historians have suggested that the high frequency of postpartum sepsis in mothers and the associated infections in their newborn infants was in large part responsible for the demise during the 1890s of rooming-in of infants with their mothers and the replacement during the early 1900s of this practice with centralized hospital nursery care (1,2). In the intervening years delivery of infants has become much safer and currently relatively few infections in infants are acquired from the mother during delivery or postnatal care. The incidence of nosocomial (of hospital origin) acquisition of disease has varied considerably over the years, however, with gastroenteritis being a common problem during the 1940s and staphylococcal disease being epidemic during the 1950s and 1960s. Several investigators state that had centralized nurseries been eliminated and rooming-in required for all healthy infants and mothers, the frequency of these infections in newborn infants might have been markedly reduced (3,4). Because of fear of serious infection in infants many hospital nurseries in this country have been slow to modify practices and have remained tightly controlled and highly centralized. Part of the responsibility for the slow change in nursery routines belongs with state and local health authorities who have established inflexible regulations for operation of hospital nurseries, primarily to assist in control of infections. Many of these regulations, however, do not reflect current knowledge and practice.

Prior to the early 1970s only a few pioneering efforts at reinstituting rooming-in or initiating other innovative obstetric and newborn care practices have been recorded in the medical literature. The last 10 to 15 years have witnessed a significant revolution in obstetric and neonatal care which has developed in two separate directions. The more obvious trend has been the proliferation of sophisticated electronic and biochemical monitoring of the fetus and laboring mother, the development of regionalized transport and hospital facilities to care for high risk obstetric and newborn patients, and the rapid growth of neonatal intensive care units (5-11).

The other trend which is becoming increasingly vocal, has been the development of alternative methods of birth, including family oriented methods such as the Lamaze method, the Leboyer technique, rooming-in, birthing centers, and home deliveries (12-13). One early group of proponents for hospital

James R. Allen, M.D., M.P.H., is a researcher with the Hospital Infections Branch, Bacterial Diseases Division, Bureau of Epidemiology, Center for Disease Control, Public Health Service, U.S. Department of H.E.W., Atlanta; he is a pediatrician and an authority on hospital infections, particularly those associated with a newborn nursery.

rooming-in have described this movement as a "joint psychologic and maternal protest against the harsh denial of parental privileges which the usual present day maternity ward procedures and hospital nursery care of newborns entail" (2).

Physicians, nurses and others in hospitals frequently have resisted strongly the trend toward liberalizing maternity practices and have demanded proof that the new practices are safe before allowing them to be adopted. As with other new techniques introduced into medical practice, it is imperative that these be assessed carefully for their safety, efficacy, and impact on the patient and the medical care system. Because of the paucity of well designed studies in which the relative risk of various techniques of delivery and infant care have been compared, however, proof of the safety of these programs is difficult to find. Although many comparisons need to be made between the alternative birth methods and more standard obstetric and nursery care, this paper will address only the relative risk of infection in infants delivered by different techniques and cared for during the first days of life in different ways.

### Bacterial Colonization of Newborn Infants

Newborn infants are susceptible to infection for a variety of reasons, including the developmental immaturity of their immune response (14). Of major importance also is that most infants at birth move from a sterile environment to one teeming with bacteria and other microorganisms. The skin, umbilical stump, mouth, nose, gastrointestinal tract and other sites rapidly become colonized with a variety of microorganisms, some of which are potentially highly pathogenic. Because of the absence of a balanced normal flora to inhibit further bacterial growth, the colonizing bacteria may proliferate rapidly to dense populations, and disease may result. These colonizing bacteria are obtained from several sources: 1. Some are obtained from the mother at the time of delivery or in subsequent handling, 2. some from the hospital attendants or other persons caring for and handling the infant; and 3. some from contaminated items in the infant's environment. In the absence of serious infection in the mother, the colonizing bacteria she is likely to transmit to her infant frequently are less potentially virulent than are bacteria acquired from hospital personnel or other sources within the hospital. This is particularly true if the mother is breast feeding her infant, since colostrum and breast milk contain secretory immunoglobulin A, which is protective against many of the bacteria which the mother is likely to transmit to the infant (15-19). We can postulate, therefore, that rigid practices in hospital nurseries which minimize maternal-infant contact might not provide the optimum care to prevent infection in newborn infants. Certainly, few people would argue that they provide the best psychological support for infants or promote maximum development of maternal-infant bonding (1,20,21).

### Rooming-In for Infants

The medical literature contains few articles describing alternative methods of obstetric care, deliveries and neonatal care. Of these, most are anecdotal and are not carefully designed clinical trials which attempt to control the variables affecting outcome. Despite this, however, all the studies suggest the relative safety and low rates of infection of the alternative birth and neonatal care methods used.

Jackson and her colleagues (2) note that by the late 1930s parents were more frequently demanding rooming-in units for neonatal care in hospitals, and that a few hospitals attempted to meet this need by developing small, experimental rooming-in units. General acceptance of the idea was slow, however. Therefore, during the mid-1940s they established for study purposes a rooming-in unit in a community hospital affiliated with Yale University. They state that "one of the most important considerations in constructing the rooming-in unit was that of making it as attractive and home-like as possible, in conformity with the ideal of comfort and ease in the treatment plan" (2). In contrast with standard nurseries of the day which isolated infants in the nursery and limited mothers with premature infants only to viewing them in the nursery through glass windows, a limited number of visitors were allowed to visit with the mothers and infants in the rooming-in unit. Fathers and other visitors were allowed to hold the infant after washing and gowning, although those with upper respiratory or other infections were excluded from the unit. During the 8 months of the study period covered in the report, none of the 116 infants had to be removed from the unit and isolated because of diarrhea or skin infection, even though the standard period of confinement was 8 days.

Subsequently, in 1947, McBryde (3) succeeded in establishing compulsory rooming-in for infants on the ward and private newborn service at Duke Hospital. All infants were taken from the delivery room to the mother's room or ward and remained with her for the duration of her hospitalization unless the infant was abnormal or the mother's condition was critical or she had an infection. Over 90 percent of the infants born during a 3-year period were able to room-in. Interestingly, the stated reason for instituting compulsory rooming-in was "not primarily for its psychological advantages but in order to avoid the possibility of nursery epidemics" (3). Since a primary objective of the system was to limit contact of the infants with hospital personnel, a combined obstetric-newborn infant nursing service was started with one nurse during each shift being responsible for 4 to 6 infants and mothers. Over the 3-year period, only 5 (0.3 percent) infants developed infections that required isolation — an unusually low rate of infection. The multiple factors which could have contributed to the low rate of infection were not specifically studied in this anecdotal report, but probably include factors such as minimal handling of the infants by only a small number of hospital personnel and an increased frequency of breast feeding of infants by the rooming-in mothers. Visitors were limited to the father and grandparents, although they were allowed to visit whenever they wished if they were free of respiratory, skin and intestinal infections. These family visitors were encouraged to assist in the care of the infant.

Montgomery (4) established a rooming-in unit for ward mothers at Jefferson Medical College in 1947 because of the fear of infectious disease among newborn infants in the central nursery and because of inadequate numbers of nurses to staff the nursery. After the first 1200 infants had been cared for in the new unit, they had observed "no instances of diarrhea or impetigo." Visitors during the 5-day stay of the mother and infant were limited to the maternal grandmother and the father of the infant, but they were allowed to wash, gown, and hold the infant. Part of the subjective evaluation of the program was that mothers were more interested in the care of their infants than when they were housed in the regular nursery, and the frequency of breast feeding was greater.

## Early Discharge and Family-Centered Care
It was only during the early 1960s that hospitals began evaluating the

feasibility of discharging postpartum patients and their infants within 72 hours of delivery. Hellman, et al. (22), in a widely quoted controlled trial discharging obstetric patients within 72 hours after delivery noted that there was no statistically significant difference between the study and control mothers or infants. This study provided the incentive for others to examine the safety and feasibility of alternative delivery methods with early discharge of the mothers and infants. Yanover and his colleagues (13) at the Kaiser-Permanente Medical Center in San Francisco selected a group of low-risk women during pregnancy who agreed to participate in a voluntary study. The families were randomly assigned to traditional perinatal care or family-centered perinatal care study groups. The family-center perinatal care program included an expanded prenatal education program; collaborative perinatal care by nurse practitioners, obstetricians, pediatricians and others; integral participation by the father in all aspects of perinatal care; early discharge from the hospital following birth if both mother and infant were healthy and the family was ready; and, following discharge, home visits by the perinatal nurse practitioner. Of the families in the special program, 46 percent were discharged between 12 and 24 hours postpartum, and an additional 40 percent were discharged between 24 and 48 hours after delivery. Approximately 4 percent of the infants required readmission, most of them for observation and treatment of hyperbilirubinemia. The incidence of superficial skin infection and other measures of morbidity during hospitalization and the first 6 weeks after delivery was comparable in the two study groups for both infants and mothers.

Kerner and Ferris (12) have taken the in-hospital alternative birth center one step further by providing a room for labor and delivery which incorporates both a home-like atmosphere and essential equipment for care of the mother and infant available in an inconspicuous place. To provide a margin of safety for unexpected complications, the room is located adjacent to the regular labor and delivery and nursery areas, but it is furnished attractively and is provided with a standard king-sized bed with a firm mattress for labor and delivery. The father and other persons are encouraged to provide support throughout labor and delivery, and nurses skilled in alternative methods of birthing provide one-to-one nursing. Preparation for delivery in the birth center requires that the patient be at low risk for developing complications, have received acceptable prenatal care, and attended prenatal classes and orientation in preparation for childbirth. Following birth, the infant is examined by a pediatrician before continuing rooming-in with its mother. Both mother and infant are again examined before discharge and are followed at home by the nurse practitioner. Siblings of the new infant are permitted to be present at the birth as part of the carefully supervised program. Although the study is uncontrolled, the outcome for both infants and mothers has been very good. Because of the standard labor and delivery facilities adjacent to the birthing center, the staff are able to transfer easily patients with complications developing during labor. Many of these women are returned to the birthing center after the problem resolves to continue with their planned method of birthing.

### Evaluation of Alternative Methods

These limited studies provide an initial basis for believing that family-centered delivery practices or alternative birthing methods are inherently no more likely to result in maternal or neonatal infections than is standard obstetric and newborn care, and in other factors such as encouraging family support and maternal-infant bonding are definitely superior. The converse of this statement, that alternative birthing methods and perinatal care will result in a lower rate of neonatal and maternal infections than standard obstetric care in a comparable population, might be true, but the carefully designed studies to prove it have not been conducted.

Because of the current interest in family-centered maternity and perinatal care, the Committee on Fetus and Newborn of the American Academy of Pediatrics has included a chapter entitled "Family Participation in the Care of the Newborn Infant" in the Sixth edition of its manual, Standards and Recommendations for Hospital Care of Newborn Infants published in 1977 (23). This chapter strongly supports the birth of an infant as a family event. and encourages prenatal planning and education and parental contact with the infant starting at the time of delivery. Although several alternative methods of family participation are discussed, including rooming-in and short-term hospitalization for labor and delivery, the manual includes a strong statement that since "life threatening problems cannot always be predicted during the perinatal period . . . optimum care for the mother, fetus, and newborn infant can be provided only in a hospital equipped to deal with all perinatal emergencies" (23).

The main question, then, is what methods of care can be provided for the mother during and after labor and delivery and for the infant to make a hospital environment more like home? The studies reviewed strongly suggest that rooming-in, whether continuous or intermittent, is highly desirable. For selected families, discharge within the first 12 to 24 hours following delivery appears to be safe if home follow-up is provided and access to medical care is available. Hospitals should be encouraged to experiment with a variety of facilities and methods for birthing as long as they carefully select patients for admission to these facilities, provide careful prenatal instruction and post-natal follow up, have contingency plans for emergencies, and follow generally accepted aseptic techniques during delivery.

In specific terms, there is no reason to restrict the type of furniture, drapes, carpeting, wallpaper and pictures, radio or television, and other amenities as long as the potential medical needs of the mother and baby are not compromised. Allowing the mother to be with her family or supporting persons or allowing her to visit a labor lounge or family waiting room if she desires should not increase the risk of infection. The equipment for delivery could be any of a wide variety of acceptable types, including a modern hospital bed or a specially designed bed which allows the mother to assume a semi-sitting position for delivery, since these factors probably are not associated with a risk of infection. Sterile equipment and drapes and an adjustable lamp to provide sufficient light must be available, but equipment necessary only for medical emergencies can be unobtrusively stored in the room or available on carts immediately outside the room. Although every effort should be made to allow the infant to remain with the mother immediately after delivery for as long as possible, consideration must be given to maintaining the infant's body temperature, and a heated infant examination and resuscitation unit should be readily available.

The father or another person of the mother's choosing should be allowed to provide support and assistance throughout labor and delivery. The presence in the birthing room of healthy children of the family who have been instructed in what to expect and how to behave should not increase risk of infection or other complications. Persons with an acute infectious illness, particularly an upper respiratory tract infection, purulent or draining skin infection, or infectious diarrhea should be excluded from the room. It is unknown whether requiring family members and others in the birthing room to wear a hospital scrub suit or clean gown over regular clothing, a cap and a mask will reduce the incidence of infections compared with only requiring them to wear clean street clothes. The program described by Kerner and Ferris (24) only requires observers to wear clean clothes or a scrub suit; persons assisting at delivery do not gown but simply use sterile gloves and optionally use caps and masks. Because of the close contact of the delivery assistant with the mother and infant, until alternative methods have been proved acceptably safe, I would recommend that all persons directly assisting with delivery wear a cap and mask, scrub, and don a sterile gown and sterile gloves. Family members or hospital personnel must wash their hands carefully and should put on a clean gown before holding or caring for the infant.

Following delivery, rooming-in of infants with their mothers should be encouraged following guidelines established by the American Academy of Pediatrics (23). The father or another adult family member selected by the mother should be allowed extended visiting privileges to assist in the care of the infant and mother to the extent desired by the mother. The other children in the family may require reassurance from their mother, and reasonable visiting of the entire family should not be restricted by age or routine hospital visiting hours. The family visiting could be in the private room of a mother and infant or in a special family lounge if the mother is sharing a room. More distant family members and casual friends might interfere with the emphasis of a private family experience, and visitors of this type should be restricted in number and duration of visits. In general, the number of persons allowed to hold or care for the infant during its hospital visit should be as restricted as possible; parents, however, should be encouraged to provide as much of the care as possible for their infant.

### Family-Centered Central and Premature Nursery Care

Not all families are able to or desire to use an alternative type of birthing facility. Hospitals should be encouraged to be innovative in making standard labor and delivery facilities as attractive and home-like as possible within the limits imposed by function and need for asepsis. Mothers should be encouraged to hold their infants immediately after delivery and breast feeding should be strongly supported. Rooming-in should be encouraged for all mothers if their condition permits, including mothers who deliver by cesarean section. A flexible approach would allow a mother to initiate rooming-in at any time during her hospital stay if either she or her infant is not able to start rooming-in immediately after delivery.

Currently little information is available on the risk of infection in infants cared for or nursed by mothers who have low-grade post-partum fever or who are under treatment for a known infection such as a urinary tract infection. Progress in developing rational recommendations will depend on careful documentation of extent of contact, type of exposure and subsequent outcome. Although there are numerous questions of this type for which no satisfactory answer is available, it is known that mothers with certain infections, such as mastitis, should not breast feed their infants until the infection has resolved. Although mothers receiving many types of antibiotics probably may breast feed their infants without worry, mothers receiving antibiotics which either reach concentrations in milk similar to maternal serum levels or which are known to be potentially toxic to infants (for example, tetracyclines or sulfonamides) should not breast feed their infants (25).

Parents should be encouraged to visit an infant requiring premature or intensive care or isolation, and within the limits of the medical and nursing needs of the infant should be encouraged to feed it or otherwise assist in its care. The American Academy of Pediatrics has clearly stated that "visiting and physical contact with sick infants does not increase the risk of infections when parents follow the same handwashing and gowning procedures as the nursery personnel. When possible, parents are encouraged to help with their infant's care. Rooming-in before discharge is desirable when parents have only occasionally visited their hospitalized infant. Parents should be given the opportunity to arrange for siblings to visit sick infants when they are in the intensive care area" (23).

## Clinical Evaluation of New Methods

Changes in standard routines in newborn nurseries and premature nurseries have only been made slowly and after multiple trials of different techniques to establish their relative safety (26-29). In retrospect, as we have better understood the epidemiology of certain infectious diseases or the physiology or immunology of the problems, the reluctance to change more rapidly is difficult to understand. Nevertheless, it is reasonable to expect proof that a change in technique or practice is both safe and effective. Unevaluated developments or change frequently result in unexpected complications, as occurred with scalp abscesses complicating a change in fetal monitoring techniques (30) or respiratory distress syndrome developing in newborns following elective delivery of presumed term infants (31-32). It is imperative that the changes in obstetric and neonatal care being introduced with the alternative birthing programs be assessed as carefully as possible.

The types of randomized, controlled clinical studies necessary to document adequately the different outcome variables which should be measured (including maternal and infant morbidity and mortality, family satisfaction, use of analgesic or anesthetic drugs, frequency of operative delivery or cesarean section, length of stay and utilization of hospital and home-care resources, and dollar cost) are complex and time-consuming but extremely important (34). The rapidity and enthusiasm with which family centered and alternative birthing practices are accepted by the medical community depends not only on the demand for such services by families but also on the clear demonstration that such techniques are superior in outcome and costs. Documentation of the feasibility and safety of alternative birthing programs in hospitals and demonstration of optimum techniques and procedures for use in these programs will provide a solid foundation for the subsequent adoption of these programs by hospitals throughout the country and acceptance of them by health care providers and families using the services.

## REFERENCES

1. Klaus MH, Kennell JH: Mothers separated from their newborn infants. Pediatr Clin North Am 17:1015, 1970
2. Jackson EB, Olmsted RW, Foord A, et al: A hospital rooming-in unit for four newborn infants and their mothers. Pediatrics 1:28, 1948
3. McBryde A: Compulsory rooming-in in the ward and private newborn service at Duke Hospital. JAMA 145:625, 1951
4. Montgomery TL: Bedside care of the newborn by the parturient mother. Med Clin North Am 32:1699, 1948
5. Committee on Perinatal Health: Toward Improving the Outcome of Pregnancy. White Plains, NY: The National Foundation-March of Dimes, 1976
6. Swyer PR: The regional organization of special care for the neonate. Pediatr Clin North Am 17:761, 1970
7. Segal S, Pirie GE: Equipment and personnel for neonatal special care. Pediatr Clin North Am 17:793, 1970
8. Adamsons K, Myers RE: Perinatal asphyxia: causes, detection and neurologic sequelae. Pediatr Clin North Am 20:465, 1973
9. Dorand RD: Neonatal asphyxia: an approach to physiology and management. Pediatr Clin North Am 24:455, 1977
10. Butterfield LJ: Regionalization for respiratory care. Pediatr Clin North Am 20:499, 1973
11. Shott RJ: Regionalization: a time for new solutions. Pediatr Clin North Am 24:651, 1977
12. Kerner J, Ferris CB: An alternative birth center in a community teaching hospital. Obstet Gynecol 51:371, 1978
13. Yanover MJ, Jones D. Miller MD: Perinatal care of low-risk mothers and infants: early discharge with home care. N Engl J Med 294:702, 1976
14. Miller ME: Host defenses in the human neonate. Pediatr Clin North Am 24:413, 1977
15. Goldman AS, Smith CW: Host resistance factors in human milk. J Pediatr 82:1082, 1973
16. Hanson LA, Winberg J: Breast milk and defense against infection in the newborn. Arch Dis Child 47:845, 1972
17. Goldman AS: Human milk, leukocytes, and immunity. J Pediatr 90:167, 1977
18. Cunningham AS: Morbidity in breast-fed and artificially fed infants. J Pediatr 90:726, 1977
19. Larsen SA, Homer DR: Relation of breast versus bottle feeding to hospitalization for gastroenteritis in a middle-class U.S. population. J Pediatr 92:417, 1978
20. Klaus MH, Jerauld R, Kreger NC, et al: Maternal attachment: importance of the first postpartum days. N Engl J Med 286:460, 1972
21. Minde K. Trehub S, Corter C, et al: Mother-child relationships in the premature nursery: an observational study. Pediatrics 61:373, 1978
22. Hellman LM, Kohl SG, Palmer J: Early hospital discharge in obstetrics. Lancet 1:227, 1962
23. American Academy of Pediatrics Committee on Fetus and Newborn: Standards and Recommendations for Hospital Care of Newborn Infants (6th ed). Evanston, IL: AAP, 1977

24. Kerner J: Personal communication, 1978
25. McCracken GH Jr: Clinical pharmacology of antibacterial agents, in Remington JS, Klein JO (eds): Infectious Diseases of the Fetus and Newborn Infant. Philadelphia, WB Saunders Company, 1976, pp 1020-67
26. Williams CPS, Oliver TK: Nursery routines and staphylococcal colonization of the newborn. Pediatrics 44:640, 1969
27. Forfar JO, MacCabe AF: Masking and gowning in nurseries for the newborn infant: effect on staphylococcal carriage and infection. Br Med J 1:76, 1958
28. Silverman WA, Sinclair JC: Evaluation of precautions before entering a neonatal unit. Pediatrics 40:900, 1967
29. Evans HE, Akpata SO, Baki A: Bacteriologic and clinical evaluation of gowning in a premature nursery. J Pediatr 78:883, 1971
30. Winkel CA, Snyder DL, Schlaerth JB: Scalp abscess: a complication of the spiral fetal electrode. Am J Obstet Gynecol 126:720, 1976
31. Kafka H, Hibbard LT, Spears RL: Perinatal mortality associated with cesarean section. Am J Obstet Gynecol 105:589, 1969
32. Hack M, Fanaroff AA, Klaus MH, et al: Neonatal respiratory distress following elective delivery: a preventable disease? Am J Obstet Gynecol 126:43, 1976
33. Maisels MJ, Rees R, Marks K, Friedman Z: Elective delivery of the term fetus: an obstetrical hazard. JAMA 238:2036, 1977
34. Byar DP, Simon RM, Friedewald WT, et al: Randomized clinical trials: perspectives on some recent ideas. N Engl J Med 295:74, 1976

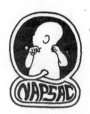

230

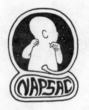

# CHAPTER TWENTY TWO

## FAMILY CENTERED CARE FOR THE HIGH RISK

### By Murray W. Enkin, M.D.

One of the basic tenets of NAPSAC - and of all of us who are participating in this conference - is that the vast majority of births are normal, and that nature, left to her own devices, will usually produce a healthy baby to a healthy mother. If 80 percent or 90 percent, or whatever figure one chooses, of births are normal, why do we need all the fancy space age technology? Are we producing people who think like machines, when we make machines that think like people?

I am well aware of the dehumanization of childbirth which is going on in our society. In other meetings, in other settings, I have spoken to the best of my ability, with all the eloquence at my command, about the harm, both physical and emotional, both personal and social, that can come from the overuse, or the abuse of technology.

This session here at NAPSAC is somewhat different. Those of us here are all aware that the current, unthinking overemphasis on high risk pregnancy is doing more harm than good, and this is not the place to reiterate the obvious. Today, I would like to concentrate on two equally important issues.

The first is, that if a majority of childbirths are normal, a minority are not. Nature is on the side of the species, but not of the individual. Nature is not always kind - sometimes she is cruel. Nature does not have to be good - she just has to be good enough to ensure the survival of the species. If the occasional mother dies, or the occasional baby doesn't make it, nature doesn't really care. But the individual mother, or father does care, and cares very deeply.

The exact percentage, or number of women with high risk pregnancies is not really that important. The important issue is that there are some pregnancies which, without aggressive management and meticulous care, will not result in a happy outcome. Those mothers love their babies, want their babies - and those babies have just as much right to live, and be loved - as the babies born naturally to a healthy, well nourished mother who carries her baby for a full nine months, and goes into labor at her full term.

The second vital issue I would like to address today, is that hospitals and machines do not depersonalize or dehumanize childbirth. People dehumanize childbirth. It is possible for unfeeling attendants to make childbirth a demoralizing experience in any setting, without any technology, in home as well as in hospital. It is equally possible for sensitive, empathetic birth attendants to make childbirth a self-fulfilling, beautiful experience in any setting. It is possible to use the most modern space age technology as an aid to communication with mother, baby and family, to make childbirth a warm, human, safe experience for all concerned.

With the present conflict between an obstetric establishment using scare

---

Murray W. Enkin, M.D., F.A.C.O.G., is a professor of obstetrics at McMaster University, Hamilton, Ontario, Canada; Board member and former vice president, ICEA.

tactics, and exponents of non intervention over-reacting with equally indiscriminate rhetoric, the only real losers can be the unfortunate mothers and children caught in the no man's land. The innocent victims in the middle are burned when there is so much heat, so little light.

High risk mothers need all the benefits of modern technology. They also need, in an ultrasophisticated hospital setting - intensive family centered maternity care. Not just as much family centered care as a mother with a normal pregnancy, but even more. Fortunately, even with the worst abuses of modern obstetrics, under the most adverse conditions, most families turn out pretty well. When the pregnancy is not progressing normally, the risk of an ego damaging, family shattering experience is increased. Normal maternal infant bonding may not occur. This risk is just as great as is the risk of physical damage to mother or baby, and must be just as carefully monitored and managed.

Perhaps, first, we should take a look at what we mean by high risk, because the term is often bandied about rather loosely. We can recognize some situations, fortunately rare, in which the risk is great - severe hypertension, insulin dependant diabetes, extreme prematurity - perhaps 1 or 1½ percent of all pregnancies. These mothers need all the intensive care which is available, in order to give them a chance for a happy outcome. Left to nature, the likelihood of a safe birth and well child is virtually non existent.

Some others may be considered moderate risk, where the hazards to mother or baby are moderately increased - a mild to moderate toxemia, or gestational diabetic, or birth between, let us say 32 and 36 or 37 weeks - perhaps about 15 percent of all pregnancies. These mothers may greatly improve their chance of a happy outcome by skilled care, to meet their individual needs during pregnancy and birth, and in the care of their newborn.

### What Constitutes High Risk Care?

First, high risk care must include meticulous preconceptual and prenatal screening. A careful history must be taken, looking for factors which may influence the outcome. An equally careful physical examination is required, and then ongoing evaluation of the pregnancy. At the same time as encouraging the normal progress of the pregnancy, ensuring adequate nutrition and education, there must be careful vigilance, and watching for significant deviations from normal. If deviations from the normal are observed, they must be evaluated, and if intervention is necessary, it must be properly timed and carried out to give the most benefit, with the least risk and the least interference with the physical, emotional and social well being of the mother, infant and family. No easy task.

Sometimes the intervention may be minimal - no more than advice about proper health habits, or a need for increased rest. Sometimes much more aggressive intervention is required to prevent a tragic outcome. And when this is the case, sometimes there is an emphasis on the physical needs, with a devastating disregard for the equally important emotional and social factors. This disregard is as unnecessary as it is dangerous. High risk centers can, and must be centers for family centered maternity care. If a hospital takes on the responsibility for the care of a woman with a high risk pregnancy, it takes on the responsibility for all aspects of that care, to the best of its ability. The birth of a child is the birth of a family. No part of that family's needs can be ignored.

## The Example of one Canadian Regional Perinatal Program

The current debate about regionalization is a bitter one. The motives of some of the participants in that debate are perhaps suspect, and much harm has been done in the name of regionalization. And yet, much good can be done. I would like to talk a little about our center; its aims and its accomplishments. It is, as yet, far from perfect, but that is not surprising in a far from perfect world. Last July, we had the pleasure of David and Lee Stewart's company in Hamilton, and spent a long and active evening at our home with them and the chairman of our department, our perinatologists, and our nursing patient care co-ordinator. It was an exhausting evening, exchanging experiences and insights. David mentioned after, that he had never had a group of obstetricians listen to him so attentively, for so long. We went on and on, and it was hard to leave. His visit, I might add, left an indelible mark on our community, and birthing practices have never been the same since. But the important thing was, the ground was already prepared. We were already on the way, and ready for further improvement.

McMaster University Medical Center's Obstetric Department was set up with the dual role of serving as a model of family centered maternity care for all births, and as a regional referral center for high risk. The Hamilton and District Regional Perinatal Program commenced in 1973, comprising an area of 12 counties, with a little over 27,000 births per year. It was estimated that if all the babies needing intensive care were referred, we would have, from those 27,000 births, about 900 babies per year admitted. Recognizing that all would not be referred, preparations were made for about 600 admissions per year to the intensive care nursery.

The result has been a reduction in neonatal mortality in the entire region from 12.7 per thousand to 7.7 per thousand.

The basic philosophy of the unit is that parents must take the responsibility for their own care. They may make any choice they choose, except the choice not to make a choice. The professional's role is to advise, and to provide the facilities for optimal care.

Because of the dual role it set for itself, the patient mix has been an interesting one. Many women come expressly for the purpose of having a real say in the management of their childbirth, with the safety of the hospital facilities present. One doctor who is actively practicing home births in the not too far distant city of Toronto was recently asked bluntly, if he was having a baby himself, what would he choose - home or hospital? He replied promptly - "neither, I'd move to Hamilton and have my baby at McMaster."

The majority of the women are referred, however, because of a recognized high risk situation. In 1977, 18 percent of the women were coming without any high risk; 42 percent fell into the moderate risk category, and 40 percent were classified as ultra high risk - the most common being extreme prematurity. Forty-seven percent of the patient days in the hospital were antepartum, mainly the stopping of premature labor.

Statistics are dry, however, and not very informative. Besides, like many of you, I have a healthy disregard for them. Figures may not lie, but liars can figure, and statistics can be selected, or manipulated, to serve any end. It might be more productive, then, to talk about some of our recent clients, and let their stories tell a little about our aims and procedures.

### Meredith - A Vaginal Birth after previous Cesarean

Meredith - for example - and let me digress for a moment. I am going to use first names, partly for the obvious reason of not identifying the person - but also because, in addition to being patients, they are friends - and while there are many exceptions, most of our patients call the nurses and doctors by first names as well.

Meredith lived in Toronto, and had had a Cesarean birth in Toronto for her first pregnancy. It had been a rather bad experience - a long labor, fetal distress, a crash section - general anesthetic - her husband excluded. She woke angry, frustrated, and swore never again. When she became pregnant again, she came to McMaster, and we agreed that she would have a trial of labor, a normal birth if it all possible, and if a Cesarean was necessary, she would meet the anesthetist first, have an epidural anesthetic, and of course her husband could remain with her.

Unfortunately, about her fifth month, she began to have some bleeding, and discussing the whole problem together, we felt that the long drive for prenatal visits, and in labor was not worth the risk. With some difficulty, we found a doctor in Toronto who agreed to let her try for a vaginal birth, and who managed to prevail on his hospital to - just this once - let a husband in for a Cesarean if it should be needed. All went well until she went into labor.

She phoned her obstetrician who was out of town; also his partner was out of town, and the obstetrician on call listened to her story, and said "Yes dear, I understand. Now come down to the hospital right away, and we'll do a Cesarean immediately. And forget about your husband being with you. That's against hospital regulations."

At first, she felt she had no choice but to agree - but then she thought of phoning me in Hamilton for advice. Need I say more? I was out of town too. But her call was put through to the Perinatologist, Pat, who was on call. Pat listened to her carefully, and offered her an option to get into her car and come down to McMaster. An hour later she was examined, her cervix was five cm. dilated, the baby's head well in the pelvis. Labor progressed normally; she was carefully monitored; the operating room was set up for a possible emergency Cesarean, and she had a beautiful spontaneous birth a few hours later. Two days later still, she was home with an eight pound baby boy.

### Mary - A Case of Long Antepartum Hospitalization

Mary didn't have quite so simple or straightforward a story. Her first two pregnancies, 10 and 11 years ago, had gone well. Then her world fell apart. She was divorced and remarried. Two years ago she had her third pregnancy, complicated by an incompetent cervix. She gave birth to a two pound baby, anoxic, retarded, who will probably never walk, and still requires tube feeding, chest suctioning, and constant care. When she became pregnant a fourth time, her second husband left her, and she required welfare assistance. She had a suture placed in her incompetent cervix, but her uterus was irritable and she kept going into premature labor, requiring almost constant hospitalization and intravenous medication to prevent another disastrously premature birth.

It wasn't too hard to make good arrangements for the two healthy older children. But the two year old was another matter. So she was brought into the hospital with her mother. Mary was able to look after her daughter, herself, and give her the care she needed during the prolonged hospitalization; during the times when she was confined to bed, the nurses cared for the two year old. The older children came in to visit regularly, and Mary had a healthy baby near term. The family was kept intact through what might have been a shattering experience to a family whose coping mechanisms had already been strained to capacity.

### Esther - An Orthodox Jewish Diabetic

Esther gave birth to a healthy baby in April. She was a brittle, juvenile diabetic, who required frequent adjustments of her insulin dosage, and extremely careful management of her diet. Well, we have lots of those, but Esther had an extra problem. She was the wife of a rabbi, extremely orthodox, and unwilling to eat hospital, non Kosher food under any circumstances. For a while, attempts were made to have her husband bring food in for her, but this didn't work. So she got her own fridge, her own food, her own dishes and cooking utensils, and under the careful supervision of the dietitian, prepared her own food. And of course, she was allowed home for Sabbath, returning Saturday night right after sundown.

### Lynn - A case of Prematurity and Survival at 24 Weeks

Lynn was transferred to McMaster from another hospital in active labor at 24 weeks gestation. She was contracting every two minutes, and her cervix was fully dilated with membranes bulging. She was immediately put in bed with her head down, given intravenous isoxuprine, and the labor stopped. This was maintained for six days, before her membranes finally ruptured and she gave birth to a seven hundred and twenty gram infant - just a bit over two pounds - who was rushed to the intensive care nursery next door. It was touch and go for awhile - tubes from every orifice. Lynn spent most of her days in hospital in the nursery touching and watching her little one. She expressed her milk, and learned to tube feed the baby.

After five days she was discharged from the hospital, but she remained in the bunk room near the nursery, going out for her meals, but remaining close to her baby. Eventually, the baby was able to breast feed and two months later, Lynn took her baby home, nursing, loving someone she had known from birth, not a stranger from whom she had been separated.

### Total Patient Care vs. Physical Care Alone

These examples perhaps serve to illustrate that care must be for the total patient, not for her physical needs alone. Care must be individualized, because every person's needs are different. And yet many generalizations can still be made.

The high risk patient has many special needs. She has great anxiety as to the outcome of the pregnancy, and is worried about her unborn child. This, in turn, leads to a delay or distortion of the normal steps in bonding.

The prolonged hospitalization, so often necessary, brings with it many problems in itself. There is a loss of self esteem, a tendency to dependence. There is great strain on the family. Separation from other children is painful. Separation from the marital partner is hard for both partners. There are sexual difficulties, and added responsibilities.

It isn't easy for the staff either. It is hard to switch one's thinking and feeling quickly from the happy, healthy mother and baby to the overwhelming problems of the high risk. Special skills, special attitudes, and constant reinforcement are necessary.

A number of mechanisms must be built into the system to satisfy the special needs of patient, family, and staff. These are not costly, but they must be thought of, carefully planned and carried out.

## Programs to Promote Independence and Self-Esteem

At McMaster, in order to foster her feeling of independence and self worth, a variety of programs have been arranged for the woman. She is encouraged to take as much responsibility for her own care as possible.

A self medication program is utilized. A pharmacist explains to the woman what medication is prescribed, its purpose, the timing and doses required. The reason for each drug is explained, its side effects; which drugs are for symptoms to be taken when she feels need, and which are for a therapeutic effect and must be taken at special times. The medications are then left at her bedside, to be taken by herself as needed.

The woman is encouraged to do those tests which she can do herself, like weighing herself, urinalysis, etc. and chart them. Her progress chart is kept at her bedside. All tests are carefully explained to her, including the reasons why they are done, and the significance of the results.

Some of the more frequently encountered conditions have special groups set up. A diabetic day care center helps mothers take care of their own diets and insulin requirements. A twins club meets regularly (and triplets are not excluded).

Antepartum patients meet regularly as a group, with a nurse as facilitator and unofficial ombudsman. These group meetings serve often as bitch sessions, where the women can express some of their frustrations, and where they complain about the consultants, or the interns, or the food or whatever else is making them unhappy. Where problems are identified, attempts are made to help the situation. Where nothing can be done, at least the problem is ventilated.

Whenever possible, patients are encouraged to be active. If they can be up, they attend prenatal classes. Craft sessions run by the hospital volunteers are popular. When possible, patients may go home at night to be with their families, or are taken out for drives or outings.

For out of town patients, or others where families are not available, hospital volunteers meet on a one to one basis with the woman, so that she will not feel friendless or alone. Often a nonprofessional can add a dimension to care that a professional cannot begin to give.

## Inclusion of the Family

The rest of the family is not forgotten. As I mentioned, if it is possible for the woman to go out from time to time, this is encouraged. If not, the family is encouraged to come in. Visiting hours are open 24 hours per day and unrestricted; other children are of course welcome. Depending on the circumstances, sometimes a crib or cot is brought in, and the child may stay with his mother. A cot is also available for the husband or partner, or he may share the bed with his wife. Do not disturb signs hung on the door are respected.

The partner's anxieties are respected and understood as well. Tests and their results are explained to him, as well as his wife. If it is expected that the baby will have to go to the intensive care nursery, husband and wife are taken on a tour of the nursery together, so they can meet with the pediatric staff, and become familiar with the unit and its equipment.

Normal life events are maintained. There is a family room for birthday parties, and baby showers, as well as informal get togethers. Life need not stop because one is in hospital.

## Family Centered Birth - Regardless of Circumstances

Birth is managed in the most appropriate manner considering the circumstances. Most normal births occur in the woman's own bed in the labor room. If difficulties are expected, then a delivery room with better facilities for early newborn care is used. Appropriate technology is of course utilized for the safety of mother and baby, but is hopefully, not used without a valid indication. The woman may have with her for all births, spontaneous or operative, the companion or companions of her choice.

The problems involved in bonding with a tiny premature, or ill infant are great. Often it is necessary to take the baby immediately to the intensive care nursery. Whenever possible, the parents become familiar with the nursery, and its personnel before the birth. In any case, the father is encouraged to go to the nursery as soon as he can leave his wife, and the mother is taken as soon as possible. Both parents are helped to touch and hold the newborn as soon as possible, and to learn to take at least partial care of him. As soon as possible, he is taken to the mother's room if she is still in hospital.

If the mother is discharged from hospital, we have a bunk room, not far from the nursery, where the mother, or mother and father may stay, nearby the baby, to allow them to continue the interaction. The mother is encouraged to express her milk to tube feed the baby, until he is strong enough to suckle.

Sometimes, despite encouragement to early contact, the observant nurse will notice a failure of bonding behaviour. Child abuse of the premature or separated newborn is sadly not rare. Sometimes a mother's fears and anxieties for her newborn do not permit normal attachment to take place. Careful note is made of parents' behaviour with the ill or extraordinary baby, and if necessary, a skilled social worker will try to help the parents cope with their fears, or marshal community resources to help them. A mothering role day care program is available, and Parents Anonymous has a 24 hour line, manned by volunteers, to help the mother who is at the end of her tether.

Often increasing the contact between mother and baby is enough. Twenty-four hour rooming in is especially encouraged if there has been separation at birth. If photo therapy is needed for jaundice, it is carried out in the woman's room.

The nurses and other personnel in a unit where family centered care for the high risk birth is paramount, work under extreme tension at times, and need support and care themselves. We hold weekly team rounds, attended by consultants, house staff, nurses, social workers, nutritionists, home care coordinators; all those concerned with the care of mother or newborn. At these meetings, patients with problems are discussed and the team pools the resources of its members to find the best possible way to help the woman achieve her goals. Regular meetings between the obstetrical and pediatric staff, between nurses and physicians maintain the communication so vitally needed.

### Conclusion

To conclude then - may I repeat - all births are not normal; family centered maternity care is not only necessary for the high risk family - it is possible, and we have models to prove it. McMaster is only one such model - there are many.

If our aim is to truly bring the best care to the birthing women of our society and to their offspring, parents and professionals must truly become partners, in developing and utilizing the safest alternatives in childbirth possible, to all mothers.

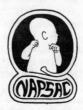

Want to Write to a Particular Author?
All of Their Addresses Are on Page 281.

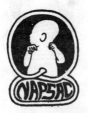

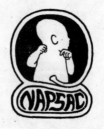

# CHAPTER TWENTY THREE

## BLUEPRINT FOR THE REHUMANIZATION
## OF AMERICAN OBSTETRIC PRACTICE
### (Costs, personnel and floor plans)

**By Loel Fenwick, M.D.**

---

"Doctor, before we begin, there's a form we want you to sign. These are things we want to be guaranteed. We insist that you agree not to submit us or our baby to any unnecessary procedures; we want your promise there will be no routine enemas or shaves; we want to be assured a comfortable room and bed and the promise that our new baby will not be separated from us."

"And Doctor, please understand that we appreciate your knowledge and your skill, but we want your promise that you will intervene to help only if nature fails. We don't want routine medications and episiotomy-- we want the chance to work with our healthy bodies and enjoy the experience of normal childbirth."

---

More and more frequently, parents are stating this position to their doctors. Perhaps you said something similar to your doctor and were surprised at the angry response you received, and you wondered how parents ever got into this position in the first place.

While I wasn't present when healthy American women first decided that hospitals were the place to have their babies, I could follow the re-creation of this process on a geographic time machine, as I attended both home and hospital births on the tip of Africa. It has been said that passengers approaching Johannesburg are told to fasten their seatbelts and set their watches back 30 years, but this is not a fair comment as far as South African hospitals are concerned. Leading the world in fields as diverse as neonatology and heart transplantation, their medical centers are not to be outdone in the battle against that dread disease, pregnancy. Technology notwithstanding the maternity care system resembles the situation as it was in America 30 years ago. Most children are born at home, delivered by midwives. Home childbirth is an extended family occasion and children, friends, relatives all share in the experience. Neighbors tell of niagara-like hemorrhages and 10-day labors to reassure the mother-to-be; menfolk are sent to boil water and do other unrelated errands. As guardian of community health and morality, the midwife quietly and confidently dispenses advice and admonition to the assembled gathering while taking the delivery in her stride.

---

Loel Fenwick, M.D., A.C.O.G., is an obstetrician in private practice in Spokane, WA, and is a consultant to insurance companies and manufacturers of medical equipment and was an assistant in the design of a special birthing bed, eliminating the need for a delivery table. Dr. Fenwick was formerly in hospital practice in South Africa where he provided backup for homebirth programs there.

Occasionally, very occasionally, things do go wrong, in spite of a searchingly thorough screening program and the vast experience of the midwife. Heralded by wailing sirens and flashing lights, the frightened mother is thrust into the hospital emergency room, and gone is the comforting, confident expectancy. Gone is the familiar surroundings of home, family, and friends, replaced by stainless steel, tile and white coat.

### How Obstetrics Became Dehumanized

Dealing daily with high risk pregnancies screened into the hospital and the occasional unsuccessful homebirth, the obstetric specialists saw nature as an antagonist, or at best a capricious ally. Women, capable of fathomless treachery, were to be regarded with suspicion at all times, for without any warning, the nicest of ladies could present them with a most horrible emergency. Anticipating the worst, the hospital personnel were in strong contrast to the confident caring midwife. Not that they didn't care, but caring was of a different order. Caring was winning the battle against shock, sepsis, and hemorrhage; and to win, one had to outwit and control nature. Procedures developed for the sick were applied to the well. Defenses were in place against the probability, not possibility, of complications. Caring was relentless vigilance and the use of every known gadget and potion which might sway the odds in favor of a healthy mother and baby. This too, was caring.

Hospital birth was the alternate then, available only to the high risk mother. Partly from a fear of the unknown, but also from a fear of the known, anxious mothers embellished their risks of complicated birth in an attempt to gain a coveted place in the hospital. Fearful of the infrequent but tragic price exacted by nature, parents saw hospitals as security and comfort. There would be no pain. There would be no strain. There would be no remembrance. There would be no responsibility. The hospital would care for everything. In time the hospital would become a standard for all, as it was in this country, where by and large, the American arrangement appeared to be working well as the baby boom produced healthy young citizens in record numbers.

Admittedly there were some problems. Sedated women would vomit and fall over, so they were kept in bed, starved and given IVs. Because sedated women, lying in bed, tended to have prolonged and ineffectual labors, we had oxytocin and artificial rupture of the membranes — then fetal monitors to warn of their effects. Because our sedated woman, lying flat on her back, found she couldn't deliver in that position, the problem was solved by transferring her to a mini-operating room where episiotomy and forceps made delivery a rapid and sure thing. Because fathers and friends could be upset by the profusion of technology, overwhelmingly arranged as if to challenge nature to do her worst, and because delivery was now a mechanical surgical procedure with its great vulnerability to infection, fathers were excluded from the labor and delivery rooms.

The newborn nursery took care of the baby after delivery—mother was still strapped in stirrups having her perineum reconstructed. Not surprisingly mother and baby needed time to recover from their surgery and medications. Two or four or more days in the hospital would give strength enough to take a wheelchair ride to the front door. Naturally all the resting was considered beneficial, as it prepared the mother for the task of caring for a baby whom she had hardly even met.

Technology and inventiveness provided a solution to every problem. Although there was some complaint about the high cost, and grumbles of assembly-line procedures, it was generally considered to be a reasonable price for safety, if it was considered at all. Childbearing lost its sinister reputation. It became a time for knitted booties and Dr. Spock. Doctors were justifiably self-congratulatory that this care had brought the lowest infant and maternal mortality rate of all time.

## The Beginning of Public Disenchantment

Then in a cosmic moment, dissatisfaction led to questions, to challenges, to accusations, and to widespread rejection of much of both the good and the bad of standard American maternity care.

The wave of protest caught the maternity establishment by surprise. Childbearing had been made safe for their patients who now refused even to be called patients; laymen recklessly disputing the sacred and proven tenants of proper maternity care. Doctors responded with anger, rejection, disappointment, and muttered fears of the return of the dark ages. But parents continued to back their demands with arguments that required academic acceptance. These were as much the result of scientific investigation as they were a statement of humanity.

Yet the professionals remain cautious and divided many recognizing the need for change but seeing no clear direction. Some would like to save people from themselves by limiting alternatives and enforcing the status quo. Others are cautiously supporting birthing rooms, alternate birth centers, and supervised homebirths. Each of these alternatives has a legitimite place among the choices available to intelligent and informed parents. But each is the answer for only a few. We still need to have a mainstream maternity system to bring family centered care to all mothers in all risk categories.

## Balancing Rights and Responsibilities

At NAPSAC a wide and healthy range of opinions has been expressed. We are unanimously aware of the inappropriateness of standard hospital maternity care — we don't want it. Informed and aware, we know what we want and are in a better position than most to get it. We are able to prepare ourselves educationally, philosophically, and physically for alternate birth styles, and be responsible for our choices. We represent the vanguard, not the main body of public opinion. We are a sophisticated minority in a culture characterized by the abdication of personal responsibility. Most people have willingly handed over control of the most important personal areas of their lives to an all-caring bureaucracy and "rights to expect" everywhere replace personal "responsibility to provide."

Comfortable standardization requiring minimum initiative is the American Way. Not surprisingly only a small percentage of deliveries are performed at home. For home delivery to be successful, it requires initiative, motivation, preparation, and a healthy body. It also requires a skilled attendant, for nature, to quote Dr. Ratner, "only works for the most part." (1)

## Humanistic Care for the Average Unaware Family

Even if home delivery were to be encouraged, as it should be, rather than suppressed as it is, how many families would have these qualities in sufficient measure? Similarly, birthing rooms represent an alternate within the standard system, reserved for those fortunate women of low risk who have demonstrated sufficient preparation, motivation, and assertiveness. The majority remain in the conventional multi-transfer system. Even admission to the birthing room doesn't guarantee a humanistic delivery, for all too often traditional attitudes and procedures prevail, and deviation from normal course of labor will banish a mother into the conventional system. Home birth and birth room are available to healthy, aware, educated parents. But who has been the advocate for the average, twinky-eating, TV watching, beer drinking, suburban-living conventional-thinking American family who needs humanistic childbearing at least as much as we do?

If we believe that the advantages of family-centered care should be brought to all women, we must look beyond the alternates we seek ourselves. Everybody deserves better, more responsive care. Where and how will it be provided?

It will not be in the average home. Although I accept the figures for the safety of home delivery, I attended enough home births to know that these figures do not mean that houses are inherently safer places to have babies than are hospitals. Rather they mean that the things that happen to mothers and babies at home may be less harmful than the things that happen to mothers and babies in hospitals. Each has advantages. While home is home, where the family is paramount, hospitals have the tools that occasionally make the difference between health and lifetime disability or even death. Optimally, the best of each should be combined in safe places, and perhaps controlled by parents and professionals together. This could be a free-standing maternity care center, or it could be a separate area of the hospital. As we have collectively paid for a great abundance of underutilized hospitals and staff to fight disease, the latter would appear the logical way to go.

### Separating Health Care from Sickness Care

First hospitals must be aware of the magnitude of change required and prepared to make the basic attitudinal adjustment needed. The conventional system, designed during the twilight sleep era for yesterday's anesthetized patient won't lose its character by putting posters on the wall and plastic flowers on the window shelves. It requires recognition of the competence of nature and the rejection of childbirth as a pathologic process. Whether childbearing centers are located in hospitals or not isn't as important as that they should be separate entirely from the management of disease.

In a childbearing center, parents should be provided with a secure environment they can call their own, free of the proscriptions and protocols that replace judgment. They need only to be secure in the knowledge that support is available if the need arises. As professionals we have an obligation to our generation to share with them the results of cumulative experience. When called upon, we should be competent to use every skill and device that could have, as its result, satisfied and healthy parents and children.

### What is "Natural Childbirth?"

In designing a support system using our understanding of the needs of families, we would be wise not to rely on established notions of what procedures and protocols are necessary. We should first understand the innate ability for childbirth that has existed in humans since the origin of our species. We should deepen this understanding by the study of the basic anatomical, physiological, psychological and spiritual requirements of childbirth. This doesn't require another experimental research program. Nature did it long before the first accoucheur claimed credit for performing the first delivery. We should humble ourselves and take our lessons not from academic ivory towers alone but also from natural childbirth around the world and through the ages. Then we should individually, and with proper justification, take of those safeguards that are of indisputable benefit and use them judiciously only when nature fails in her purpose.

If we would do so, we would see that in almost every society a woman in early labor is ambulatory which in turn produces more effective labor (2,3). Nearing delivery, we would see that she takes to the quiet company of people she trusts. She most likely delivers in a reclining, squatting or sitting position (2,4,5,6), where spine and sacrum form a continuous downward curve, and she is free to use her arm, chest, and abdominal muscles to full advantage. She is also able to see and assist at her delivery. She is spared the constriction, indignity and separation of the lithotomy position, and labor is both more tolerable and more frequently successful (7,8,9,10). We would see that she very seldom requires medications, forceps or surgery. Surely today's better nourished, better educated and healthier American women could do even better.

Of course she can — and given the opportunity, will do so. To quote Dr. Ratner again: (1)

"The introduction of routine episiotomy and outlet forceps led to the dehumanization of the American obstetrical delivery. Its introduction is reminiscent of the account of the loss of the battle of Waterloo; for loss of a nail, the shoe was lost, for loss of the shoe the horse was lost, for loss of the horse the courier was lost and the message never delivered and the battle lost.

"Routine episiotomy and outlet forceps led to the routine lithotomy position, led to routine stirrups, shackled legs and strapped wrists--the mother spread-eagled or trussed up like a Thanksgiving turkey--led to routine anesthesia, led to postpartum incapacity and distress from anesthesia and episiotomy.

"Whereas nature intended that the mother be an active participant for she is the one intended by nature to be the deliverer of her baby, the technologic delivery either robbed her of her consciousness or with the introduction of regional and local anesthesia made her more like a spectator than a participant because of the paralysis of the lower half of her body."

This has been entirely ignored by our obstetric departments as we imitated the specialists handling emergencies, then applied it to the normal, thus making it abnormal, too. Technology, usually overwhelming in its profusion, for once was found entirely lacking in providing a maternity bed designed for normal delivery, and birth chairs appear to have gone the way of the buggy whip.

## Home Birth as the Model for Hospital Care

Delivery tables, designed to handle the need for occasional mechanical surgical delivery, dictated by their design that all deliveries be done this way. To allow natural forces to operate, this cycle had to be broken. The solution is to start with the concept of a normal home bed and birth chair, a simple support for comfortable childbirth which would free the mother from routine mechanical-surgical positions and give her every opportunity to deliver spontaneously in the normal sitting or reclining position. Leg supports are reserved for those deliveries where surgical intervention is really necessary.

To make this arrangement available for all mothers, high or low risk, all the

## COST COMPARISON
### Hospital Childbearing Center
### vs. Conventional Multiple-Transfer System

> **Data Below Based On Both Units Having the Following:**
> - 180 Babies Born Each Month (Or 6 Per Day Average)
> - All-Risk Population Served at Level III Capability
> - One Mother in 6 Delivered By Cesarean Section
> - Intensive Care for 6 Babies, Mothers Not in Hospital

| CONVENTIONAL SYSTEM | | | CHILDBEARING CENTER | | |
|---|---|---|---|---|---|
| **Number of rooms that must be set aside for the use of the 6 women admitted today:** | | | | | |
| Labor rooms | 4* | 8** | Childbearing rooms | 6* | 6** |
| Delivery rooms | 2 | 4 | Delivery rooms | 1 | 2 |
| Nursery cribs | 6 | 6 | Nursery cribs | 2 | 2 |
| **Rooms needed for the 6 mothers & babies delivered yesterday, now on their:** <br> **First Post-Partum Day** | | | | | |
| Post-partum beds | 6 | 6 | Childbearing rooms | 6 | 6 |
| Nursery cribs | 6 | 6 | Nursery cribs | 2 | 2 |
| **Rooms needed for the 6 mothers & babies who delivered 2 days ago, now on their:** <br> **Second Post-Partum Day** | | | | | |
| Post-partum beds | 6 | 6 | Childbearing rooms | 1 | 1 |
| Nursery cribs | 6 | 6 | Nursery cribs | 1 | 1 |
| **Rooms for those delivered 3 days ago, all of whom have gone home except C-Sections:** <br> **Third Post-Partum Day** | | | | | |
| Post-partum beds | 1 | 1 | Childbearing rooms | 1 | 1 |
| Nursery cribs | 1 | 1 | Nursery cribs | 1 | 1 |
| **Fourth Post-Partum Day** | | | | | |
| Post-partum beds | 1 | 1 | Childbearing rooms | 1 | 1 |
| Nursery cribs | 1 | 1 | Nursery cribs | 1 | 1 |
| Neonatal Intensive Care | 6 | 6 | Neonatal Intensive Care | 6 | 6 |
| Assumes: Vaginally delivered mothers stay day of delivery & 2 more days. <br> Mothers stay 4 days after C-Section. <br> All babies have a nursery crib. | | | Assumes: Vaginally delivered mothers stay day of delivery & 1 more day. <br> Mothers stay 4 days after C-Section. <br> Only 2 babies have nursery crib (C-Section & 1 baby on 1st day.) | | |
| **Nursing Staff Requirements to Provide Basic Care:** | | | | | |
| 8 Labor rooms & 6 mothers with 4 Delivery rooms | 4 Nurses | | 14 Childbearing rooms (Each nurse has one mother in labor) | 7 Nurses | |
| 14 Post-partum rooms | 4 | | No Post-partum rooms | 0 | |
| 20 Nursery cribs for well babies | 4 | | 4 Nursery cribs for well babies | 1 | |
| 6 Neonatal Intensive Care cribs | 3 | | 6 Neonatal Intensive Care cribs | 3 | |
| | **15 Nurses** | | | **11 Nurses** | |

\* Beds physically occupied on average day.   \*\* Beds to be available for possible peak periods.

| CONVENTIONAL UNIT | CHILDBEARING CENTER |

| CONVENTIONAL UNIT | | CHILDBEARING CENTER | |
|---|---|---|---|
| 8 | Labor Rooms | 2 | Delivery Rooms |
| 4 | Delivery Rooms | 14 | Childbearing Rooms |
| 14 | Post-Partum Rooms | 4 | Well-Baby Cribs |
| 1 | Fathers' Waiting Room | 6 | NICU Cribs |
| 20 | Well-Baby Cribs | 11 | Nurses |
| 6 | NICU Cribs | | |
| 15 | Nurses | | |

| C | Childbearing Room | L | Labor Room |
|---|---|---|---|
| D | Delivery Room | P | Post-Partum Room |
| FWR | Fathers' Waiting Room | O | Nurse |

ROOM & PERSONELL REQUIREMENTS
FOR CONVENTIONAL MATERNITY UNIT
AND CHILDBEARING CENTER MODEL

critical care capabilities of a delivery table and delivery room were inconspicuously incorporated but only used when necessary. When problems arise, they can be handled without transfer. Breaking free from a routine mechanical surgical approach while retaining capability for emergency intervention is the key to providing safe family centered childbearing support as standard, family centered maternity care.

## Changing Hospitals into Birth Centers

We have yet to establish centers where all families — sophisticated or underserved, rich or poor, high risk or low — can enjoy the rich experience we want for ourselves. Childbearing centers not limited to low risk are the logical replacement of the conventional hospital system. For these childbearing systems to be established in hospitals would require that hospitals and personnel redefine their roles. They will have to stop seeing themselves as ministers to the sick and become guardians of the well.

The biggest changes would be philosophical rather than architectural. The average hospital maternity department could be changed readily to a childbearing center. Most hospital labor rooms, postpartum room and general ward rooms can be converted to rooms or suites for the use of families. The initial cost of conversion would be offset by the continued savings brought about by instituting a childbearing room system. Additional space is not required because parents having natural childbirth tend to spend far less time in hospitals. Fewer and larger rooms replace the multiplicity of room necessary in the multitransfer system.

A few women who would require delivery by cesarean section would be the only ones to use the conventional delivery rooms or surgical suites. As childbearing suites replace maternity units a few delivery rooms could be retained for this purpose. While well babies remain with their parents, nursery space is reserved for those babies who need special medical attention. Well babies are not intermingled with the sick, and family togetherness and bonding is not interrupted. Secure in a single room throughout their stay, parents have a chance to establish a rapport and cooperation with their attendants and support persons, who in turn enjoy the privilege of contributing to the growth of the family rather than providing a fragment of total care.

## Costs, Personnel and Floor Plans

What will childbearing centers cost compared to the present hospital based system? There are no childbearing rooms using the single room concept available to the general population, so a hypothetical childbearing center must be compared to a competent hospital unit that it will replace. In these projections, both the hospital maternity unit and the childbearing center care for 2200 deliveries each year. Each is equipped to handle the needs for normal, high risk, and complicated pregnancy.

In our 180 delivery-a-month unit, childbearing rooms would have 8 labor rooms, 2 delivery rooms, and 16 nursery cribs. It would also free 5 nurses for other duties, possibly to spend more time with parents teaching ante natal care, child care and parenting. The logistics of single room care are simple compared to the need to transfer between and supply a prep room, labor room, delivery room, post-partum room and nursery crib for each family.

While these figures apply to a large facility, relative gain in efficiency and cost control potential are greater when applied to smaller units, where normal fluctuations in patient load cause greater under and overstaffing problems. As an exercise, you could calculate the potential savings to any unit by following the steps on the previous page, using figures relevant to the situation you are studying.

## Conclusion

So we see that it can be both practicably and economically advantageous to provide for people the type of care that they want.

Childbearing centers can replace the standard hospital multiple transfer system as the mainstream approach to providing safe maternity care to the American population. By so doing, better more responsive care can be provided for less cost, childbearing centers offer an unusual opportunity in medical care.

## References

1. Ratner, Herbert, M.D., A.C.H.O., in 21st Century Obstetrics, Stewart & Stewart, eds., vol. 1, pp. 116 and 138.
2. Jarcho, Julius, M.D., F.A.C.S. Postures & Practices During Labor Among Primitive Peoples.
3. Clark, A.P. The influence of the position of the patient in labor in causing uterine inertia and pelvic disturbances. J.A.M.A., 1891, 16:433.
4. Howard, F.H. The physiologic position for delivery. Am. J. Obstet. Gynecol, 1959, 78:1141.
5. Naroll, F., Naroll, R., and Howard, F.H. Position of women in childbirth. Am J. Obstet. & Gynecol, 1961, 82:943.
6. Porteus, J.L. Posture in parturition. N.Y. State J. Med., 1892, 56:153.
7. Markoe, J.W. Practical experience with the obstetric chair. Bull. Lying-In Hosp. N.Y., 1916, 10:95.
8. Montgomery, T.L. Physiologic considerations in labor and the puerperium. Am. J. Obst. & Gynec. 76:706, 1958.
9. Newton, M. The effect of position on the course of the second stage of labor. Surgical Forum 7:517, 1957.
10. Newton, M. and Newton N. The propped position for the second stage of labor. Am. J. Obstet. & Gynecol. Vol. 15, No. 1, 1960.

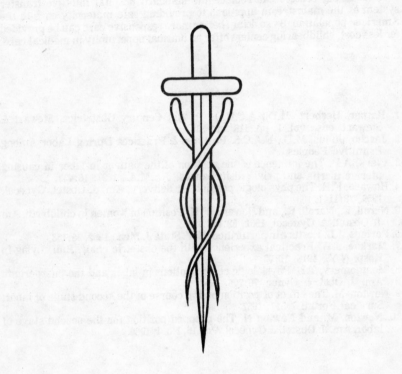

# Model Programs & Other Topics

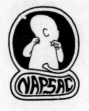

# CHAPTER TWENTY FOUR

## A SOCIOLOGIC VIEW OF BIRTH:
### Physiologic Reality vs. Peoples' Interpretations of that Reality

### by Barbara Katz Rothman

The sociologist's perspective on birth is very different than the medical view. We focus not on what is happening physiologically, but rather on the interpretations that people have of what is happening. Their behavior and interactions depend on these interpretations. In this paper, I intend to look at the way we define, understand and organize the birth experience, and in particular the importance of the hospital and of childbirth education in the social construction of birth.

Human beings live in a social as well as a physical world. We do not simply see, hear, feel, smell and taste; we interpret what our senses take in, and our interpretations are based on what we have learned from other people (1). When we talk to one another, we do not hear just sounds, we actually hear words. As you read this page, you do not see the texture or designs of ink on paper, but recognize these as symbols, as words. This social process of interpretation goes on not only for highly abstracted things like language, but for physical objects as well. A chair, for instance, is seen and recognized as a chair, its purpose seemingly obvious. Yet if we brought in a Martian and showed her a chair, there is nothing about it that proclaims its use. That it exists is its physical reality; but what it exists as, what its meaning and purpose are, that is something that we have created socially in our interaction with one another.

From a symbolic interactionist perspective, birthing is a social as well as a physiological event, a process which is socially constructed and socially defined. In any social situation the possibility exists for alternative definitions of the situation, alternative social realities. Which version is accepted and acted upon is a reflection of the power of the participants. The consequences are of course dependant on the definition of the situation which has been arrived at. Those who define, control.

The prepared childbirth movement, under which heading I am including Dick-Read, Lamaze, Bradley and assorted other modes of preparation, have in common a desire to define childbirth as a "natural" and "healthy" phenomenon. This definition of a universal physiological event occurring preponderantly in healthy women would not seem to be unreasonable. However, even a cursory reading of obstetric texts and the history of obstetrics,

---

### Acknowledgement
This paper was originally presented at the 72nd annual meeting of the American Sociological Association, Chicago, September, 1977.

Barbara Katz Rothman is a Ph.D. candidate in Sociology, New York University, an instructor at Brooklyn College, author of several articles on childbirth.

shows that childbirth in the hands of doctors is perceived as a crisis situation, needing careful medical evaluation and control (2). This is an example of alternative social definitions of a physical event or state.

David Sudnow has pointed out that death, clearly a physical state, nonetheless is socially determined and acknowledged, to the extent that two persons in similar physical condition may be differentially designated as dead or not (3). The same physical signs may be death or not-death, depending on what happens next. People who are revived, were never dead. Dead people are those who stay dead.

Pregnancy too is a socially determined as well as a physical state (4). The very way pregnancy is dated by the medical profession is an interesting example of a retroactive social definition. A woman who is menstruating considers that menstrual period a sign of her non-pregnant state. Yet if two weeks later she conceives, her pregnancy will be dated from the first day of her last menstrual period. The very date on which she knows she is not pregnant becomes, retroactively, the first day of pregnancy. It is not possible to socially enter a pregnancy before the sixth week, the earliest time to get a positive pregnancy test. Further, the pregnancy is always approximately two weeks older than the fetus whose existence presumably determines the pregnancy. This is a professional definition, not particularly well-suited to the needs or perceptions of women viewing their own pregnancies.

Let us apply this concept of socially determined reality to the physical reality of childbirth, and take as an example the situation of a woman at term having painful contractions at ten-minute intervals, who has not yet begun to dilate. Whether she is in labor or not in labor will depend on whether she then begins to dilate or the contractions stop and begin again days or weeks later. Whether a woman is in labor or "false labor" at Time 1 depends on what will have happened by Time 2.

Inevitably, applying social definitions to physical states will involve a certain amount of bargaining or negotiating between the people involved. If a woman comes to a hospital claiming that she is in labor, that she needs help and must be admitted, and yet by professionally established judgments of what is and what is not labor she is not in labor, the client and the professional are going to attempt to reach an agreement. On the side of the professional is expertise and authority, and on the side of the client is the physical reality of what is happening to her. Perhaps if she cries and pleads the professional will come to think that with so much pain evidenced something must indeed be happening, and so she will not be sent directly home. Similar negotiating processes take place in mental hospitals where patient and doctor negotiate competence (5) and in tuberculosis hospitals when patients claim that they really are cured enough for a weekend pass (6).

The definition of the situation that participants arrive at through their negotiations becomes the reality with which they have to work. Let us return to the example of a woman having regular contractions without dilatation. If admitted when she first comes requesting admission, and she does not begin to dilate for 24 hours, and then 12 hours after that — 36 hours after her admission — she delivers, that woman will have had a 36 hour labor. On the other hand, if she is denied or delays admission, and presents herself at the hospital 24 hours later for a 12 hour in-hospital labor, she will have had a 12 hour labor preceded by a day of discomfort. The physical sensations are precisely the same in this hypothetical example. But the social definitions, calling it labor or not, make the difference between a terribly long labor or a pretty average labor with some strange contractions beforehand.

What difference would it make in this situation if we did not have to consider the issue of hospital admissions? In a situation in which women are not admitted to hospitals, but midwife-neighbors are birth attendants in the home, the midwife comes to see the woman when asked. If nothing much other than the woman's discomfort is happening, perhaps the midwife makes her a cup of tea and goes on about her business as the woman goes on about hers. The midwife drops in now and again to see how things are going. She stays when needed to stay. It is never necessary to tell a woman that she is not in labor if she thinks she is, or is if she thinks not. It is only necessary to come to a firm definition of her condition when that definition makes a difference in the way she will be handled. Take away the issue of hospital admission, and the question of when labor begins is no question at all. It is a situation without consequences.

It becomes important for the pregnant woman to be accurate about defining her labor for the following reasons: if she gains early admission, she will have helped to create the social situation of an overly-long labor. In addition to the stress inherent in thinking oneself to be in labor for 36 hours, hospital treatment of long labor is problematic. Laboring women are routinely confined to bed in hospitals, a situation which is as psychologically disturbing as it is physically. Not only is the labor perceived as being longer, but the horizontal position physically prolongs labor, as may the routine administration of sedatives during a long hospital stay. In addition to variations in treatment during those first 24 hours, treatment is different in the last hours when the woman is hospitalized in either case. Women who have been in a hospital labor room for 30 hours receive different treatment than women who have been there for only six hours, even if both are equally dilated and have had identical physical progress. The account of physical sensations preceding admission is virtually discounted in exchange for the professional view of what is happening.

Secondly, it is important for the pregnant woman to be accurate in identifying labor because if she presents herself to the hospital and is denied admission, she is beginning her relationship with the hospital and her birth attendant from a bad bargaining position. Her version of reality is denied, leaving her with no alternative but to lose faith in her own or the institution's ability to perceive accurately. Either has negative consequences for the eventual labor and delivery situation.

The same issue arises again when a decision has to be made about when a woman should be moved from a labor to a delivery room. In American hospitals, unlike most hospitals in the world, the first and second stages of labor are seen as sufficiently separate as to necessitate separate rooms and frequently separate staff. Women attended by nursing and house staff throughout labor may first see their private physician in the delivery room. Since a woman will be moved from one room to another to mark the transition from one stage of labor to another, the professional staff has to make a distinction between laboring and delivering, and then apply that distinction to the individual woman. A cut-off has to be named at which point a woman is no longer laboring but is actually delivering. If the point is missed, and the woman delivers in the hall, then she is seen as having "precipped," having had a precipitous delivery. If it is called too soon, if the staff decides that the woman is ready to deliver and the physical reality is that she has another hour to go, then concern is aroused about the length of her second stage because she has spent that extra hour in a delivery rather than a labor room.

The hospital makes necessary arbitrary decisions defining labor and its stages, if only because the use of the facilities requires scheduling. For that reason it becomes necessary to periodically examine women internally, to judge cervical dilitation and to predict delivery time. It is usually the function of the nursing staff to make the appropriate predictions in order that staff and facilities be ready. Some examinations may be necessary to evaluate the physical condition of the laboring woman and fetus, but repeated examinations of cervical dilitation are equally important for scheduling purposes. Since such examinations are usually quite painful, childbirth education classes teach specific breathing techniques to use for the examination, as well as the transfers from bed to table. The American Society for Psychoprophylaxis in Obstetrics, ASPO, is the original Lamaze organization in the United States, and a major source of childbirth education. An early 1970's Guidelines for ASPO Teachers states:

> It should be pointed out to patients that internal examinations during labor in the hospital can be performed by the patient's own physician, by a resident physician, an intern or a nurse. This depends on the procedures established by hospital policy. Examinations will be given either rectally or vaginally, again depending on hospital rules or individual physicians, but it is not for the parturient to decide who should, or should not, examine her during labor.(7)

Interestingly, this is in direct opposition to the legal rights of hospital patients. According to George Annas in the ACLU handbook, The Rights of Hospital Patients, "All patients have a right to refuse to be examined by anyone in the hospital setting."(8)

Nancy Stoller Shaw, in her study of maternity care, Forced Labor, notes that for a woman giving birth in a hospital, childbirth involves "a continual inability to protect herself and control the access of others to her body."(9) Standard "prepping" procedures, like the admissions procedures to any total institution, reinforce the idea that the woman loses control over her body and herself, including "a systematic removal of all personal effects as well as parts of the body (hair, feces) and its extensions (eyeglasses, false teeth)."(10) The perineal shave has been repeatedly demonstrated to serve no medical purpose at all, having developed from the clipping of any very long pubic hairs with a scissor to a full shave with the invention of the disposable razor (11). While it is a pointless, humiliating, depersonalizing and irritating experience, this same ASPO teacher guideline states that "it is not worth while to make an issue out of this." Similar arguments can be made for each of the prepping procedures, with similar ASPO responses in this early 1970's guideline.

Health professionals are used to hospitals, adjusted to the sights and sounds and smells. Many childbirth educators are also nurses or other health professionals. Admission to some Lamaze teacher training courses frequently requires an R.N. (although this is not so for Bradley teacher training). To the woman in labor, the hospital environment is foreign, and quite possibly threatening. When a laboring woman is wheeled and moved around from one unfamiliar room to another, perhaps entering the situation from the Emergency Room, she is confronted with strange sights, strange noises and strange smells. She has limited knowledge of which are relevant to her and which are not, which are threatening and which are not. She may not even know how to sort out which uniform stands for which kind of worker, does not know if the person entering her room is there for good (i.e. bringing ice chips) or evil (i.e. doing a painful physical examination). The sounds of a big cart coming down the hall may be intended for her or may be just linens for the closet next door. She is not familiar enough with the situation to sort out the legitimate anxiety-provoking cues from those that would not produce anxiety if she understood them. And it is particularly important to realize that one's grasp of reality may be a little fuzzy when in labor to start with, and there is just so much of which one can keep track. Interpreting her environment is at best an added stress, at worst a continual source of anxiety.

For the most part, rather than teaching in detail about hospital facilities and personnel, many childbirth preparation classes teach ways to avoid dealing with external events. For example, with Lamaze training, the woman may be taught to distract herself, to take a focal point, a picture or flower she brings with her from home, or simply a spot on the wall, and focus on that alone, blocking out all other happenings during a contraction. By contrast, with Bradley training, the woman is not taught to distract herself, but is taught to deal directly with events. In any case, most childbirth preparation classes spend a great deal of time in preparation, not for childbirth, but for the hospital — a social institution.

To the woman laboring at home, the background stimuli, far from being anxiety provoking, are actually reassuring. She hears sounds like the refrigerator opening, children playing, someone calling their dog. The sounds are not threatening, they have nothing to do with her labor, and she can make that distinction. She smells chicken cooking, not medicine and disinfectants. If she takes in external events, she is provided with messages of normality.

The cues available to us in a situation include not only physical objects and sensations, but perceived behavior, and even the way we see ourselves acting. One of the basic contributions of symbolic interactionist thinking is to point out that human beings can and do take objective account of themselves, and that the cues we get from our own behavior are an important part of how we understand what is happening to us. This has interesting implications for childbirth.

Margaret Myles is a British midwife, author of one of the most widely used textbooks of midwifery in the world. Speaking at the Maternity Center Association of New York in 1976, she said that it was her experience that no matter what childbirth preparation breathing techniques a woman used, as long as it was a regular pattern of breathing, it worked. Fancy Lamaze puff-pants, plain puh-puh-puhs, or no special breathing at all such as in the Bradley method, they all worked. The usual explanation for the effectiveness of these methods is that the concentration on breathing blocks out the sensations of pain. However, women practice their breathing exercises while driving, or watching television, or reading, all activities that themselves require some level of concentration. Can it be that the breathing is distracting enough to take your mind off pain, but not distracting enough to take your mind off the road or a television program? Hardly likely.

I suggest that the reason that breathing exercises can work in the control of pain in childbirth is that they are presenting the woman with positive cues regarding her situation. If she were not doing the breathing, she might very well be crying or even screaming. Her ability to objectively evaluate her own situation, taking cues from her own behavior as well as that of others, becomes very important. The woman who has just gotten through a contraction without crying out has presented herself with evidence that it is bearable. If it were not bearable, after all, she knows she would be crying. Cognitive dissonance theory offers a framework in psychology with which to understand this process (12). In a sense, it is a more structured version of "Whenever I feel afraid, I whistle a happy tune."

When a woman is laboring in her own home, perhaps her cat on her lap or watching her older child play, some nice music in the background, and she is concentrating on her Lamaze breathing pattern, all the cues available to her are that all is well. It would be difficult to reconcile all that normality with the idea that something terrible is happening.

If, however, that woman is in a hospital bed, with an IV in her arm, listening to doctors being paged, having strangers coming in and out, then the cues available to her are objectively no different than the cues she could expect if she were dying. You do not put someone in hospital gowns on hospital tables under hospital lights with little bracelets on so that you can always tell whose body it is whether they are socially present or not, and not create the image of patient. You cannot maintain a definition of self-as-healthy with all the external cues reading illness. All you can work for is control over pain and the expression of pain.

The messages that the birthing woman picks up from the cues available to her are not limited to the normality, health and relative pain of her situation. The definition of the situation goes much deeper than that, to the very heart of what is happening and who controls what is happening. This is best exemplified by the use of the word "deliver." Both mothers and birth attendants are said to deliver babies. When the mother is seen as deliverying, then the attendant is assisting, aiding, literally attending. But when the doctor or midwife is delivering the baby, the mother is in the passive position of being delivered. The words used are of course the least of the cues that the laboring woman receives regarding the importance of her contribution to the activity taking place, the delivery of her baby.

### The Active-Passive Model

Szasz and Hollender suggested that there are three basic models of patient-practitioner relationships (13). Let us consider each with regard to childbirth. The first is the Active-Passive relationship, particularly applicable to the unconscious patient in an emergency situation. The doctor makes all decisions, and the patient is "worked on" in much the same way one does mechanical repairs. In the childbirth situation this relationship is typified by the doctor using forceps or surgery to pull a baby out of an unconscious mother. What is particularly important to note is that the doctor not only has complete control once the mother is unconscious, but it is the physician who has the authority to define normal, variations from normal, and obstetric emergencies, as well as the "state" of the patient. The physician in a hospital birth always holds the power to create an Active-Passive relationship by having the mother anesthetized. In the original ASPO teacher training course, written by Elizabeth Bing and Marjorie Karmel, published in 1961, they state, "If your doctor himself suggests medication, you should accept it willingly — even if you don't feel the need for it — as he undoubtedly has very good reasons for his decision."(14) The 1970's teacher training guideline states that "The final decision on the use of drugs has to be with the individual physician." This policy is again in contradiction to the legal rights of patients to refuse "any medical or surgical procedure from being performed on them regardless of the opinions of their doctors as to the advisability of the treatment."(15)

### Guidance - Cooperation Model

The second model of practitioner-patient relationships is the Guidance-Cooperation model. The practitioner guides and directs the patient who, if she is a good patient, takes guidance and direction easily. In childbirth, I believe that this is best typified by the in-hospital "prepared" childbirth. The laboring woman is there to be coached. All the preparation she has had has taught her to work within the framework of the institutional rules. The ASPO teacher guidelines have this to say about doctor-patient relationships:

The patient should be encouraged to have a good "rapport" with her physician. If her doctor is not acquainted with the Lamaze technique, she should try and get his confidence, show that she is not fanatic and perhaps see if he will read the ASPO "Physicians Communique," or the ASPO training manual. It should be pointed out that, quite obviously, physicians do not cherish to be told by their patients how to conduct their labor and delivery. However, it can certainly be tactfully discussed, and from our experience a great deal can be gained from this.

Note that physicians' conduct labor and delivery, and if the "patient" (note too the acceptance of the patient-role for the laboring woman) makes it clear that she is not a fanatic, her labor may be conducted in accord with some of her wishes. Provided of course that she is tactful and doesn't offend anyone.

### Mutual Participation Model

The third possible relationship is Mutual Participation, in which practitioner and patient work together towards a common goal. In essence, it is a denial of the "patient" role. In childbirth it is probably possible, though very difficult, to achieve this relationship in an institutional setting. It flows naturally, however, in a home birth, where the attendant is clearly hired by and guest of the mother. The hospital patient is in no position to be an equal participant in her birthing. She is outnumbered and outpowered. She may be allowed to act as if she were an equal participant, even bringing a patient advocate (husband, coach) with her, but should she stop playing by the rules and become disagreeable, difficult or disruptive, as defined by the birth attendants and hospital staff, her true powerlessness is made clear. Her "advocate" is only there as long as the hospital attendants choose to allow him there, only so long as he continues to "coach" the woman in accord with institutional rules. Lest anyone think that the husband or friend is along as a social support, to offer loving companionship and protection for the woman at a time when she is relatively defenseless, consider ASPO teacher guidelines on the subject of husband participation:

ASPO very much encourages "Family Centered Maternity," i.e. a husband and wife team during labor and delivery when possible. It is understood, however, that only husbands who have taken a formal course with their wife in the Lamaze technique can be of real help to the wife.

It is perhaps for these reasons that so much emphasis is put on control of both pain and the expression of pain in preparation for childbirth classes. According to the rules of the game, if the laboring woman chooses to deal with her pain by crying or calling out, she has forfeited her right to decision making. Much is made in childbirth preparation circles of being in control during labor, while all that is meant by that is being in control over expressions of pain. A woman who maintains a fixed, if somewhat glazed cheerful expression, and continues breathing patterns regularly, is said to be "in control" as she is carted from one room to another and literally strapped flat on her back with her legs in the air.

Certainly a woman who was unconscious, semi-stuperous, amnesiac or simply numb from the waist down cannot have experienced giving birth as an accomplishment, something over which she had conscious control. But what of the woman who is encouraged in childbirth preparation classes to see herself as a member of a "team" delivering the baby? Though she may help, and watch in a mirror, she is not the primary locus of action. Positioning her and draping her in such a way that she cannot directly see the birth, and not allowing her to touch her genitals and the forthcoming baby tells the mother that the birth is something that is happening to her, or being done to her, and not something that she is doing. The birth is managed, conducted, by the other members of the team, the ones who are telling her what to do, and using their hands on her and the baby.

A birth is an exciting, a thrilling thing to see. But it is an even more exciting and thrilling thing to do. Encouraging a woman to watch herself give birth in a mirror moves her from participant to observer of the birth. The emphasis on "seeing" the birth comes out of the context of prepared, in-hospital doctor-directed births. The woman is awake, encouraged to see herself as part of the team and help the doctor by following suggestions and direction. But the hospital members of that team have had most of their experience delivering babies without the active participation and help of the mother. They know that they will get that baby delivered with or without the woman's cooperation. If she wants to be awake, "be there" for the birth, then the only role that they have to offer her is as observer. She can watch the birth like anyone else. Her head is there and her genitals are there, but as in the gynecological examination, it is hard for doctors to see them both as belonging to the same person at the same time.

The implications of an Active-Passive or Guidance-Cooperation model for birth extends beyond the birthing experience and into the relationship with the baby. When the hospital staff is perceived as having delivered the baby, then it is the responsibility and privilege of the staff to present the baby to its mother. The mother thus becomes the recipient rather than the producer of the child. The less active the mother was in the birth and the more time that has elapsed between the birth and the presentation, the more clearly the baby is a product of the hospital. The very miracle of birth is that the baby is at the same time part of the mother's body and yet a separate person. This is not the place to discuss the psychological effects on maternal-infant bonding (16) and the physiological effects on lactation of alternative treatments of the newborn. But I ask you to consider the implications for control over the baby, for whose baby it really is, in the various ways newborns are processed.

A mother unconscious for the birth and presented 6 or 12 or 24 hours later with a baby understandbly has a hard time grasping and dealing with what has happened to her. Her pregnancy terminated. She has a baby. Those two facts are clear enough, but the relation between them is submerged.

Even women conscious for the birth, but who do not perceive it as something which they have done by their own efforts may have some difficulty in assimilating what has happened. As one mother, awake but unable to feel the birth, has said, "It's like seeing a rabbit pulled out of a hat." Being the hat is a far cry from being the magician. It is the sleight of hand that makes a magic trick, things done that the audience cannot see. Similarly, continuity is lacking in a birth in which the baby is held up for the mother to see but not touch and then taken out of her sight for processing, recording and prophylactic treatment. When the baby is returned, wiped off and swaddled, in hospital "uniform" it is one step further removed from the immediate product of birth. The newborn is abruptly changed from being part of its mother's body to a standard-issue hospital baby.

But when the mother feels herself giving birth to her baby by her own efforts, with whatever help she needs, when she holds the baby while the cord still physically connects it to her, the full reality of the birth is before her. Nancy Mills, a lay midwife who has done hundreds of home births, now encourages women to touch the baby's head when it is crowning, to feel it emerge with their hands. One woman later told her, "I felt I was giving birth to myself and my baby."(17) The baby is part of the mother. The acceptance of the baby as a separate person can follow slowly, during a period of psychological weaning, and not as a fait accompli.

The issue of control over the baby continues in the days after birth. A baby in a hospital nursery is controlled by the nursery. The mother has access to it only with the approval of the nursery staff. I once saw a mother, her face pressed against the nursery glass, say to her crying infant, "It's ok, baby, I'm here." The baby is brought to the mother but returned to the nursery. Consider the classic scenario of the mother being wheeled to the front door of the hospital and handed her baby to take home. In more or less subtle forms, the message is that the baby is a product of the hospital which the parents bring home with them. After three or five days or more of being cared for by the professionals and experts, the baby is entrusted to the parents. It enters the mother's life not as a continuation of the pregnancy and birthing experience, still more or less a part of her, but as a stranger.

## Conclusion

It has been the goal of this paper to point out the ways in which the birth experience is socially constructed, from the acknowledgement of labor to the care of the newborn, and to consider the agents which control the definitions used in the childbirth situation. Childbirth education, in order to gain the wide acceptance which it has received, has had to accept the bulk of professional-medical definitions of childbirth. The "preparation" has therefore been for the hospital experience and not for the birth itself. Unlike the current home birth movement and the return to lay or empirical midwives, the "natural childbirth" movement's simple desire that the parturient be awake, "be there" for the hospital birth, even with husband, is not a particularly radical request. Recent consumer pressure for more home-like labor rooms, more comfortable labor-delivery beds, and for rooming-in go a long way toward making birth in hospitals a more pleasant experience. But these changes, even if they were all made, would not change the fundamental balance of power between the individual and the institution. The struggle for individual control against institutional demands is not a problem unique to childbirth.

## References

1. For a more complete discussion of this perspective in sociology, see Herbert Blumer, Symbolic Interaction, (Englewood Cliffs, New Jersey: Prentice Hall, 1969).
2. For a review of contemporary American obstetrical practices, see Doris Haire, The Cultural Warping of Childbirth (International Childbirth Education Association, 1972). For a historical review, see G.J. Barker-Benfield, Horrors of the Half-Known Life (New York: Harper and Row, 1976) Part II: From Midwives to Gynecologists) and Frances Kobrin, "The American Midwife Controversy," (Bulletin of the History of Medicine, 40, 1966).
3. David Sudnow, Passing On: The Social Organization of Dying, (Englewood Cliffs, New Jersey: Prentice Hall, 1967).
4. Rita Seiden Miller, "The Social Construction and Reconstruction of Physiological Events: Acquiring the Pregnant Identity," in Denzin, editor, Studies in Symbolic Interaction, JAI.
5. Erving Goffman, Asylums, (New York: Anchor Books, 1961).
6. Julius Roth, Timetables, (Bobbs Merrill, 1965).
7. ASPO teacher training guidelines, unpublished, c. 1970. N.Y.
8. George Annas, The Rights of Hospital Patients, (New York: Discus Books, 1975) p 147.
9. Nancy Stoller Shaw, Forced Labor: Maternity Care in the United States, (New York: Pergamon Press, 1974) p 62.
10. Shaw, p 69.
11. Burchall, "Predelivery Removal of Pubic Hair," Obstetrics and Gynecology, 1964).
12. Leon Festinger, A Theory of Cognitive Dissonance, (New York: Row, Peterson, 1957).
13. T.S. Szasz and M.H. Hollender, "A Contribution to the Philosophy of Medicine: The Basic Models of the Doctor-Patient Relationship," (A.M.A. Archives of Internal Medicine, 97, 1956).
14. Bing, Elizabeth, Marjorie Karmel and Alfred Tanz, A Practical Training Course for the Psychoprophylactic Method of Childbirth, (New York: ASPO, 1961). p 33.
15. Annas, p 80.
16. Marshall H. Klaus and John H. Kennel, Maternal-Infant Bonding. (St. Louis: C.V. Mosby, 1976).
17. Nancy Mills, "The Lay Midwife," in Stewart and Stewart, editors, Safe Alternatives in Childbirth, (Marble Hill, MO: NAPSAC, 1976).

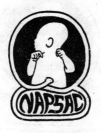

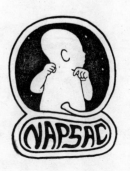

# CHAPTER SEVENTY THREE

## SYNOPSIS OF AN OPTIMAL MATERNITY PLAN
### by David Stewart, Ph.D.

### Perinatal Regionalization: Hospitals For All?

There is a current plan in the United States to regionalize maternity services. The thrust of the program is to consolidate all of the high-risk care into a few "tertiary" centers in each state where high risk mothers and infants would be transported. Current available technology, as well as teams of medical specialists, would be concentrated in these tertiary centers. For those of intermediate risk, there would be "secondary" centers and for those of low risk, "primary" facilities in local areas. Presumably, mothers would be screened as to which level of care would be appropriate and, whenever possible, this screening would be done in prenatal care. When high risk factors appear intrapartum or post partum, arrangements for rapid transport of mothers and-or babies would be available.

### The Problem with Perinatal Regionalization

There are many problems with the perinatal regionalization plan as it is now being implemented. A basic problem is that the plan is in the control of the tertiary centers and the specialists in high risk. At present, almost all efforts are toward developing the high risk centers, at the expense of neglecting the primary care. The rationale is that the tertiary centers must come first and that primary care will come later. But this argument ignores that fact that by slighting primary care, a greater incidence of high risk is created and if one concentrated on primary care first, the extent to which tertiary centers would be needed would be reduced.

Another problem with regionalization is its enormous cost. There is also the incurable propensity of medical specialists and technologically equipped hospitals to use their technology for educational and instructional purposes, for research purposes, to justify the expense, and out of sheer habit. Technology is there to be used, but prevailing philosophy is that it is to be used because it is there.

Perinatal regionalization also fails to recognize the efficacy of out-of-hospital alternatives and does not acknowledge the fact that hospitals have never been proven to be the safest place for most mothers to give birth. It ignores the body of published data that strongly suggests that the opposite may be true. Dr. Belton Meyer, Co-Director of the Arizona State Newborn Transport and Intensive Care Program stated at the 1977 Annual Meeting of the Southern Perinatal Association that "tertiary and secondary centers have a vested interest in utilization and, therefore, advertising and promotion must be parts of their programs." (quote taken from my notes). To a consumer, this is a chilling statement, indeed.

---

Based on a somewhat longer paper prepared for the 105th Meeting of the American Public Health Association, October 31, 1977, Washington D.C. The other paper contains 67 cited references.

---

David Stewart Ph.D., is Executive Director of NAPSAC and editor, author or co-author of many publications in the area of childbirth.

From this and all other indications, it is clear that if the promoters of regionalization have their way, the majority of mothers (i.e. the low risk) will no longer be treated as low risk but will be herded into the high risk centers where they will be submitted to the hazards of unnecessary, assembly-line technology. There is a better way.

## Outline of an Optimal Maternity Plan

**Prenatal Factors**

1. Education, from upper elementary through high school, on healthful practices and wholesome attitudes leading to optimal outcomes in pregnancy (nutrition, avoidance of drugs, normality of birth as a bodily process, natural superiority of breastfeeding etc.)

2. Adequate nutrition for all pregnant mothers (principally through education).

3. Little or no use of drugs, smoking, or alcohol by women of childbearing age.

4. Training for expectant couples, by consumer-oriented teachers, in how to give birth naturally, without drugs or obstetrics.

**Intrapartum Factors**

1. Family-centered birth for all--whether high risk or low risk--including spouse or biological father, siblings, and, if desired, friends and relatives.

2. Availability of well coordinated home birth programs with birth centers working with hospitals where the majority of women may give birth outside of the hospital.

3. Availability of midwives for all women with specialists for back up and high risk care.

4. Natural, educated childbirth.

**Postpartum Factors**

1. Close, immediate, and continuous maternal-infant contact, skin to skin, as well as paternal-infant contact and sibling-infant contact. (This is automatic in home birth.)

2. Breastfeeding for all babies beginning right after birth.

3. Postpartum followup by public health nurses in the home.

## General Philosophy of the Optimal Plan

The emphasis would be on prevention through nutrition, education, exercise, and mental preparation for birth to eliminate the deleterious effects of fear, ignorance and physical unpreparedness during labor. The primary responsibilities would be on parents who would seek the advice and counsel of professionals, but who would be educated by consumer oriented groups to make their own decisions. With adequate screening and preventive measures, the need to spend millions on hospitals, technology, and in the training and hiring of medical specialists would be reduced to a fraction of the apparent need today.

## Advantages of the Optimal Program

1. Safer.

2. Better long and short term outcomes, both in terms of the mother and baby, but also the family and, therefore, society at large.

3. Less costly, directly, in terms of less expensive alternatives.

4. Less costly, indirectly, in terms of special schools and custodial care for life-time obstetrically damaged children.

5. Eliminates the need for so many OB-GYN Departments in training centers and medical universities and turns a shortage of obstetricians into a surplus.

6. More personal care, more appropriately geared to various individual needs.

7. Happier families and a healthier, more intelligent, better balanced society.

### How to be Implemented?

Such an optimal program with both in and out-of-hospital options can be implemented through the existing Health Service Agencies.

### Will It Work?

One can justifiably question if all of the advantages stated above would, in actuality, be realized. This is a good question and the answer is a matter of speculation until the plan is tried. However, the outcome of perinatal regionalization is also a matter of speculation. One can, however, speculate based on existing data and the fact is that there is little or no scientific data favoring most mothers giving birth in hospitals. There is also little or no scientific data favoring the practice of most mothers being attended by an obstetrician, or even a physician. The evidence is to the contrary on both counts. The data, both historical and current, strongly suggests that the safest plan would be one that offered freedom of choice between in and out-of-hospital birth and between midwives and physicians.

### Is There a Risk?

Birth is not without risk regardless of where accomplished or by whom attended. There are no guarantees in or out of the hospital, with or without a physician or midwife. The question is not "how to eliminate risk?" because this is impossible. The question is "how to reduce risk to a minimum compatible with gleaning the greatest emotional, mental, and social benefits from birth." Life itself is a risk--daily and unavoidably. Riding in a car, taking a shower, walking down steps, eating a steak, swimming, mountain climbing--all are risks. To take an unnecessary risk with little potential for benefit would be reckless. But to comprehend and accept a small risk when the potential benefit is very great is only good judgment and a mark of maturity. The potential life-time benefits to baby, mother, father, family and society at large of obstetrically unhampered home birth are so great that some increased risk would even be warranted, if indeed, there were an increased risk. But relative to the hospital regimen, there is no increased risk with a well planned home birth. A comprehensive plan as outlined above with home births, birth centers, and hospitals working together with educated parents, would, in one stroke, optimize the benefits and reduce the risks to the inevitable minimums of nature.

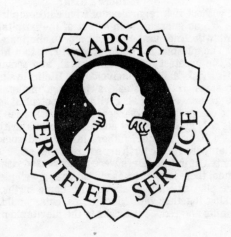

# CHAPTER SEVENTY FOUR

## WHAT IS A NAPSAC CERTIFIED MATERNITY SERVICE AND HOW CAN YOURS QUALIFY?

### by Penny Simkin, R.P.T.

---

Editors' Note: This article is a statement of official NAPSAC policy. In drawing up this statement, Ms. Simkin sought the input of all of the members of the NAPSAC Board of Directors and the NAPSAC Board of Consultants. What appears here is also a result of a presentation given by Ms. Simkin at the Third NAPSAC Conference in Atlanta, May, 1978, where NAPSAC members and others had the opportunity to discuss these points and have their input. We welcome comments from others who are interested or have ideas as well.

---

The whole concept of approval of maternity services is extremely complex. If a service is NAPSAC certified, should that mean that NAPSAC guarantees it as a safe alternative? Does it mean that NAPSAC controls the service, or enforces a particular standard of care? Does it mean that NAPSAC can control the practices of that service? As NAPSAC's Director of Maternity Standards, I have been wrestling for months with a system of certification which will be meaningful to both consumer and provider and also realistic in terms of what NAPSAC, with its limited resources, is able to do to assure a standard of care. NAPSAC would also like to avoid the common pitfalls inherent in many efforts at certification and standard-setting (e.g., becoming a "regulatory" agency, excluding capable but non-traditional people, stifling individuality). When a commitment is voluntarily made, kept and renewed by the maternity service, itself, these pitfalls can be avoided. Therefore, NAPSAC certification will be based upon voluntary committment.

NAPSAC certification will not imply that a particular maternity service does or does not offer specific services or employ specific types of personnel nor any other operational details of the practice. NAPSAC certification will imply that a particular maternity service does practice according to certain specified general principles of good care and does have a family-centered consumer orientation.

The essence of NAPSAC philosophy is one of "alternatives." There is no one type of care that is "best" for all. Different families have different needs and, therefore, need different types of birth attendants, medical treatment, and environments for birth. A great variety of services can qualify for NAPSAC certification — from single, practicing lay midwives to university hospitals, from privately practicing physicians to clinics, from birth centers operated by nurse-midwives to in-hospital centers under the direction of obstetricians.

If NAPSAC certification is to be meaningful to prospective parents, we feel that it is imperative that they have a clear understanding of the principles

---

Penny Simkin, RPT, from Seattle, Washington, is the NAPSAC Director of Maternity Standards, editor of the NAPSAC Directory of Alternative Birth Services and Consumer Guide, a member of the editorial staff of the Birth and the Family Journal, co-editor of the proceedings of the last two Biennial Conventions of ICEA, a childbirth educator, and proprietor of the Pennypress, publishers of materials on childbearing and parenting, 1100 23rd Ave. East, Seattle 98112.

guiding a particular service, as well as some recourse if they feel those principles are not being followed in their care.

NAPSAC certification can have value for providers of maternity services (such as midwives or home birth services) who are unable to gain certification from the usual sources — medical societies, state licensing commissions, etc. NAPSAC certification will make it possible to provide meaningful credentials to their clients.

For maternity services which do have the approval of their medical societies, licensing board, etc., NAPSAC certification could represent assurance to the consumer that NAPSAC's principles are also theirs and that they do represent an alternative to conventional medical care in childbearing.

Before introducing the NAPSAC Principles of Maternity Care, I would like to discuss some of the reasoning behind their establishment.

- There is real need for promotion of the concepts that pregnancy is a normal state and that excellent physical and emotional health during childbearing is extremely important to the quality of life.
- There is also real need for a restructuring of priorities in maternity care, placing prevention far ahead of treatment. Today the emphasis is on "rescue" measures — detecting conditions after they have developed and then "saving" mother and-or baby. Many of these dangerous conditions (e.g., toxemia, fetal alcohol syndrome, some prematurity) can be prevented through education, good nutrition and other health measures.
- The environment for birth, including the people present, is extremely important to the childbearing couple. Because there is no one universally "correct" environment for everyone, and because birth is a highly personal event for any woman or couple, there should be choices of environment available to all childbearing couples — choices which suit their individual wishes and needs. A compromise in safety for mother or child is not necessary in order to achieve personally satisfying circumstances for birth.

Following is a statement of the NAPSAC Principles of Maternity Care, after which I will conclude by discussing how these Principles can be incorporated in maternity care for the benefit of both consumers and providers.

## The NAPSAC Principles of Maternity Care

1. **Childbearing as a normal physiologic process — not a medical one.**

Pregnancy and parturition are unique in health care in that they are natural functions. They are events of profound and lasting significance in the lives of the families involved. Maternity policies and procedures should provide for both the physical safety of mother and baby and for the important psychological and spiritual needs and desires of family and baby. These needs can be met safely in a variety of environments, depending on the circumstances and preferences of the individual: hospital, home, clinic, or birth center.

## 2. Parent Responsibility.

The responsibilities of pregnancy, childbirth, baby and child care ultimately lie with the parents. Providers of maternity care give advice, accurate information (both general and specific as it relates to the individual), support and care, which can be helpful to parents in exercising their responsibilities, and in making choices best suited to their individual circumstances.

## 3. Essentials of Maternity Care.

A program of maternity care includes the following:

-Positive prenatal, intranatal, and postpartum care geared to individual preference and need, and emphasizing good health, prevention, and, if necessary, referral of problems which require high risk care.

-Preparation for natural childbirth and breastfeeding.

-Nutritional counseling.

-Qualified birth attendants.

-Post-natal followup for mother and baby.

## 4. Cooperation between parents and their birth attendants.

Cooperation between parents and their birth attendants is one component of safe and successful maternity care. As a part of this cooperation, patients assume responsibility for their own good health through education, exercise, relaxation, nutrition and avoidance of drugs, tobacco and alcohol.

## 5. Informed consent.

Informed consent involves the consent of patients based on their having been fully informed of and understanding their conditions, risks and benefits of the proposed course of treatment, alternative courses of treatment and their risks and benefits, as well as the risks and benefits of no treatment at all. The use of diagnostic procedures, obstetric intervention, and medications and-or anesthesia during pregnancy, birth, and lactation may carry risk for mother, child, or both. Unless the attendant believes the benefits of such procedures, intervention or medication will outweigh the possible risks, their use will not be suggested or recommended, they will not be utilized without the fully informed consent of the mother-couple, and their use will take place only in an environment where such procedures can best be handled.

## 6. Family unit.

The family is a unit and its members should not be separated without justification during the period of childbirth and afterwards. The period immediately after birth is a particularly important one for the bonding of family members. Time alone together is encouraged.

## 7. Limits of care and back-up.

Prospective parents should know the background, training, and experience of those providing their care throughout pregnancy, birth and postpartum. They should know any limitations on the care offered by that person or facility, as well as back-up plans for cases or circumstances that cannot be handled by that person or facility. From the outset of the relationship between provider and client, the client should be informed of any criteria for receiving care (health standards, financial standards, attitudinal standards).

What do the NAPSAC Principles have to do with NAPSAC Certification of Maternity Services and how can one qualify? The plan is that NAPSAC Certification will be available to anyone adhering to the above principles, who discusses the principles fully with each client, and gives each client a signed copy.

Maternity services may apply for certification by writing to NAPSAC, P.O. Box 267, Marble Hill, Missouri 63764. When a service has voluntarily declared in writing that they support and adhere to these principles, they will be granted provisional NAPSAC Certification Status. They will be sent a high-quality printed parchment copy of the principles for viewing by the clients of the service. Depending on whether the service be a hospital, birth center, private practitioner, midwife, etc., the certificate may be posted in a waiting room, living room of the provider, or rolled up and carried to the places where clients are met. In addition to the Principles, the certificate will contain the following:

(To appear at the top of the certificate)

**CERTIFICATE OF COMMITMENT
TO NAPSAC PRINCIPLES OF MATERNITY CARE**

This is to certify that ___(name of birth service)_____

is committed to the care of expectant families according to the NAPSAC Principles given below:

---

(A listing of the NAPSAC principles to appear here)

---

(To appear at the bottom of the certificate)

**NOTICE TO CLIENTS OF THIS MATERNITY SERVICE**

If, at any time, you feel that the above principles have not been followed in your care, or if you have any other objections to the practices of this maternity service, please discuss it with the personnel involved and notify NAPSAC, Director of Maternity Standards, P.O. Box 267, Marble Hill, MO 63764 (314) 238-2010. An inquiry will be conducted.

Signature(s) of the provider(s) of the service

Signature(s) of appropriate NAPSAC officer

Date of this agreement and its expiration date

**"A COPY OF THIS STATEMENT IS ON FILE
AT NAPSAC HEADQUARTERS"**

NAPSAC Certified Services will see that each client is given a signed and dated copy of the Statement of Principles after discussion of each principle. Copies of the Statement of Principles are available from NAPSAC and can be used only by NAPSAC Certified Maternity Services. If there are problems, and NAPSAC is asked to investigate, an inquiry, fair to both client and provider, will be conducted with the main goal being to correct any misunderstandings and resolve the difficulty. If, however, NAPSAC deems the provider does not adhere to the Principles, then renewal will be denied for the following year.

NAPSAC Certified Services will be listed in the NAPSAC Directory of Alternative Birth Services in a special way to indicate their special status.

We in NAPSAC believe that adherence to these Principles and a full discussion of them with each client will promote trust and a mutually beneficial and rewarding relationship. It provides an opportunity for providers of maternity care to take a clear stand on the normalcy of childbearing, its importance to family life, and the importance of an honest, cooperative relationship between parents and provider.

There will be a fee charged by NAPSAC for application and for maintaining NAPSAC Certification. This article outlines the basic concepts of the NAPSAC Certification Program. For a full set of details, write to NAPSAC.

In conclusion, the answers to the questions at the beginning of the paper as to what NAPSAC approval really means are as follows:

1. While NAPSAC cannot guarantee safety, this system of announcing the standards of maternity care of the service will guarantee an opportunity for parents to learn and discuss the services offered, and decide whether they are adequate in terms of what is important to them. Parents are encouraged to make a critical evaluation based on their discussions with the providers, and on reading, discussion with other parents, and also on their own individual wishes, feelings, and needs.

2. NAPSAC does not control the service or enforce a particular standard of care. However, NAPSAC will hear and investigate complaints, and, on the basis of what is learned about the complaints, either grant or withhold renewal of NAPSAC Certification.

3. We in NAPSAC feel that any maternity service which voluntarily subscribes to the NAPSAC Standards, announces this fact and discusses the Standards with all clients, is offering honesty, openness, good basic health and maternity care, a respect for the family unit and each member's individuality, as well as an opportunity for the clients to know them well enough to know before it is too late whether this is the service desired by them.

4. While NAPSAC Certification does not specify the particulars of a given service, it does specify the presence of an attitude of consumer orientation.

---

NOTE: To obtain details and application form for NAPSAC Certification, write NAPSAC, Director of Maternity Standards, P.O. Box 267, Marble Hill, Missouri 63764, or call (314) 238-2010. Copies of the "Statement of Principles" for mutual signing and distribution to clients to be used by NAPSAC Certified Services are available only from NAPSAC and cannot be used by any services other than those with current NAPSAC Certification.

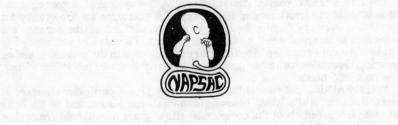

# CHAPTER TWENTY SEVEN

## FORCED LABOR OR FREE CHOICE: WHICH WILL IT BE?
(closing address at the 3rd NAPSAC conference)

### Robert S. Mendelsohn, M.D.

I am going to give an historical analysis of forced labor and free choice. Four thousand years ago, a small group of Jewish midwives, Shiphrah and Puah were their leaders, rejected the edict of an Egyptian pharoah and his powerful doctors. The ultimate result of the defiance of these courageous midwives was the liberation of 600,000 Hebrew slaves from Egyptian forced labor. For this act, the Bible tells us, the midwives were especially blessed. (Exodus, chapter 1, verses 15-21).

A hundred years ago, one brave physician rose and commanded his hostile colleages to wash their hands before entering the delivery room after they left the autopsy room. Thus, Ignacz Semmelweiss brought an end to the high mortality rate caused by doctors over the centuries for which they never took the blame. And Semmelweiss achieved immortality for lowering the death rate for which doctors ever since have claimed the credit.

Twenty-one years ago, a small band of determined women brought everlasting fame to a small midwestern suburb — some of you may have heard of Franklin Park in Illinois — by replacing the stupidity of modern doctors with the sage advice of experienced mothers. The La Leche League, led by Marion Tompson, already a legend in her own time, aimed to promote good mothering through breastfeeding. They have brought better mothering to millions of families now and in the future throughout the world.

Finally, four years ago, a geophysicist-seismologist and his wise wife created a new national organization dedicated to repeating the Biblical exodus, and again bringing freedom — this time to the slaves of American obstetrics.

Lee Stewart set the example by ignoring the doctors and by voting with her feet, rejecting the iron stirrups. Her husband, David, previously skilled in predicting earthquakes, now leads in producing earthquakes that shake the entire country, converting forced labor into free choice throughout America. Rejected by the Goliath's of the academic world in the past, David is destined to be offered their future honorary degrees. Here, at this 3rd NAPSAC conference the Carter family, first families of the land, honored all of us, as well as themselves, by their inspiring and tremendously moving appearance.

The message is clear. As important as it is to be reborn, it is even more important to be born right the first time. We are now emerging as free men and women from the decades of bondage under a forced labor and the tyranny of modern medicine. No longer will we sacrifice our children's lives and health to the false gods of Columbia, Harvard, Yale, Cornell, Stanford and the other

---

Robert S. Mendelsohn, M.D. is a pediatrician and family physician; Vice President, SPUN, Board of Advisors, LLLI, and editor of the newsletter and syndicated column entitled, "The People's Doctor."

temples of idolatry that have enslaved our minds and our bodies, and that have given us, not higher education, but longer education.

As you can see from the excitement of this meeting, we still have many problems to solve. And we must remember that the first generation of freedom, as it was in Biblical times, must always travel through the wilderness in order to purify their ideas and emotions.

It is indeed appropriate that this third NAPSAC Conference is being held in Atlanta, the home of a great leader of a people bent on finding freedom. I believe that if Martin Luther King were here today, he would be blessing Lee and David and all of us gathered here in this noble cause. Our present journey through the wilderness leads, as we all know, to the promised land where our own children and grandchildren, liberated from previous oppression, can live their lives together with their families in freedom and peace.

EDITORS NOTE: Dr. Mendelsohn is the author of an excellent newsletter called THE PEOPLE'S DOCTOR. There are 12 issues a year containing invaluable information concerning every sort of health or medical field. It could well be entitled, "Everything Your Doctor Should Have Told You, But Didn't." Every issue also contains a page length article by Marian Tompson, President of La Leche League International and a writer of considerable insight into family health. $18 per year. Send check and request for subscription to: THE PEOPLE'S DOCTOR, 664 N. Michigan Ave., Suite 720, Chicago, IL    60611

You may also be interested in reading Dr. Mendelsohn's best selling book, CONFESSIONS OF A MEDICAL HERITIC, published by Contemporary Books, 1979, hard cover, $9.95, available in bookstores.

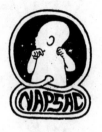

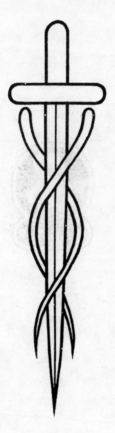

Appendices

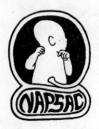

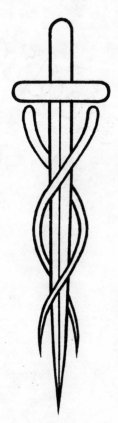

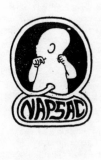

# ADDRESSES OF CONTRIBUTORS
## TO VOLUME ONE

James R. Allen, MD, MPH
Center for Disease Control
Hospital Infections Branch
Bureau of Epidemiology
Atlanta, GA 30333

Susan M. Basham, MA
67 Montcalm
Brighton, MA 02135

Yvonne Brackbill, PhD
Department of Psychology
University of Florida
Gainesville, FL 32611

Carol Brendsel, RN
Center for Research on Birth
2340 Ward Street
Suite 105
Berkeley, CA 94705

Lynn R. Browne
Cesarean Educational Alliance
Journey's End Road
Francestown, NH 03043

Susan Doering, PhD
Department of Social Relations
Johns Hopkins University
Baltimore, MD 21218

Murray Enkin, MD
Department of Obstetrics & Gyn
McMaster University
Hamilton, Ontario L8S 4J9
Canada

Loel Fenwick, MD
The Cybele Society
Suite 414, Peyton Building
Spokane, WA 99201

Asher Galloway, MD
755 Columbia Drive, Suite 601
Decatur, GA 30030

Linda Goodman, CNM
755 Columbia Drive, Suite 601
Decatur, GA 30030

Ann Gray
Federal Monitor
Drawer Q
McLean, VA 22101

Albert Haverkamp, MD
333 Jersey Street
Denver, CO 80220

W.B. Jarzembski, PE, PhD
4208 49th Street
Lubbock, TX 79408

Sheila Kitzinger
Standlake Manor
Standlake
Nr. Witney, Oxon.
England

Judith Dickson Luce
92 Claybourne Street
Dorchester, MA 02124

J.R. McTammany, MD
620 Walnut Street
Reading, PA 19601

Lewis Mehl, MD
Center for Research on
Birth & Human Development
2340 Ward Street, Suite 105
Berkeley, CA 94705

Robert Mendelsohn, MD
664 N. Michigan, Suite 720
Chicago, IL 60611

Judy Norsigian
Boston Women's Health
  Book Collective, Inc.
Box 192
West Somerville, MA 02144

Gail Peterson, MSSW
Center for Research on
Birth & Human Development
2340 Ward Street, Suite 105
Berkeley, CA 94705

Robbi Pfeufer
Boston Women's Health
  Book Collective, Inc.
Box 192
West Somerville, MA 02144

Barbara Katz Rothman
827 East 21st Street
Brooklyn, NY 11210

George Ryan, Jr., MD, MPH
Department of OB/Gyn
Center for Health Science
University of Tennessee
800 Madison
Memphis, TN 38163

Madeleine Shearer, RPT
Birth & Family Journal
110 El Camino Real
Berkeley, CA 94705

Penny Simkin, RPT
1100 23rd Avenue East
Seattle, WA 98112

David Stewart, PhD
Lee Stewart
NAPSAC
P.O. Box 267
Marble Hill, MO 63764

Richard Stewart, MD
755 Columbia Drive, Suite 601
Decatur, GA 30030

Muriel Sugarman, MD
15 Chatham Street
Brookline, MA 02146

Norma Swenson, MPH
Boston Women's Health
  Book Collective, Inc.
Box 192
West Somerville, MA 02144

Diony Young
43 Oak Street
Geneseo, NY 14454

NOTE: Some of these addresses may change in time. If you have found this to be so for a particular person above, contact NAPSAC for a current address. If you wish to obtain a phone number for any of the above, contact NAPSAC for that also.

## SELECTED RESOURCE ORGANIZATIONS

| | |
|---|---|
| **AAHCC**<br>American Academy of<br>Husband-Coached Childbirth<br>P.O. Box 5224<br>Sherman Oaks, CA 91413<br>(213) 788-6662 | *Certifying and Training Agency for childbirth educators in the Bradley Method.* |
| **ACHI**<br>Assoc. for Childbirth at Home Intern'l<br>1675 Monte Cristo<br>Cerritos, CA 90701<br>(714) 994-5880 | *Instruction on home birth for couples, with or without a birth attendant; trains and certifies teachers.* |
| **ACHO**<br>Am. College of Home Obstetrics<br>2821 Rose Street<br>Franklin Park, IL 60131<br>(312) 642-7472 | *Support, information, and training for physicians in home birth; certifies home obstetricians.* |
| **ACNM**<br>Am. College of Nurse-Midwives<br>1012 14th St. NW, Suite 801<br>Washington, DC 20005<br>(202) 347-5445 | *Certifying agency for nurse-midwives, both in home and in hospital practice.* |
| **ASPO**<br>American Society for<br>Psychoprophylaxis in Obstetrics<br>1411 K Street NW<br>Washington, DC 20005<br>(202) 783-7050 | *Certifying and Training Agency for childbirth educators in the Lamaze Method.* |
| **CEA**<br>Cesarean Educational Alliance<br>Journey's End Road<br>Francestown, NH 03043<br>(603)547-2095 | *Education on vaginal birth after previous cesarean, avoiding primary cesareans, emotional support for anticipated or past cesareans.* |
| **C/SEC**<br>Cesareans/Support, Education<br>and Concern<br>66 Christopher Road<br>Waltham, MA 02154<br>(617) 547-7188 | *Emotional and educational support for cesarean parents via phone, correspondence, literature, audio-visual material, hospital workshops.* |
| **HOME**<br>Home Oriented Maternity Experience<br>511 New York Avenue<br>Takoma Park, Washington, DC 20012<br>(301) 587-4664 | *Instruction on home birth for couples, emphasis on medically attended birth; trains and certifies leaders.* |

## SELECTED RESOURCE ORGANIZATIONS

| | |
|---|---|
| ICEA<br>Internat'l Childbirth Education Assoc.<br>P.O. Box 20852<br>Milwaukee, WI 53220<br>(612) 881-9194 | *All aspects of childbirth education; emphasis on birth preparation and family-centered hospital care.* |
| IH<br>Informed Homebirth<br>P.O. Box 788<br>Boulder, CO 80302<br>(303) 444-0434 | *Instruction for couples desiring birth at home or other alternative environments; trains and certifies teachers.* |
| LLLI<br>La Leche League, International<br>9616 Minneapolis Avenue<br>Franklin Park, IL 60131<br>(312) 455-7730 | *Support and information on breast feeding; distributes scientific reprints; trains and certifies leaders.* |
| NAPSAC<br>Nat'l Assoc. of Parents/Professionals<br>for Safe Alternatives in Childbirth<br>P.O. Box 267<br>Marble Hill, MO 63764<br>(314) 238-2010 | *All aspects of birth; emphasis on providing coordinated alternatives both in and out-of-hospital; certifies maternity services.* |
| NMA<br>National Midwives Association<br>P.O. Box 163<br>Princeton, NJ 08540<br>(915) 533-8142 | *An association of practicing midwives, largely lay midwives, but nurse-midwives also.* |
| SPUN<br>Society for the Protection of the<br>Unborn Through Nutrition<br>17 N. Wabash, Suite 603<br>Chicago, IL 60602<br>(312) 332-2334 | *Education in nutrition in pregnancy; training seminars, brochures on benefits and specifics of good diet; trains and certifies nutrition counselors.* |

NOTE: Parents and professionals can find valuable assistance from the above organizations. There are also many others too numerous to list here. For a more comprehensive listing, as well as a more complete and thorough description of the functions of each organization, obtain a copy of the *NAPSAC Directory of Alternative Birth Services and Consumer Guide.* It, as well as the other NAPSAC publications, is described near the end of this volume.

## ACRONYMS AND ABBREVIATIONS
## FOR ORGANIZATIONS, AGENCIES, DEGREES & MEDICAL TERMS

| | |
|---|---|
| AAFP | American Academy of Family Physicians |
| AAHCC | American Academy of Husband-Coached Childbirth |
| AAP | American Academy of Pediatrics |
| ABC | Alternative Birth Center (usually implies within a hospital) |
| ABOG | American Board of Obstetricians & Gynecologists |
| ACHI | Association for Childbirth at Home International |
| ACHO | American College of Home Obstetrics |
| ACNM | American College of Nurse-Midwives |
| ACOG | American College of Obstetricians & Gynecologists |
| ACOMEH | Accreditation Committee on Medicl Educatn & Hospitls(AMA) |
| ACOOG | American College of Osteopathic Obstetricians & Gynecologists |
| ACS | American College of Surgeons |
| AFMCH | American Foundation for Maternal Child Health |
| AG | Affinity Group |
| AHA | American Hospital Association |
| AIP | Annual Implementation Plan |
| AMA | American Medical Association |
| ANA | American Nurses Association |
| APA | Allopathic Practice Act |
| APA | American Psychiatric Association |
| APHA | American Public Health Association |
| ASPO | American Society for Psychoprophylaxis in Obstetrics |
| BC | Birth Center (usually implies out-of-hosital) |
| BWHBC | Boston Women's Health Book Collective |
| BSN | Bachelor of Science in Nursing |
| CC | Cesarean Concern, Inc. |
| CCE | Certified Childbirth Educator |
| CBC | Childbearing Center (out-of-hospital) |
| CBS | Community Birth Service |
| CDC | U.S. Center for Disease Control (Atlanta) |
| CE | Childbirth Educator |
| CEA | Childbirth Education Association |
| CF | Client Feedback |
| CHOICE | Consumer Health Options & Information for Client Education |
| CHP | Comprehensive Health Planning |
| CNM | Certified Nurse-Midwife |
| CNS | Central Nervous System |
| CPD | Cephalopelvic Disproportion |
| CR | Community Review |
| CRBHD | Center for Research on Birth & Human Development |
| C/SEC | Cesareans/Support, Education & Concern , Inc. |
| CWPEA | Childbirth Without Pain Education Association |
| CWPEL | Childbirth Without Pain Education League |
| DC | Doctor of Chiropractic |
| DES | Diethystilbestrol (a synthetic estrogen) |
| DHEW | U.S. Department of Health, Education & Welfare |
| DIY | Do It Yourself (refers to an unattended home birth) |
| DO | Doctor of Osteopathy |
| DBA | Doctor of Business Administration |
| DPH | Department of Public Health |
| DrPH | Doctor of Public Health |

| | |
|---|---|
| ECG | Electrocardiogram |
| EEG | Electroencephalogram |
| EFM | Electronic Fetal Monitor |
| EKG | Electrocardiogram |
| EM | Empirical Midwife (also Lay Midwife) |
| EMG | Electromyogram |
| EMIC | Emergency Maternity & Infant Care |
| EMR | Electromagnetic Radiation |
| EMS | Emergency Medical Service |
| ER | Emergency Room |
| FAAFP | Fellow of the AAFP |
| FAAP | Fellow of the AAP |
| FACOG | Fellow of the ACOG |
| FCMC | Family-Centered Maternity Care |
| FDA | U.S. Food & Drug Administration |
| FHM | Fetal Heart Monitor |
| FHR | Fetal Heart Rate |
| FM | Fetal Monitor |
| FNP | Family Nurse Practitioner |
| FNS | Frontier Nursing Service (Kentucky) |
| FWHC | Feminist Women's Health Center |
| HCMC | Home Centered Maternity Care |
| HEW | U.S. Department of Health, Education & Welfare |
| HMO | Health Maintainance Organization |
| HOME | Home Oriented Maternity Experience, Inc. |
| HPC | Health Planning Council |
| HRS | Health Responsibility System |
| HSA | Health Systems Agency |
| HSP | Health Systems 'Plan (long range) |
| IC | Informed Consent (a formal written document) |
| ICEA | International Childbirth Education Association |
| ICN | Intensive Care Nursery |
| ICU | Intensive Care Unit |
| IFGO | International Federation of Gyneclogists & Obstetricians |
| IM | Intramuscular |
| ISPO | International Society for Psychoprophylaxis in Obstetrics |
| ISPOG | International Society for Psychosomatic Obstetrics & Gynecology |
| IV | Intravenous |
| IH | Informed Homebirth, Inc. |
| IMR | Infant Mortality Rate |
| JAMA | Journal of the American Medical Association |
| JD | Doctor of Jurisprudence |
| LLLI | La Leche League International (also LLL) |
| LM | Lay Midwife (also Empirical Midwife) |
| LPN | Licensed Practical Nurse |
| MA | Master of Arts |
| MCA | Maternity Center Association (New York City) |
| MCH | Maternal Child Health |
| MD | Doctor of Medicine |
| MDiv | Master of Divinity |
| MHA | Master of Hospital Administration |
| MMR | Maternal Mortality Rate |
| MPH | Master of Public Health |
| MS | Master of Science |
| MSN | Master of Science in Nursing |
| MSSW | Master of Science in Social Work |
| MOD | National Foundation of the March of Dimes |

| | |
|---|---|
| MPA | Medical Practice Act |
| MMWR | Mortality & Morbidity Weekly Report (from the CDC) |
| NAACOG | Nurses Association of the ACOG |
| NAPSAC | Natl Assoc of Parents & Professionls for Safe Alternativs in Childbirth |
| NASPOG | North American Society for Psychosomatic Obstetrics & Gynecology |
| NCHPD | National Council on Health Policy & Development |
| ND | Doctor of Naturopathy |
| NFMOD | National Foundation for the March of Dimes (also MOD) |
| NICU | Neonatal Intensive Care Unit |
| NIH | U.S. National Institutes of Health (part of DHEW) |
| NINCDS | Natl Institute of Neurological & Communicative Disorders & Stroke |
| NMA | National Midwives Association |
| NMR | Neonatal Mortality Rate |
| NOW | National Organization for Women |
| NP | Nurse Practitioner |
| NWHN | National Women's Health Network |
| OCT | Oxytocin Challenge Test |
| OR | Operating Room |
| OTA | U.S. Office of Technology Assessment (part of DHEW) |
| PA | Physician's Associate |
| PAST | Practitioners Audited Statistics |
| PC | Professional Corporation |
| PDR | Physician's Desk Reference |
| PE | Professional Engineer |
| PhD | Doctor of Philosophy |
| PHM | Popular Health Movement |
| PKU | Phenylketonuria |
| PL | Public Law |
| PMR | Perinatal Mortality Rate |
| PNP | Pediatric Nurse Practitioner |
| PSRO | Professional Standards Review Organization |
| RADS | Resource & Development Services |
| RCT | Randomized Clinical Trial |
| RDS | Respiratory Distress Syndrome |
| RHNI | Resources in Human Nurturing, International, Inc. |
| RMP | Regional Medical Program |
| RN | Registered Nurse |
| RPT | Registered Physical Therapist |
| SAC | Subarea Council |
| SC | Solo Corporation |
| SHCC | Statewide Health Coordinating Council |
| SHPDA | State Health Planning & Development Agency |
| SIDS | Sudden Infant Death Syndrome |
| SMA | Standard Statistical Metropolitan Area (also SSMA) |
| SPUN | Society for the Protection of the Unborn Through Nutrition |
| SR | Stillbirth Rate |
| SSMA | Standard Statistical Metropolitan Area (also SMA) |
| TM | Transcendental Meditation |
| UHB | Unattended Home Birth |
| VC | Voluntary Certification |
| WHO | World Health Organization |
| WIC | Special Supplemental Food Program for Women, Infants & Children |

# What Is NAPSAC ?

The National Association of Parents and Professionals for Safe Alternatives in Childbirth is dedicated to exploring, examining, implementing and establishing Family-Centered Childbirth Programs ... programs that meet the needs of families as well as provide the safe aspects of medical science.

### OUR GOALS ARE:

* To act as a forum facilitating communication and cooperation among Parents, Medical Professionals, and Childbirth Educators.

* To encourage and aid in the implementation of Family-Centered Maternity Care in Hospitals.

* To assist in the establishment of Maternity and Childbearing Centers.

* To help establish Safe Homebirth Programs.

* To provide educational opportunities to parents and to parents-to-be that will enable them to assume more personal responsibility for Pregnancy, Childbirth, Infant Care, and Child Rearing.

### ABOUT MEMBERSHIP IN NAPSAC

If you would like to receive the NAPSAC NEWS quarterly, to be kept informed of upcoming NAPSAC programs and publications, and participate in some of the NAPSAC activities - you may become a member. Annual dues: $8 (USA); $9 (Other Countries)

SEND: Name - Address - Phone - Specialty or Major Interest
With Check or Money Order payable to NAPSAC

**box 267, marble hill, mo 63764**   Phone: (314) 238-2010

If you would like to form a local NAPSAC Member Group, please write to the NAPSAC Membership Director.

# HAVE YOU READ
## THE OTHER NAPSAC BOOKS?

NAPSAC books are read the world over. Written for the public at large, they are also documented for the professional. Used by parents & childbirth educators, they are also used as texts in schools of medicine, nursing, midwifery, and public health. They are on the forefront of today's research, practice, & trends in maternity care. Unique in content & unique in approach, no one in the field of maternity care can be up to date who is not familiar with the NAPSAC publications.

SAFE ALTERNATIVES IN CHILDBIRTH won the 1976 Books of the Year Award from the American Journal of Nursing of the American Nurses' Association. 21st CENTURY OBSTETRICS NOW! has also been well received. Both are required reading for certification in several national childbirth teacher training programs. Safe Alternatives.. is on the approved library list of La Leche League International and is being translated into Swedish. Both books will soon be available in Braille.

New Age Magazine, commenting on these two books, said, "they occupy a category all of their own and represent the leading edge of thinking in the childbirth field.... scrupulously documented...the established medical community cannot dismiss them....they also present invaluable primary research. One can only hope that NAPSAC's work flourishes and that their publications become required reading for practitioners in the childbirth field."

The DIRECTORY OF ALTERNATIVE BIRTH SERVICES & CONSUMER GUIDE by Penny Simkin, RPT, is one of NAPSAC's most popular books. BIRTH GOES HOME by Lester Hazell is one of the best known studies of home birth and one of the most widely quoted.

# 21st Century Obstetrics Now!

## Volume One

THE PREGNANT PATIENT'S BILL OF RIGHTS
Doris B. Haire, DMS

CHILDBIRTH OF THE FUTURE--WHAT WILL IT BE LIKE?
Lee Stewart, BS, CCE

THE AMERICAN COLLEGE OF OB/GYN: STANDARDS
FOR SAFE CHILDBEARING
Richard Aubry, MD

A REBUTTAL TO NEGATIVE HOMEBIRTH STATISTICS
CITED BY ACOG
David Stewart, PhD, CCE, & Lewis E. Mehl, MD

POSITION PAPER ON OUT-OF-HOSPITAL MATERNITY
CARE, DISTRICT II, ACOG
Richard Aubry, MD

ICEA REPLIES TO ACOG
Peg Beals, RN, & Ted Beals, MD

NAPSAC REPLIES TO ACOG
Cedar Koons

FULFILLING THE NEEDS OF FAMILIES IN A HOSPITAL
SETTING: CAN IT BE DONE?
Ruth T. Wilf, CNM, PhD

EFFECT OF FEAR AND DISTURBANCES ON LABOR
Niles Newton, PhD

WHY WOMEN SHOULD BE IN CONTROL OF CHILDBIRTH
Suzanne Arms

THE AMERICAN COLLEGE OF NURSE-MIDWIVES: WHAT
IS THE FUTURE FOR CNM'S?
Dorothea Lang, CNM, MPH

THE IATROGENESIS OF DAMAGED MOTHERS & BABIES
David Birnbaum, BS

HISTORY OF THE DEHUMINIZATION OF AMERICAN
OBSTETRICAL PRACTICE
Herbert Ratner, MD

FETAL MONITORS, OXYTOCIN STRESS TESTS, ETC.:
DO THE BENEFITS OUTWEIGH THE RISKS?
Frederic M. Ettner, MD

HOW TO SURVIVE MEDICAL TRAINING WITHOUT BEING
DEHUMANIZED
Robert S. Mendelsohn, MD

SCIENTIFIC RESEARCH ON CHILDBIRTH ALTERNATIVES:
WHAT CAN IT TELL US ABOUT HOSPITAL PRACTICE?
Lewis E. Mehl, MD

STUDIES OF PSYCHOLOGICAL OUTCOME FOR VARIOUS
CHILDBIRTH ALTERNATIVES
Gail H. Peterson, MSSW, & Lewis E. Mehl, MD

FAMILY BONDING: WHY FAMILIES SHOULD BE TOGE-
THER AT BIRTH & WHY WE CHOSE BIRTH AT HOME
Marian & C.R. Tompson & the entire Family

SPIRITUAL & ETHICAL ASPECTS OF BIRTH
Lester Dessez Hazell, MA

## Volume Two

THE LIMITS OF SCIENCE IN CHILDBIRTH
David Stewart, PhD

IMPLEMENTING A MEDICALLY SOUND CHILDBEARING
CENTER: PROBLEMS & SOLUTIONS
Myrtle E. Hosford, CNM, MA

SETTING UP A VIABLE HOMEBIRTH SERVICE RUN BY
CNM'S, BACKED BY DOCTORS AND HOSPITALS
Janet L. Epstein, CNM

THE AMERICAN COLLEGE OF HOME OBSTETRICS:
PHILOSOPHY & PRACTICE OF PHYSICIANS
IN HOMEBIRTH
Gregory White, MD, & Mayer Eisenstein, MD

MATERNAL-INFANT BONDING: THE PROFOUND LONG
TERM BENEFITS OF IMMEDIATE, CONTINUOUS SKIN
AND EYE CONTACT AT BIRTH
Ruth Rice, PhD

WHY WOMEN MUST MEET THE NUTRITIONAL STRESS
OF PREGNANCY
Tom Brewer, MD, & Jay Hodin, AB

PREGNANT? AND WANT A HEALTHY CHILD?
(SPECIFICS OF A WELL BALANCED DIET)
Tom Brewer, MD

BREASTFEEDING, NATURAL MOTHERING, AND
WORKING OUTSIDE THE HOME
Merilyn Salomon, MA, Victoria Schauf, MD, &
Anne Seiden, MD

A WORKING LAY-MIDWIFE HOMEBIRTH PROGRAM IN
SEATTLE, WA: A COLLECTIVE APPROACH
Midwives & Physicians of the Fremont Clinic

A WORKING LAY-MIDWIFE HOMEBIRTH PROGRAM IN
MADISON, WI: AN INDIVIDUAL APPROACH
Thya Merz

THE LAY MIDWIFE: A CURRENT PERSPECTIVE
Cedar Koons

HOW TO WORK WITHIN OLD LAWS, AVOID MALPRAC-
TICE, AND INFLUENCE NEW LEGISLATION IN
MATERNITY CARE
George J. Annas, JD, MPH

THE CULTURAL UNWARPING OF CHILDBIRTH: HOW?
Doris B. Haire, DMS

BIRTH AS THE FIRST EXPERIENCE OF MOTHERING
Michelle Harrison, MD

SOCIAL IMPACTS OF UNNECESSARY INTERVENTION &
UNNATURAL SURROUNDINGS IN CHILDBIRTH
Ashley Montagu, PhD

---

21st Century Obstetrics Now! In Two Volumes.
Price: $6.50 per single volume; $11 per 2-vol set.
Order from: NAPSAC, P.O. Box 267
Marble Hill, MO 63764
Shipping: 75¢ for 1st vol, 25¢ per additional vol
Hence, for 2-vol set, add $1.00 shipg.

---

Does your library have a set?

If not, why not recommend that they purchase one.

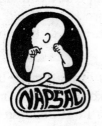

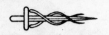
- Want to Set Up a Hospital Birthing Room, see Chapters 20, 21 & 23. pp. 215-220, 241-251.

- Should Doctors in Hospital Practice Give Prenatal Care and Back Up to Home Birth Couples? See Chapter 20, p. 177. Also see Chapters 22 & 23, pp. 231-251

- Did You Know that Cesarean Sections Occur More Frequently During the Convenient Daylight Hours In Some Hospitals? See Chapter 16. pp. 181-182.

- Is There Really a Conspiracy Among Hospital Doctors To Force All Births Into Hospitals? See Chapter 1, p. 1, as well as Chapters 9 & 10, pp. 83-118.

- Is the Natural Process of Maternal-Infant Bonding In Danger of Being Tokenized Into Another Mechnical Hospital Routine? Can Real Bonding Take Place Amidst the Disruptions of IV's, Monitors, and the Like? See Chapter 19, p. 205.

- Are Government Regulations of Health Care Always Based On Science? See Chapter 3, p. 25.

- Can Family-Centered Maternity Care Save Your Hospital Money? See Chapter 23, p. 241.

- How Should a Hospital Service Interface with a Home Birth Service for Prenatal Care & Back Up? See Chapter 20, p. 215.

- Does Your Maternity Service Qualify for NAPSAC Certification? See Chapter 26, p. 269.

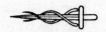

- Fearful of Being Forced into an Unnecessary Cesarean?
  See Chapters 16, 17 & 18, pp. 177-202

- Want to Have a Say in How Your Tax Dollars Are Spent
  On Health Care Planning in Your Area?
  Read Chapter 4, p. 39.

- If Your Doctor Has Misled You to Believe
  That Simple Analgesic Drugs Given During Labor
  Are Safe....
  You'd Better Read Chapter 14, p. 161.

- If your Hospital is under the Misconception
  That Fetal Monitors are Better
  Than Midwifery or Good Nursing Care....
  You'd better read Chapters 11-12, pp.  121-140.

- Want to Learn, First Hand, Why the ACOG, the
  Official Organization for American Obstetricians,
  Favors Compulsory Hospitalization?  See Chapter
  5, p. 57, written by the Secretary of the ACOG,
  Himself.

- Interested in the Politics, the Conspiracies,
  The Things Organized Medicine Does to Exploit
  The Public and What You  as a Consumer can do
  About it?  See Chapters 1, 2 & 7, pp. 1, 13, & 71.

- Are you a Member of an HSA or other Health
  Planning group?  You should read Chapters 9 & 10,
  pp. 83-120.

- Concerned about Humane Treatment and Family-
  Centered Care for High Risk Mothers & Babies?
  You should read Chapter 22, p. 231.

For A Quick Review of This Volume--
See the SYNOPSIS in the Front
Beginning on Page i.

WINNER Of The 1979

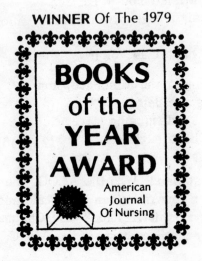

BOOKS
of the
YEAR
AWARD
American
Journal
Of Nursing

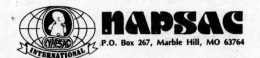

NAPSAC

P.O. Box 267, Marble Hill, MO 63764